ANTI-INFLAMMATORY DIET COOKBOOK FOR BEGINNERS

Enjoy 500 Effective, Healthy & Tasty Anti-Inflammatory Diet Recipes to Reduce Inflammation & Chronic Pain Improving Your Immune System + Meal Plan Bonus

KIMBERLY YOUNG

L.Feuerbach:

"We are what we eat"

Hippocrates:

"Let food be thy medicine and medicine be thy food"

© **Copyright 2021 Kimberly Young - All rights reserved**.

This eBook is provided with the sole purpose of providing relevant information on a specific topic for which every reasonable effort has been made to ensure that it is both accurate and reasonable. Nevertheless, by purchasing this eBook you consent to the fact that the author, as well as the publisher, are in no way experts on the topics contained herein, regardless of any claims as such that may be made within. As such, any suggestions or recommendations that are made within are done so purely for entertainment value. It is recommended that you always consult a professional prior to undertaking any of the advice or techniques discussed within.

This is a legally binding declaration that is considered both valid and fair by both the Committee of Publishers Association and the American Bar Association and should be considered as legally binding within the United States.

The reproduction, transmission, and duplication of any of the content found herein, including any specific or extended information will be done as an illegal act regardless of the end form the information ultimately takes. This includes copied versions of the work both physical, digital and audio unless express consent of the Publisher is provided beforehand. Any additional rights reserved.

Furthermore, the information that can be found within the pages described forthwith shall be considered both accurate and truthful when it comes to the recounting of facts. As such, any use, correct or incorrect, of the provided information will render the Publisher free of responsibility as to the actions taken outside of their direct purview. Regardless, there are zero scenarios where the original author or the Publisher can be deemed liable in any fashion for any damages or hardships that may result from any of the information discussed herein.

Additionally, the information in the following pages is intended only for informational purposes and should thus be thought of as universal. As befitting its nature, it is presented without assurance regarding its prolonged validity or interim quality. Trademarks that are mentioned are done without written consent and can in no way be considered an endorsement from the trademark holder.

Disclaimer Notice:

Please note the information contained within this document is for educational and entertainment purposes only. All effort has been executed to present accurate, up to date, and reliable, complete information. No warranties of any kind are declared or implied. Readers acknowledge that the author is not engaging in the rendering of legal, financial, medical or professional advice. The content within this book has been derived from various sources. Please consult a licensed professional before attempting any techniques outlined in this book.

By reading this document, the reader agrees that under no circumstances is the author responsible for any losses, direct or indirect, which are incurred as a result of the use of information contained within this document, including, but not limited to, — errors, omissions, or inaccuracies.

TABLE OF CONTENTS

INTRODUCTION 16

THE ANTI-INFLAMMATORY DIET 18

    Benefits of Anti-Inflammatory Diet 18

    Foods to Avoid 19

    Foods that Help You Fight Inflammation 21

    Anti-Inflammatory Friendly Ingredients 23

BREAKFAST 26

1. Oven-Poached Eggs 26
2. Turkey Burgers 26
3. Anti-Inflammatory Breakfast Frittata 26
4. Mediterranean Frittata 27
5. Spicy Marble Eggs 27
6. Tuna & Sweet Potato Croquettes 28
7. Veggie Balls 28
8. Salmon Burgers 29
9. Fennel Seeds Cookies 29
10. Sun-Dried Tomato Garlic Bruschetta 30
11. Coconut & Banana Cookies 30
12. Hash Browns 30
13. Mushroom Crêpes 31
14. Bake Apple Turnover 31
15. Almond Pancakes with Coconut Flakes 32
16. Breakfast Sausage and Mushroom Casserole 32
17. Maple Oatmeal 33
18. Apple, Ginger, and Rhubarb Muffins 34
19. Almond Scones 34
20. Cranberry and Raisins Granola 35
21. Breakfast Arrozcaldo 35
22. Apple Bruschetta with Almonds and Blackberries .. 35
23. Oat Porridge with Cherry & Coconut 36
24. Gingerbread Oatmeal Breakfast 36
25. Yummy Steak Muffins 36
26. White and Green Quiche 37
27. Beef Breakfast Casserole 37
28. Ham and Veggie Frittata Muffins 38
29. Tomato and Avocado Omelet 38

BRUNCH 39

30. Oats with Berries 39
31. Spinach Avocado Smoothie 39
32. Golden Milk 39
33. Granola 40
34. Overnight Coconut Chia Oats 40
35. Blueberry Hemp Seed Smoothie 41
36. Spiced Morning Chia Pudding 41
37. Green Smoothie 41
38. Oatmeal Pancakes 41
39. Anti-inflammatory Porridge 42
40. Cherry Smoothie 42
41. Gingerbread Oatmeal 42
42. Roasted Almonds 43

#	Item	Page
43.	Roasted Pumpkin Seeds	43
44.	Roasted Chickpeas	43
45.	Spiced Popcorn	44
46.	Cucumber Bites	44
47.	Spinach Fritters	44
48.	Crispy Chicken Fingers	45
49.	Quinoa & Veggie Croquettes	45
50.	Sweet Potato Cranberry Breakfast bars	45
51.	Savory Breakfast Pancakes	46
52.	Scrambled Eggs with Smoked Salmon	46
53.	Raspberry Grapefruit Smoothie	46
54.	Breakfast Burgers with Avocado Buns	47
55.	Spinach Breakfast	47
56.	Healthy Breakfast Chocolate Donuts	47
57.	Baked Eggs with Portobello Mushrooms	48
58.	Breakfast Spinach Mushroom Tomato Fry Up	48
59.	Sweet Cherry Almond Chia Pudding	48
60.	Pineapple Ginger Smoothie	49
61.	Beet and Cherry Smoothie	49
62.	Spicy Pineapple Smoothie	49
63.	Breakfast Cherry Muffins	49
64.	Breakfast Shakshuka	50
65.	Anti-Inflammatory Crepes	50
66.	No-Bake Turmeric Protein Donuts	50
67.	Breakfast Stir Fry	51

LUNCH 52

#	Item	Page
68.	Strawberries and Cream Trifle	52
69.	Maple Toast and Eggs	52
70.	Sweet Onion and Egg Pie	52
71.	Mini Breakfast Pizza	53
72.	Chicken Muffins	53
73.	Pumpkin Pancakes	53
74.	Cauliflower and Chorizo	54
75.	Carrot Bread	54
76.	Fruity Muffins	55
77.	Edamame Omelet	55
78.	Almond Mascarpone Dumplings	56
79.	Raisin Bran Muffins	56
80.	Apple Bread	56
81.	Zucchini Bread	57
82.	Sweetened Brown Rice	57
83.	Cornmeal Grits	58
84.	Grapefruit-Pomegranate Salad	58
85.	Oatmeal-Raisin Scones	58
86.	Yogurt Cheese and Fruit	59
87.	Chicken & Cabbage Platter	59
88.	Balsamic Chicken and Vegetables	59
89.	Onion Bacon Pork Chops	60
90.	Caramelized Pork Chops	60
91.	Chicken Bacon Quesadilla	60
92.	Rosemary Roasted Pork with Cauliflower	61
93.	Grilled Salmon and Zucchini with Mango Sauce	61
94.	Beef and Broccoli Stir-Fry	61
95.	Parmesan-Crusted Halibut with Asparagus	62
96.	Hearty Beef and Bacon Casserole	62

#	Title	Page
97.	Sesame Wings with Cauliflower	63
98.	Fried Coconut Shrimp with Asparagus	63
99.	Coconut Chicken Curry with Cauliflower Rice	63
100.	Pumpkin Spiced Almonds	64
101.	Tzatziki Dip with Cauliflower	64
102.	Classic Guacamole Dip	64
103.	Creamy Queso Dip	64
104.	Herb Butter Scallops	65

DINNER 66

#	Title	Page
105.	Pan-Seared Halibut with Citrus Butter Sauce	66
106.	Sole Asiago	66
107.	Cheesy Garlic Salmon	66
108.	Stuffed Chicken Breasts	67
109.	Spicy Pork Chops	67
110.	Almond Breaded Chicken Goodness	67
111.	Garlic Lamb Chops	68
112.	Mushroom Pork Chops	68
113.	Mediterranean Pork	69
114.	Brie-Packed Smoked Salmon	69
115.	Blackened Tilapia	69
116.	Salsa Chicken Bites	69
117.	Tomato & Tuna Balls	70
118.	Fennel & Figs Lamb	70
119.	Tamari Steak Salad	70
120.	Blackened Chicken	71
121.	Mediterranean Mushroom Olive Steak	71
122.	Buttery Scallops	71
123.	Brussels sprouts and Garlic Aioli	72
124.	Broccoli Bites	72
125.	Bacon Burger Cabbage Stir Fry	72
126.	Bacon Cheeseburger	73
127.	Cauliflower Mac & Cheese	73
128.	Mushroom & Cauliflower Risotto	73
129.	Pita Pizza	74
130.	Skillet Cabbage Tacos	74
131.	Taco Casserole	74
132.	Creamy Chicken Salad	75
133.	Spicy Keto Chicken Wings	75
134.	Cheesy Ham Quiche	76
135.	Feta and Cauliflower Rice Stuffed Bell Peppers	76
136.	Shrimp with Linguine	77
137.	Mexican Cod Fillets	77
138.	Simple Mushroom Chicken Mix	77
139.	Squash Spaghetti with Bolognese Sauce	78
140.	Healthy Halibut Fillets	78
141.	Clean Salmon with Soy Sauce	78
142.	Simple Salmon with Eggs	78
143.	Easy Shrimp	79
144.	Scallops with Mushroom Special	79
145.	Delicious Creamy Crab Meat	79

SNACKS AND APPETIZERS 80

#	Title	Page
146.	Candied Dates	80
147.	Berry Delight	80
148.	Blueberry & Chia Flax Seed Pudding	80

#	Item	Page
149.	Spicy Roasted chickpeas	80
150.	Berry Energy bites	81
151.	Roasted Beets	81
152.	473.Bruschetta	81
153.	Cashew Cheese	81
154.	Low Cholesterol-Low Calorie Blueberry Muffin	82
155.	Carrot Sticks with Avocado Dip	82
156.	Boiled Okra and Squash	82
157.	Oven Crisp Sweet Potato	82
158.	Olive and Tomato Balls	83
159.	Mini Pepper Nachos	83
160.	Avocado Hummus	83
161.	Flavorsome Almonds	84
162.	Chewy Blackberry Leather	84
163.	Party-Time Chicken Nuggets	84
164.	Protein-Packed Croquettes	85
165.	Energy Dates Balls	85
166.	Energetic Oat Bars	85
167.	Soft Flourless Cookies	86
168.	Delectable Cookies	86
169.	Turmeric Chickpea Cakes	86
170.	Almonds and Blueberries Yogurt Snack	87
171.	Cottage Cheese with Apple Sauce	87
172.	Cucumber Rolls Hors D'oeuvres	87
173.	Ginger Turmeric Protein Bars	88
174.	Avocado with Tomatoes and Cucumber	88
175.	Salmon & Avocado Toast	88
176.	Avocado and Egg Sandwich	89
177.	Coconut Porridge	89
178.	Almond and Honey Homemade Bar	89

SIDE DISHES 91

#	Item	Page
179.	Simply Vanilla Frozen Greek Yogurt	91
180.	Salad Bites	91
181.	Greek Chop-Chop Salad	92
182.	Cauliflower Fried Rice	92
183.	Roasted Garden Vegetables	92
184.	Asian Cabbage Salad	93
185.	Southwest Deviled Eggs	93
186.	Rajun' Cajun Roll-Ups	93
187.	Everything Parmesan Crisps	94
188.	Edamame Hummus	94
189.	Chia Chocolate Pudding	94
190.	Mashed Cauliflower	95
191.	Pickle Roll-Ups	95
192.	Baked Zucchini Fries	95
193.	Italian Eggplant Pizzas	96
194.	Tomato, Basil, and Cucumber Salad	96
195.	Roasted Root Vegetables	96
196.	Cauliflower Rice	97
197.	Tomato and Mozzarella Bites	97
198.	Homemade Potato Chips	97
199.	Brie with Apricot Topping	98
200.	Chocolate Peanut Butter Protein Balls	98
201.	Hummus	98
202.	Cheese Chips	99

203.	Caprese Salad Bites	99
204.	Kale, Butternut Squash, and Sausage Pasta	99
205.	Lemon Juice Salmon with Quinoa	100
206.	Asian Peanut Cabbage Slaw	100
207.	Cinnamon Fried Bananas	100
208.	Melting Tuna and Cheese Toasties	101
209.	Spinach and Artichoke Dip	101
210.	Slow Cooker Boston Beans	101
211.	Low Cholesterol Scalloped Potatoes	102
212.	Green Beans Greek Style	102
213.	Marinated Mushrooms	102
214.	Moch Mashed Potatoes	103
215.	No Dish Summer Medley	103
216.	Pureed Classic Egg Salad	103
217.	Maple-Mashed Sweet Potatoes	103
218.	Garlic-Parmesan Cheesy Chips	104

STAPLES, SAUCES, DIPS AND DRESSINGS ... 105

219.	Roasted Garlic Dip	105
220.	Cashew Yogurt	105
221.	Artichoke Spinach Dip	105
222.	Chickpea & Artichoke Mushroom Pâté	106
223.	Buffalo Dip	106
224.	Barbecue Sauce	107
225.	Barbecue Tahini Sauce	107
226.	Bolognese Sauce	107
227.	Chipotle Bean Cheesy Dip	108
228.	Cilantro and Parsley Hot Sauce	108

FISH AND SEAFOOD ... 110

229.	Lemon-Caper Trout with Caramelized Shallots	110
230.	Shrimp Scampi	110
231.	Shrimp with Spicy Spinach	110
232.	Shrimp with Cinnamon Sauce	111
233.	Pan-Seared Scallops with Lemon-Ginger Vinaigrette	111
234.	Manhattan-Style Salmon Chowder	111
235.	Roasted Salmon and Asparagus	112
236.	Citrus Salmon on a Bed of Greens	112
237.	Orange and Maple-Glazed Salmon	113
238.	Salmon Ceviche	113
239.	Cod with Ginger	113
240.	Rosemary-Lemon Cod	114
241.	Halibut Curry	114
242.	Lemony Mussels	114
243.	Hot Tuna Steak	114
244.	Marinated Fish Steaks	115
245.	Baked Tomato Hake	115
246.	Cheesy Tuna Pasta	115
247.	Salmon and Roasted Peppers	116
248.	Shrimp and Beets	116
249.	Shrimp and Corn	116
250.	Chili Shrimp and Pineapple	117
251.	Balsamic Scallops	117
252.	Whitefish Curry	117
253.	Swordfish with Pineapple and Cilantro	118
254.	Sesame-Tuna Skewers	118

#	Recipe	Page
255.	Trout with Chard	118
256.	Sole with Vegetables	119
257.	Poached Halibut and Mushrooms	119
258.	Halibut Stir Fry	119
259.	Steamed Garlic-Dill Halibut	120
260.	Italian Halibut Chowder	120
261.	Dill Haddock	120
262.	Chili Snapper	121
263.	Lemony Mackerel	121
264.	Honey Crusted Salmon with Pecans	121

POULTRY 123

#	Recipe	Page
265.	Basic "Rotisserie" Chicken	123
266.	Hidden Valley Chicken Dummies	123
267.	Chicken Divan	123
268.	Apricot Chicken Wings	124
269.	Champion Chicken Pockets	124
270.	Chicken-Bell Pepper Sauté	124
271.	Avocado-Orange Grilled Chicken	125
272.	Honey Chicken Tagine	125
273.	Roasted Chicken	125
274.	Chicken in Pita Bread	126
275.	Skillet Chicken with Brussels Sprouts Mix	126
276.	Spicy Chipotle Chicken	127
277.	Chicken with Fennel	127
278.	Adobo Lime Chicken Mix	127
279.	Cajun Chicken & Prawn	127
280.	Healthy Turkey Gumbo	128
281.	Chinese-Orange Spiced Duck Breasts	128
282.	Super Sesame Chicken Noodles	129
283.	Lebanese Chicken Kebabs and Hummus	129
284.	Nutty Pesto Chicken Supreme	130
285.	Delicious Roasted Duck	130
286.	Duck Breast with Apricot Sauce	130
287.	Duck Breast Salad	131
288.	Duck Breast and Blackberries Mix	131
289.	Chicken Piccata	132
290.	Honey-Mustard Lemon Marinated Chicken	132
291.	Spicy Almond Chicken Strips with Garlic Lime Tartar Sauce	133
292.	Chicken Scarpariello with Spicy Sausage	133
293.	Almond Chicken Cutlets	134
294.	Cheesy Chicken Sun-Dried Tomato Packets	134
295.	Tuscan Chicken Saute	135
296.	Breaded Chicken Fillets	135
297.	Turkey Ham and Mozzarella Pate	135
298.	Boozy Glazed Chicken	136
299.	Pan-Fried Chorizo Sausage	136
300.	Easy Chicken Tacos	136
301.	Cheesy Bacon-Wrapped Chicken with Asparagus Spears	137
302.	Delightful Teriyaki Chicken Under Pressure	137
303.	Turkey and Potatoes with Buffalo Sauce	137
304.	Exquisite Pear and Onion Goose	138
305.	Turkey Breast with Fennel and Celery	138
306.	Pancetta and Chicken Risotto	138

MEAT		140
307.	Beef with Carrot & Broccoli	140
308.	Beef with Mushroom & Broccoli	140
309.	Citrus Beef with Bok Choy	141
310.	Beef with Zucchini Noodles	141
311.	Beef with Asparagus & Bell Pepper	142
312.	Spiced Ground Beef	142
313.	Ground Beef with Cabbage	142
314.	Ground Beef with Veggies	143
315.	Ground Beef with Cashews & Veggies	143
316.	Ground Beef with Greens & Tomatoes	144
317.	Beef & Veggies Chili	144
318.	Ground Beef & Veggies Curry	144
319.	Spicy & Creamy Ground Beef Curry	145
320.	Curried Beef Meatballs	145
321.	Beef Meatballs in Tomato Gravy	146
322.	Pork with Lemongrass	146
323.	Pork with Olives	147
324.	Pork Chops with Tomato Salsa	147
SALAD RECIPES		148
325.	Loaded Kale Salad	148
326.	Avocado Kale Salad	148
327.	Broccoli Sweet Potato Chickpea Salad	149
328.	Broccoli, Kelp, And Feta Salad	149
329.	Cauliflower & Lentil Salad	149
330.	Cherry Tomato Salad with Soy Chorizo	150
331.	French Style Potato Salad	150
332.	Kale Salad with Tahini Dressing	151
333.	Almond-Goji Berry Cauliflower Salad	151
334.	Mango Salad with Peanut Dressing	152
335.	Niçoise Salad	152
336.	Penne Pasta Salad	152
337.	Maple Rice	153
338.	Rainbow Vegetable Bowl	153
339.	Red Bell Pepper Hummus	153
340.	Roasted Asparagus with Feta Cheese Salad	154
341.	Roasted Bell Pepper Salad with Olives	154
342.	Roasted Broccoli with Peanuts and Kecap Manis 155	
343.	Roasted Chili Potatoes	155
VEGETABLE AND VEGAN RECIPES		156
344.	Lentils with Tomatoes and Turmeric	156
345.	Whole-Wheat Pasta with Tomato-Basil Sauce	156
346.	Fried Rice with Kale	156
347.	Nutty and Fruity Garden Salad	157
348.	Stir-Fried Brussels Sprouts and Carrots	157
349.	Curried Veggies and Poached Eggs	157
350.	Braised Kale	158
351.	Braised Leeks, Cauliflower and Artichoke Hearts 158	
352.	Celery Root Hash Browns	158
353.	Braised Carrots 'n Kale	159
354.	Stir-Fried Gingery Veggies	159
355.	Cauliflower Fritters	159
356.	Stir-Fried Squash	159

357.	Cauliflower Hash Brown	160	383.	Athenian Avgolemono Sour Soup	169
358.	Sweet Potato Puree	160	384.	Italian Bean Soup	170
359.	Curried Okra	160	385.	Red Soup, Seville Style	170
360.	Vegetable Potpie	161	386.	Garlic Soup	170
361.	Grilled Eggplant Roll-Ups	161	387.	Dalmatian Cabbage, Potato, And Pea Soup	171
362.	Eggplant Gratin	161			
363.	Veggie Stuffed Peppers	162			

DRINKS AND SMOOTHIES ... 172

364.	Cheesy Gratin Zucchini	162	388.	Key Lime Pie Smoothie	172
365.	Korean Barbecue Tofu	162	389.	Herb And Melon Kefir Smoothie	172
366.	Fruit Bowl with Yogurt Topping	163	390.	Kefir And Yogurt Banana Flaxseed Shake	172
367.	Collard Green Wrap	163	391.	Cinnamon Roll Smoothie	172
368.	Zucchini Garlic Fries	164	392.	Strawberry Cheesecake Smoothie	173
369.	Stir-Fried Eggplant	164	393.	Peanut Butter Banana Smoothie	173
370.	Sautéed Garlic Mushrooms	164	394.	Avocado Turmeric Smoothie	173
371.	Stir-Fried Asparagus and Bell Pepper	164	395.	Blueberry Smoothie	173
372.	Wild Rice with Spicy Chickpeas	165	396.	Peanut Butter Cup Smoothies	174
373.	Cashew Pesto & Parsley with veggies	165	397.	Berry Cheesecake Smoothies	174
374.	Spicy Chickpeas with Roasted Vegetables	165	398.	Guava Smoothie	174
375.	Special Vegetable Kitchree	166	399.	Watermelon, Cantaloupe and Mango Smoothie 174	
376.	Mashed Sweet Potato Burritos	166	400.	BlackBerry & Banana Smoothie	175

SOUPS AND STEWS ... 167

			401.	Green Smoothie with Raspberries	175
377.	Spring Soup with Gourmet Grains	167	402.	Veggie-Ful Smoothie	175
378.	Spiced Soup with Lentils & Legumes	167	403.	Apple Pie Smoothie	175
379.	Lemon and Egg Pasta Soup	168	404.	Banana Almond Smoothie	176
380.	Roasted Vegetable Soup	168	405.	Protein Spinach Shake	176
381.	Mediterranean Tomato Soup	168	406.	Fresh Lemon Cream Shake	176
382.	Tomato and Cabbage Puree Soup	169	407.	Avocado Banana Smoothie	176
			408.	Banana Cherry Smoothie	176

#	Item	Page
409.	Banana and Kale Smoothie	177
410.	Blueberry and Spinach Smoothie	177
411.	Matcha Mango Smoothie	177
412.	Avocado Milk Whip	177

DESSERTS 178

#	Item	Page
413.	Carrot Cake	178
414.	Lemon Vegan Cake	178
415.	Dark Chocolate Granola Bars	178
416.	Blueberry Crisp	179
417.	Chocolate Chip Quinoa Granola Bars	179
418.	Strawberry Granita	179
419.	Apple Fritters	180
420.	Roasted Bananas	180
421.	Berry-Banana Yogurt	180
422.	Avocado Chocolate Mousse	181
423.	Anti-Inflammatory Apricot Squares	181
424.	Raw Black Forest Brownies	181
425.	Berry Parfait	181
426.	Sherbet Pineapple	182
427.	Easy Peach Cobbler	182
428.	Thar She' Salts Peanut Butter Cookies	182
429.	Almond Butter Balls Vegan	183
430.	Coffee Cream	183
431.	Almond Cookies	183
432.	Chocolate Mousse	183
433.	Raspberry Diluted Frozen Sorbet	184
434.	Chocolate Covered Strawberries	184
435.	Coconut Muffins	184
436.	Chocolate Cherry Chia Pudding	184
437.	Strawberry Orange Sorbet	185
438.	Pineapple Cake	185
439.	Mediterranean Rolled Baklava with Walnuts	185
440.	Mint Chocolate Chip Ice-cream	186
441.	Flourless Sweet Potato Brownies	186
442.	Paleo Raspberry Cream Pie	187
443.	Caramelized Pears	187
444.	Berry Ice Pops	188
445.	Fruit Cobbler	188
446.	Watermelon and Avocado Cream	188
447.	Coconut and Chocolate Cream	188
448.	Chocolate Bananas	189
449.	Watermelon Sorbet	189
450.	Cinnamon Apple Chips	189
451.	Avocado Brownies	190
452.	Fruit Salad	190
453.	Chocolate Chip Cookies	190

SLOW COOKER RECIPES 191

#	Item	Page
454.	Quinoa and Cauliflower Congee	191
455.	Zucchini and Carrot Combo	191
456.	Salmon in Dill Sauce	191
457.	Parsley Tilapia	192
458.	Cod with Bell Pepper	192
459.	Tangy Barbecue Chicken	192
460.	Salsa Verde Chicken	193

461.	Lemon & Garlic Chicken Thighs	193
462.	Chicken & Apple Cider Chili	193
463.	Buffalo Chicken Lettuce Wraps	194
464.	Cilantro-Lime Chicken Drumsticks	194
465.	Coconut-Curry-Cashew Chicken	194
466.	Turkey & Sweet Potato Chili	195
467.	Moroccan Turkey Tagine	195
468.	Turkey Sloppy Joes	196
469.	Turkey Meatballs with Spaghetti Squash	196
470.	Chimichurri Turkey	196
471.	Balsamic-Glazed Turkey Wings	197
472.	Slow Cooker Chicken Fajitas	197
473.	Spicy Pulled Chicken Wraps	197
474.	Orange Chicken Legs	198
475.	Slow Cooker Chicken Cacciatore	198
476.	Bacon-Wrapped Chicken with Cheddar Cheese 198	
477.	Slow Cooker Jerk Chicken	199
478.	Oregano Pork	199
479.	Cauliflower, Coconut Milk, and Shrimp Soup	199

LOW SODIUM RECIPES 201

480.	Pasta Primavera	201
481.	Tuscan Chicken Linguine	201
482.	Classic Beef Lasagna	202
483.	Spicy Veggie Pasta Bake	202
484.	Parmesan Spaghetti in Mushroom-Tomato Sauce 202	
485.	Mustard Chicken Farfalle	203
486.	Italian Mushroom Pizza	203
487.	Chicken Bacon Ranch Pizza	204
488.	Fall Baked Vegetable with Rigatoni	205
489.	Walnut Pesto Pasta	205
490.	Beef Carbonara	205
491.	Coconut Flour Pizza	206
492.	Keto Pepperoni Pizza	206
493.	Fresh Bell Pepper Basil Pizza	206
494.	Basil & Artichoke Pizza	207
495.	Spanish-Style Pizza de Jarmon	207
496.	Curry Chicken Pockets	208
497.	Fajita Style Chili	208
498.	Fun Fajita Wraps	209
499.	Classic Chicken Noodle Soup	209
500.	Open Face Egg and Bacon Sandwich	209
501.	Tuscan Stew	210
502.	Tenderloin Fajitas	210
503.	Peanut Sauce Chicken Pasta	211
504.	Chicken Cherry Wraps	211
505.	Easy Barley Soup	211
506.	Cauliflower Lunch Salad	212
507.	Cheesy Black Bean Wraps	212

GRAIN FREE RECIPES 213

508.	Vegan-Friendly Banana Bread	213
509.	Mango Granola	213
510.	Tomato Omelet	214
511.	Sautéed Veggies on Hot Bagels	214

#	Recipe	Page
512.	Coco-Tapioca Bowl	214
513.	Choco-Banana Oats	215
514.	Keto Chicken Enchiladas	215
515.	Roasted Whole Chicken	216
516.	Mustard Pork Mix	216
517.	Pork with Chili Zucchinis and Tomatoes	216
518.	Pork with Thyme Sweet Potatoes	216
519.	Pork with Pears and Ginger	217
520.	Parsley Pork and Artichokes	217
521.	Pork with Mushrooms and Cucumbers	217

MEAL PLANS 219

28 Days Meal Plan 219

Vegan Meal Plan 220

Paleo Meal Plan 221

Keto Meal Plan 222

Mediterranean Meal Plan 222

Time Saving Meal Plan 223

INDEX 224

CONCLUSION 231

INTRODUCTION

Do you suffer from inflammation? Did you know that the diet choices you make can have a huge impact on how your body deals with extreme stress? Anti-Inflammation Diet is a Lifestyle reveals exactly why.

The results can be life-changing. For example, we recently discovered that the quality of your sleep is totally affected by how healthy your gut is. We also learned that choosing to eat a high-quality diet is the only way you can have complete control over inflammation. Not only are meals high in anti-inflammatory foods designed to improve your health, but they are also designed to help you achieve the best night's sleep of your life.

Diet has been directly linked to a person's health. If you are looking for ways to improve your diet and reduce the inflammation in your body, an anti-inflammatory diet might be the solution that works best for you.

An anti-inflammatory diet is made up of foods that have been proven to reduce inflammation while still providing all essential nutrients. These include vegetables, fruits, nuts and seeds, whole grains and beans, healthy proteins like fish or poultry, herbs, and spices that may help fight inflammation, such as turmeric or ginger. It also includes spices like salt or pepper, which have been shown to be anti-inflammatory.

You probably don't even know what the term "inflammation" means, but if you suffer from joint pain or are trying to reduce your risk of heart disease, it's a good idea to be familiar with this word. When you injure yourself, or an external strain (like a tight muscle) causes damage to your body, a chemical reaction occurs that is known as inflammation. This allows blood vessels to dilate so that the injured area can be supplied with blood by the body's circulation system. The resulting heat and swelling are signals for the immune system to send enzymes and white blood cells to fight off infection or repair damaged cells.

Inflammation is an important indicator of the body's status. It indicates when something's wrong, but it can also be a response to a lot of foods and lifestyle changes that normal healthy people encounter every day.

The most extreme form of inflammation is Critical Diffuse Inflammatory Demyelination Disease (CDID), a rare condition in which areas of the nervous system are affected, causing problems with memory, coordination, and mood. Most people don't suffer from CDID, but there are some diseases that cause chronic inflammation that you may want to avoid. They include rheumatoid arthritis, lupus, multiple sclerosis, and irritable bowel syndrome.

Inflammation and the resulting pain are thought to be one of the factors that cause depression. And, finally – in case you didn't already know this – inflammation is a big part of weight gain, too. As I've said a number of times throughout this website (the most recent being here), excess fat cells in your body release inflammatory cytokines that can cause oxidative stress and damage your DNA. The damage caused by these chemicals is then passed down through your cell's DNA, which can lead to an increased risk of cancer.

To make matters worse, the inflammatory response is also tied to your body's stress response. When your body recognizes a stressful situation, it sends out chemicals called glucocorticoids into the bloodstream. This causes inflammation throughout the body in an attempt to increase fighting capacities by reducing pain sensitivity and increasing alertness.

Inflammation and stress go hand-in-hand. If you reduce one, you can mitigate the other.

In general, foods that are rich in pro-inflammatory agents are those that are high in fats and simple sugars. Processed foods, refined carbs, and non-organic dairy products are also extremely inflammatory. On the other hand, foods loaded with anti-inflammatory agents are those that are anti-oxidant rich (like grapefruits and blueberries), have anti-inflammatory properties (like ginger), or contain a lot of omega-3 fatty acids.

For the most part, diet is one of the best ways to decrease inflammation. Not only do you avoid eating inflammatory foods like refined sugar, but you can also substitute in foods that contain ingredients that invoke an anti-inflammatory response in your body. Combined with a regular exercise routine, you can expect to see an improvement in your overall health.

As I've already mentioned, there are certain foods that have properties that fight inflammation. In the following list of foods, you'll find examples of foods high in omega-3s (like salmon), anti-oxidants (like blueberries), and anti-inflammatory spices (like ginger).

THE ANTI-INFLAMMATORY DIET

Do you know how much inflammation your diet may be causing? New research has found that eating less red meat reduces your body's levels of inflammation. The anti-inflammatory diet includes vegetables, whole grains, fruits, legumes and nuts as well as healthy fats like those found in avocado or salmon.

Some of the foods that reduce inflammation are beans (but not soy), berries, carrots, celery, tomatoes, cabbage, leeks and parsley.

Yes you too can eat less inflammation! Try the infographic below for some recipes to try. Allergies can be caused by diet as well as lifestyle and many people who suffer from chronic health issues may be able to improve their condition by changing their diet.

You can't talk about how to deal with inflammation and chronic health issues without talking about stress. Chronic stress plays a big role in contributing to the development of many chronic lifestyle diseases. If you are under stress, your immune system becomes compromised and inflammatory responses are triggered all day every day. If you don't want to be sick, eating less inflammation is a great place to start!

The most common symptoms of inflammation include allergies, asthma, eczema, rheumatoid arthritis, joint pain and fatigue. Inflammation is also the underlying cause of many heart attacks, strokes, type 2 diabetes and cancer.

The inflammatory response causes more blood to flow through the affected area and once there, white blood cells can fight off unwanted foreign invaders like microbes and clean up debris from damaged cells. There are good forms of inflammation that are essential for our survival and keeping us healthy but there are also other forms that can lead to chronic health issues when we don't manage it properly.

How do you know if you have too much inflammation?

You should ask your doctor about specific biomarkers for inflammation to see if yours are within normal range. Some of the signs and symptoms of elevated inflammatory responses include fatigue, mood changes, dry skin, abdominal cramping or bloating, swelling of hands or feet and excessive thirst.

Inflammation can be reduced by eating an anti-inflammatory diet that is high in omega 3's found in fish, flaxseeds and walnuts as well as eating plenty of vegetables. It is also important to control your stress levels because anxiety can cause a release of hormones that initiate an inflammatory response.

Benefits of Anti-Inflammatory Diet

Less Inflammation, Less Pain, Other symptoms improved. By eliminating the right foods you might find relief from other autoimmune disease symptoms, like tendinitis and (as in my case) even asthma, eczema, and rhinitis.

I developed sciatica after my sacrum twisted out of alignment a year ago and even though it's back in alignment the nerve pain, shooting pain, and numbness have continued and worsened significantly.

I did the anti-inflammatory diet. Worked so good I was able to put off my double knee replacement surgery for three years

Chronic inflammation is the root cause of many serious illnesses - including heart disease, many cancers, and Alzheimer's disease

Learning how specific foods influence the inflammatory process is the best strategy for containing it and reducing long-term disease risks

My own doc told me to eat an anti-inflammatory diet because of my degenerative bone disease and to help prevent DVT

The Anti-Inflammatory is **NOT A DIET BUT AN HEALTHY LIFE STYLE!**

Foods to Avoid

Inflammation in the body is a normal immune response to injury or infection. Acute inflammation brings white blood cells and chemical substances called cytokines into the injured area, along with fluids and compounds like nitric oxide that dilate (widen) blood vessels to bring more nutrients, oxygen, and other chemicals needed for healing.

Chronic inflammation is different because it occurs as a reaction to bodily stressors, such as allergens or toxins. This response can last for months or years without going away completely. Meanwhile, chronic inflammation damages tissues in those injured areas by preventing cells from regenerating properly.

In addition to the damage that chronic inflammation does, some of the inflammatory compounds involved in this type of response can damage the liver. In some cases, chronic inflammation is also associated with other conditions like cardiovascular disease and cancer.

Chronic inflammation can be triggered by a number of foods or components in foods that contain substances called proinflammatory compounds. While we need these chemicals to respond to injury or infection, too much exposure causes inflammation. Here are five foods and components that have been linked to higher levels of chronic inflammation:

Starch: When consumed in excess, it triggers an immune response that leads to tissue damage and excessive production of inflammatory compounds in the body.

When consumed in excess, it triggers an immune response that leads to tissue damage and excessive production of inflammatory compounds in the body. Sugar: It causes a spike in triglyceride levels in the blood, which increases chronic inflammation.

It causes a spike in triglyceride levels in the blood, which increases chronic inflammation. Omega-6 Fatty Acids: These are found mainly in animal proteins, oils from seeds and nuts like canola and corn, and fish oil supplements. They are considered proinflammatory because they cause an increase of inflammatory compounds like cytokines and nitric oxide in the body with each meal that contains them.

These are found mainly in animal proteins, oils from seeds and nuts like canola and corn, and fish oil supplements. They are considered proinflammatory because they cause an increase of inflammatory compounds like cytokines and nitric oxide in the body with each meal that contains them. Sodium: It triggers an increase in a chemical called bradykinin in the body, which has been linked to chronic inflammation as well as asthma.

It triggers an increase in a chemical called bradykinin in the body, which has been linked to chronic inflammation as well as asthma. Saturated Fatty Acids: These are found mainly in meat products such as red meat and eggs, as well as seafood like fish, oysters, and bacon. They are associated with chronic inflammation because they suppress the ability of white blood cells to break down and remove harmful toxins.

Other common triggers that lead to inflammation are dairy products, alcohol, coffee, processed food, and other chemicals found in plastics.

Although there is no specific cause for every individual's inflammation levels aside from genetics in most cases it is possible to prevent the problem by making dietary changes and incorporating supplements that fight back against this condition.

How Food Contributes to Inflammation

Inflammation is one of the most important measures for determining health and wellness. It impacts everything from your general mood to your cardiovascular health. And it can be brought on by a wide variety of things both inside and outside our bodies, including certain foods we eat.

Top five foods that have the potential to contribute to inflammation:

1. Animal products – Meat, poultry, fish and dairy are all good at contributing to inflammation in your body. The reason is two-fold: First, these foods contain saturated fats that are known triggers for inflammation in your system. Second, they're also loaded with sodium, which raises blood pressure and contributes to an unhealthy heart rate. If you're eating animal products a lot it's important to limit your intake of these foods as much as possible so you can enjoy optimal health while enjoying some healthy meaty carby goodness!
2. Processed foods – Though there are a few exceptions (like canned tomatoes, or packaged plain dried beans), most processed foods contain ingredients that are nowhere near their natural state. For example, if you buy a package of "peanut butter," it won't actually be ground up peanuts – instead, it'll probably be heavily processed peanut oil, sugar and salt. Additionally many processed foods contain high fructose corn syrup and other artificial ingredients that your body doesn't recognize as real food. If you're eating too much of this type of food you're very likely contributing to inflammation in your body (and setting yourself up for some serious health issues down the road).
3. Trans fats – A lot of people don't realize that the "trans" in trans fat actually stands for "transported." Trans fats are all about the oil companies creating cheaper oils that are dirtier and less healthy for you than oils made from wholesome plant sources. Because they're cheaper to produce, these oils are also more commonly used in processed foods.
4. Refined grains – They're linked to some serious health problems like inflammation, type 2 diabetes and bowel disorders such as leaky gut syndrome (which can lead to autoimmune diseases). It's best to limit the amount of these types of foods you're eating to a small serving (ideally less than one cup per day) so you can enjoy optimal health while eating some carby goodness.
5. Artificial sweeteners – As I've previously mentioned before, artificial sweeteners are very different from natural sugars that come from fruits and other plants. Artificial sweeteners are known to contribute to

obesity and digestive problems and some studies have even linked them to cancer and premature death in lab animals. The liver goes into overdrive when you consume artificial sweeteners, spiking insulin levels which can lead to chronic inflammation in the body.

Other factors that contribute to inflammation:

– Mercury in fish: Fish are an incredibly important source of protein and rich in omega-3 fatty acids, which may help improve inflammatory conditions like acne. However, they can also be contaminated with mercury, which can contribute to inflammation.

– Genetics: While there's not solid evidence linking certain genes to inflammation, it's still an indisputable fact that some people do suffer from excessive inflammation due to various genetic factors. For more information see here .

– Physical activity: There are tons of studies and scientific articles documenting the health benefits of physical activity, but despite this fact many individuals still don't exercise enough. This is because sometimes people just think their health problems will go away if they stop exercising, or that it's somehow "bad" for them to get exercise. But this simply isn't true! In fact, the benefits of exercise are pretty amazing and can help keep chronic inflammation at bay. For more information see here.

– Stress: Chronic stress may contribute to elevated levels of inflammation within your body. The hormone cortisol caused by stress can have some nasty effects on your body both mentally and physically, including increasing the formation of free radicals that contribute to inflammation in the body.

Foods that Help You Fight Inflammation

Inflammation is the body's natural defense mechanism and when it is inflamed, the immune system protects your body from harmful bacteria or allergens. Inflammation occurs when you have an overreaction of the immune system to a particular foreign substance.

What are foods that help with inflammation? These are foods that can help to lower levels of inflammation in your body. A few options are blueberries, spinach, and strawberries. Sometimes whole grains may be less inflammatory than refined grains as well as nuts, legumes (dried beans), and green tea products like matcha powder or even green tea extract supplements! The last option is to reduce chronic stress in your life which can contribute greatly to inflammation.

Some foods that can help with inflammation:

Blueberries are full of antioxidants and anti-inflammatory properties. They lower the level of "bad" LDL cholesterol, they improve blood sugar control and they reduce oxidative stress in your body. They help to protect against colon cancer, breast cancer, prostate cancer and lung cancer.

Spinach is a great source of Vitamin K which helps to prevent excessive blood clotting. It also helps to lower blood pressure levels and it protects against cardiovascular disease too! It's a great source of Lutein and Zeaxanthin which is important for vision health. Studies have shown that spinach helps to improve memory retention in the brain and it lowers oxidative stress too!

Strawberries are great for improving brain health and preventing cognitive decline. They contain a significant amount of Vitamin C, Bromelain, Potassium, Vitamin A and Vitamin K which all contribute to better brain function and protecting your nervous system. They are a member of the "Brain Berry" family with blueberries and acerola cherries.

Some healthy fats may also help to reduce inflammation:

Avocado has monounsaturated fat and Omega 3 fatty acids. Omega 3 fatty acids are critical for neurological health and they are also a key component for maintaining a healthy blood pressure level too! Avocados contain compounds called carotenoids which help to improve eye health, skin health and may even be an effective treatment for macular degeneration.

Olive oil can be a good source of Monounsaturated fats. Monounsaturated fats have been shown to be beneficial for cardiovascular health as they skip the cholesterol pathway and go directly to the artery wall. There is some evidence that olive oil may also lower LDL cholesterol levels.

Even if you don't eat much healthy fat, you can add a little extra fish oil or flax seed oil to your diet which is also good for inflammatory health. You can even add flaxseed oil, chia seeds or hemp seeds to smoothies and other foods.

Reducing chronic stress is another way to lower inflammation. You don't need to go on a strict diet to do this. Just make a plan for how you will manage your stress levels in your life and try to stick with it! Meditation, yoga, exercise, social support, positive self-talk and regular sleep are all good ways of taking back control of your life from stress.

Anti-Inflammatory Foods and Spices

Inflammation is caused by free radicals in the body. Free radicals damage your cells and cause great pain when these damaged cells call for help from white blood cells. White blood cells come to battle against the viruses or bacteria causing inflammation which leads to fatigue, muscle pain, asthmatic symptoms, mood fluctuations as well as many others problems.

Vitamins B1 and B6 supplements can help by increasing the blood flow to the brain and to inflammation. Inhaling steam from a fresh lemon or drinking a glass of warm water with lemon juice will help your body fight against inflammation. Turmeric powder is another option that fights inflammation in the body. Turmeric's anti-inflammatory properties come from curcumin, which is the main component found in turmeric powder. A cup of hot tea made with one teaspoon of turmeric powder has anti-inflammatory properties that can fight inflammation at a cellular level.

Zucchini, broccoli, cauliflower are also rich in Vitamin C which reduces free radical damage. Try adding them to your meals.

Foods high in fiber also often have anti-inflammatory properties due to their ability to reduce blood sugar levels. Foods high in fiber include dark green leafy vegetables, beans, lentils, oats, brown rice and nuts.

Spices are rich source of antioxidants making them an effective way to fight inflammation in the body. Turmeric powder is a great source that can be added to almost any dish or used as a tea or powder itself.

Anti-Inflammatory Friendly Ingredients

It is important to understand what anti-inflammatory foods are. They can be identified by their special plant compounds with which they have the ability to slow down inflammation in our body. We will teach you about the main anti-inflammatory food groups as well as give you a list of their most common health benefits.

Some Anti-Inflammatory Foods:

Broccoli

Broccoli is a fruit vegetable that contains high levels of vitamins, minerals, and antioxidants. The sulfur compounds presentin broccoli are believed to be a big benefit for people who have rheumatoid arthritis as they help boost their immune system.

Fish

Fish has omega 3 fatty acids. These fatty acids help cut down the effect of inflammation in our body. They are believed to have anti-inflammatory effects by lowering the production of inflammatory markers like C-reactive protein, IL-1, and TNF-alpha. Omega 3s help prevent the oxidation of LDL cholesterol which is otherwise known as bad cholesterol. There is also a reduction in triglycerides levels and blood pressure due to the consumption of fish regularly.

Onions

Onions are rich in an ingredient called quercetin. Quercetin is a compound that has anti-inflammatory effects in our body because it helps reduce inflammation in our arteries. It also reduces the risk of rheumatoid arthritis as well as osteoarthritis. Onions also contain vitamin C and manganese which help fight off free radicals in our body.

Tomatoes

Tomatoes has antioxidant called lycopene. It is believed that lycopene helps lower down the risk of cardiovascular diseases such as stroke and heart attack by acting as a free radical scavenger. Lycopene has also been shown to help boost men's sperm count by enhancing overall reproductive health.

Turmeric

Turmeric has curcumin is one of the main ingredients in turmeric and it also has an anti-inflammatory effect. It can also help protect our cells against free radicals.

Pumpkin Seeds

Pumpkin seeds are a great snack food and they are loaded with essential nutrients such as vitamin E, iron, magnesium, zinc, and protein. They also have a very high level of zinc which is needed for normal cell function in our body. Pumpkin seeds are also able to reduce inflammation in our body by helping boost the production of tissue-repairing cytokines.

Healthy Fats

Healthy fats can help lower down the risk of inflammation and protect our cells from damage caused by oxidative stress. These fats also help our body generate hormones which produce anti-inflammatory chemicals.

Berries

Berries. There is a reduction in overall oxidative stress levels in our bodies due to their antioxidant properties present in berries.

Coconut oil

Coconut oil is a fat that is high in lauric acid, which has anti-inflammatory properties. Lauric acid is known to be a mild nerve gas that could theoretically cause temporary problems for your body. It could cause some symptoms of a "Head Spinner" in some people, and though it may be impossible to test for your own sensitivity, you can take precautions against the possible negative effects: making sure that you don't have too much coconut oil or any other oils of high lauric acid content and avoiding heating coconut oil at very high temperatures.

Supplemental fish oil

It is thought that fatty acids and certain fats known as EFAs that are found in fish oils serve a variety of functions in the body. One of them being that they are anti-inflammatory.

Bananas

A potassium-rich fruit, bananas are naturally anti-inflammatory if eaten in moderation (one level medium banana per day) as they contain a chemical compound called bromelain that inhibits an enzyme called COX-2. Consuming more than the recommended amount may actually increase inflammation due to excess bromelain affecting the production of prostaglandins. It's also important to note that the risk of high blood pressure increases by up to 60 percent when bromelain is consumed with low sodium intake (in other words, a diet high in potassium and low in sodium).

Dark chocolate

High in magnesium and antioxidants, dark chocolate is a great snack choice for anyone who is looking to lower their blood pressure. It can also help suppress immunity-boosting inflammation, which is why a boost of immunity from dark chocolate on an empty stomach can help you preserve energy levels after exercise or an intense workout routine.

Cucumber

Low salt cucumbers are high in lycopene, an antioxidant that helps ward off the effects of oxidative stress - which causes inflammation and aging. This low-salt food type also contains manganese, which aids weight loss by boosting insulin sensitivity and reducing inflammation.

Eggs

Eggs feature an impressive combination of nutrients and vitamins, which are necessary for the body to maintain optimal health. They also contain choline, which helps boost the production of glutathione, an antioxidant that can help block free-radical damage to cells and mitochondria by preventing lipid peroxidation.

Plant-based protein (nuts, hemp seeds, quinoa)

Eating foods rich in protein reduces the risk of chronic inflammation from lifestyle factors such as stress or excess sugar consumption. Protein-rich foods work by triggering an immune response to produce anti-inflammatory compounds to flush harmful inflammation out of the body and prevent its damaging effects. Proteins also supply amino acids, which stimulate the synthesis of anti-inflammatory enzymes such as COX-2 inhibitors such as bromelain.

Prunes

Prunes are an excellent way to receive a boost of nutrition and make your kidneys happy at the same time. Prune juice contains a natural fiber called pectin, which helps lower bad cholesterol levels in the body. It also contains niacin, or vitamin B3, which plays a key role in regulating hormones like insulin and stress response hormones like cortisol, both of which are associated with chronic inflammatory diseases.

Walnuts

Another healthy food choice, walnuts are the perfect snack for anyone trying to lose weight as they help increase lean muscle mass by boosting insulin sensitivity. Studies have shown that walnuts can also help reduce appetite and fight inflammation due to their high omega-3 content. Omega-3 fats are important for the body's inflammatory response as they promote healthy blood clotting, which in turn helps prevent chronic inflammation.

Fish and seafood (herring, salmon, tuna)

Many people live on a diet of fast food and processed foods that contain high amounts of salt. At the same time, modern diets are deficient in bioavailable calcium and vitamin D, both of which are vitally important for bone health. The negative effects of high salt intake cannot be overlooked when it comes to obesity, heart disease or stroke risk. A diet rich in low-mercury omega-3 fatty acids and vitamin D can help lower inflammation and boost immune functions.

Oysters

Oysters has zinc, which is essential for the production of white blood cells that help form a protective barrier against bacterial invasion. A diet rich in zinc has been shown to help protect against chronic inflammation, as it helps protect brain cells, joints, skin and bone from the damaging effects of free radicals. Every part of the oyster contains zinc - nacre (the oyster's coating), meat and milk.

BREAKFAST

1. Oven-Poached Eggs

Preparation Time: 2 minutes
Cooking Time: 11 minutes
Servings: 4
Ingredients:
- 6 eggs, at room temperature
- Water
- Ice bath
- 2 cups water, chilled
- 2 cups of ice cubes

Directions:
1. Set the oven to 350°F. Put 2 cups of water into a deep roasting tin, and place it into the lowest rack of the oven.
2. Place one egg into each cup of cupcake/muffin tins, along with one tablespoon of water.
3. Carefully place muffin tins into the middle rack of the oven.
4. Bake eggs for 45 minutes.
5. Turn off the heat immediately. Please take the muffin tins from the oven and set them on a cake rack to cool before extracting eggs.
6. Pour ice bath ingredients into a large heat-resistant bowl.
7. Bring the eggs into an ice bath to stop the cooking process. After 10 minutes, drain the eggs well. Use as needed.

Nutrition: Calories: 357 kcal | Protein: 17.14 g Fat: 24.36 g | Carbohydrates: 16.19 g

2. Turkey Burgers

Preparation Time: 15 minutes
Cooking Time: 8 minutes
Servings: 5
Ingredients:
- 1 ripe pear, peeled, cored, and chopped roughly
- 1-pound lean ground turkey
- 1 teaspoon fresh ginger, grated finely
- 2 minced garlic cloves
- 1 teaspoon fresh rosemary, minced
- 1 teaspoon fresh sage, minced
- Salt, to taste
- Freshly ground black pepper, to taste
- 1-2 tablespoons coconut oil

Directions:
1. In a blender, add pear and pulse till smooth.
2. Transfer the pear mixture to a large bowl with remaining ingredients except for oil and mix till well combined.
3. Make small equal-sized 10 patties from the mixture.
4. In a heavy-bottomed frying pan, heat oil on medium heat.
5. Add the patties and cook for around 4-5 minutes.
6. Flip the inside and cook for approximately 2-3 minutes.

Nutrition: Calories: 477 | Fat: 15g | Carbohydrates: 26g | Fiber: 11g | Protein: 35g

3. Anti-Inflammatory Breakfast Frittata

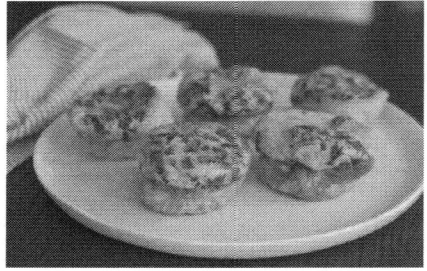

Cooking Time: 40 minutes
Servings: 4
Ingredients:
- 4 large eggs
- 6 egg whites
- 450g button mushrooms
- 450g baby spinach
- 125g firm tofu
- 1 onion, chopped
- 1 tbsp. minced garlic
- ½ tsp. ground turmeric

- ½ tsp. cracked black pepper
- ¼ cup water
- Kosher salt to taste

Directions:
1. Set your oven to 350F.
2. Sauté the mushrooms in a little bit of extra virgin olive oil in a large non-stick ovenproof pan over medium heat. Add the onions once the mushrooms start turning golden and cook for 3 minutes until the onions become soft.
3. Stir in the garlic, then cook for at least 30 seconds until fragrant before adding the spinach. Pour in water, cover, and cook until the spinach becomes wilted for about 2 minutes.
4. Take off the lid and continue cooking up until the water evaporates. Now, combine the eggs, egg whites, tofu, pepper, turmeric, and salt in a bowl. When all the liquid has evaporated, pour in the egg mixture, let cook for about 2 minutes until the edges start setting, transfer to the oven, and bake for about 25 minutes or until cooked.
5. Take off from the oven, then sit for at least 5 minutes before cutting it into quarters and serving.
6. Enjoy!
7. Baby spinach and mushrooms boost the nutrient profile of the eggs to provide you with amazing anti-inflammatory benefits.

Nutrition: Calories: 521 kcal | Protein: 29.13 g | Fat: 10.45 g | Carbohydrates: 94.94 g

4. Mediterranean Frittata

Preparation Time: 5 minutes
Cooking Time: 20 minutes
Servings: 6
Ingredients:
- 6 Eggs
- ¼ cup Feta cheese, crumbled
- ¼ tsp. Black pepper
- Oil, spray, or olive
- 1 tsp. Oregano
- ¼ cup Milk, almond, or coconut
- 1 tsp. Sea salt
- ¼ cup Black olives, chopped
- ¼ cup Green olives, chopped
- ¼ cup Tomatoes, diced

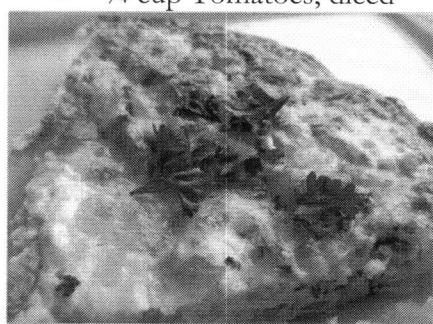

1. Heat oven to 400. Oil one eight by eight-inch baking dish. Beat the milk into the eggs, and then add other ingredients. Pour all of this mixture into the baking dish and bake for twenty minutes.

Nutrition: Calories 107 | 2 grams' sugars | 3 carb grams | 7 fat grams | 7 grams' protein

5. Spicy Marble Eggs

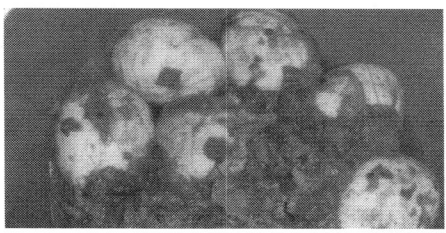

Cooking Time: 2 hours
Servings: 12
Ingredients:
- 6 medium-boiled eggs, unpeeled, cooled
- For the Marinade
- 2 oolong black tea bags
- 3 Tbsp. brown sugar
- 1 thumb-sized fresh ginger, unpeeled, crushed
- 3 dried star anise, whole
- 2 dried bay leaves
- 3 Tbsp. light soy sauce
- 4 Tbsp. dark soy sauce
- 4 cups of water
- 1 dried cinnamon stick, whole
- 1 tsp. salt
- 1 tsp. dried Szechuan peppercorns

Directions:

1. Using the back of a metal spoon, crack eggshells in places to create a spider web effect. Do not peel. Set aside until needed.
2. Pour marinade into large Dutch oven set over high heat. Put lid partially on. Bring water to a rolling boil, about 5 minutes. Turn off heat.
3. Secure lid. Steep ingredients for 10 minutes.
4. Using a slotted spoon, fish out and discard solids. Cool marinade completely to room proceeding.
5. Place eggs into an airtight non-reactive container just small enough to snugly fit all this in.
6. Pour in marinade. Eggs should be completely submerged in liquid. Discard leftover marinade, if any. Line container rim with generous layers of saran wrap. Secure container lid.
7. Chill eggs for 24 hours before using.
8. Extract eggs and drain each piece well before using, but keep the rest submerged in the marinade.

Nutrition: Calories: 75 kcal | Protein: 4.05 g | Fat: 4.36 g | Carbohydrates: 4.83 g

6. Tuna & Sweet Potato Croquettes

Preparation Time: 15 minutes
Cooking Time: 12 minutes
Servings: 8
Ingredients:
- 1 tablespoon coconut oil
- ½ large onion, chopped
- 1 (1-inch piece fresh ginger, minced
- 3 garlic cloves, minced
- 1 Serrano pepper, seeded and minced
- ½ teaspoon ground coriander
- ¼ teaspoon ground turmeric
- ¼ teaspoon red chili powder
- ¼ teaspoon garam masala
- Salt, to taste
- Freshly ground black pepper, to taste
- 2 (5 oz.) cans of tuna
- 1 cup sweet potato, peeled and mashed
- 1 egg
- ¼ cup tapioca flour
- ¼ cup almond flour
- Olive oil, as required

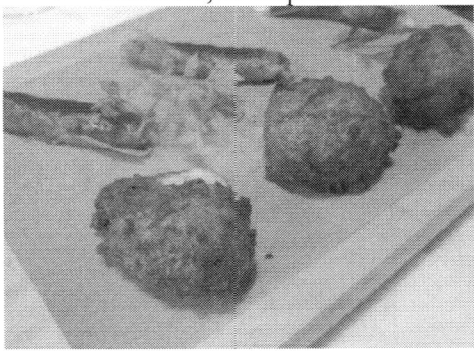

1. In a frying pan, warm the coconut oil on medium heat.
2. Put onion, ginger, garlic, and Serrano pepper and sauté for approximately 5-6 minutes.
3. Stir in spices and sauté approximately 1 minute more.
4. Transfer the onion mixture to a bowl.
5. Add tuna and sweet potato and mix till well combined.
6. Make equal sized oblong shaped patties in the mixture.
7. Arrange the croquettes inside a baking sheet in a single layer and refrigerate overnight.
8. In a shallow dish, beat the egg.
9. In another shallow dish, mix both flours.
10. Heat enough oil in a big skillet.
11. Add croquettes in batches and shallow fry for around 2-3 minutes per side.

Nutrition: Calories: 404 | Fat: 9g | Carbohydrates: 20g | Fiber: 4g | Protein: 30g

7. Veggie Balls

Preparation Time: 15 minutes
Cooking Time: 25 minutes
Servings: 5-6
Ingredients:
- 2 medium sweet potatoes, cubed into ½-inch size
- 2 tablespoons coconut milk
- 1 cup fresh kale leaves, trimmed and chopped
- 1 medium shallot, chopped finely

- 1 tsp. ground cumin
- ½ teaspoon granulated garlic
- ¼ tsp. ground turmeric
- Salt, to taste
- Freshly ground black pepper, to taste

Ground flax seeds, as required

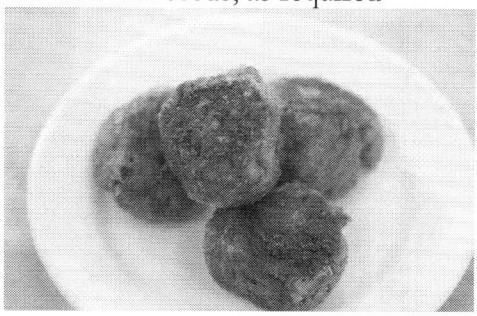

1. Set the oven to 400°F. Line a baking sheet with parchment paper.
2. In a pan of water, arrange a steamer basket.
3. Bring the sweet potato to a steamer basket and steam for approximately 10-15 minutes.
4. In a sizable bowl, put the sweet potato.
5. Add coconut milk and mash well.
6. Add remaining ingredients except for flax seeds and mix till well combined.
7. Make about 1½-2-inch balls from your mixture.
8. Arrange the balls onto the prepared baking sheet inside a single layer.
9. Sprinkle with flax seeds.
10. Bake for around 20-25 minutes.

Nutrition: Calories: 464 | Fat: 12g | Carbohydrates: 20g | Fiber: 8g | Protein: 27g

8. Salmon Burgers

Preparation Time: 15 minutes
Cooking Time: 8 minutes
Servings: 3
Ingredients:
- 1 (6-oz. can) skinless, boneless salmon, drained
- 1 celery rib, chopped
- ½ of a medium onion, chopped
- 2 large eggs
- 1 tablespoon plus
- 1 teaspoon coconut flour
- 1 tablespoon dried dill, crushed
- 1 teaspoon lemon
- Salt, to taste
- Freshly ground black pepper, to taste
- 3 tablespoons coconut oil

Directions:
1. In a substantial bowl, add salmon and which has a fork, break it into small pieces.
2. Add remaining ingredients, excluding the oil, and mix till well combined.
3. Make 6 equal-sized small patties from the mixture.
4. In a substantial skillet, melt coconut oil on medium-high heat.
5. Cook the patties for around 3-4 minutes per side.

Nutrition: Calories: 393 | Fat: 12g | Carbohydrates: 19g | Fiber: 5g | Protein: 24g

9. Fennel Seeds Cookies

Preparation Time: 10 minutes
Cooking Time: 20 minutes
Servings: 5
Ingredients:
- 1/3 cup coconut flour
- ¼ teaspoon whole fennel seeds
- ½ teaspoon fresh ginger, grated finely
- ¼ cup coconut oil softened
- 2 tablespoons raw honey
- 1 teaspoon vanilla extract
- Pinch of ground cinnamon
- Pinch of salt
- Pinch freshly ground black pepper

Directions:
1. Set the oven to 360°F. Line a cookie sheet that has parchment paper.
2. In a substantial bowl, add all together with the ingredients and mix till an even dough forms.
3. Form a small ball in the mixture made onto a prepared cookie sheet inside a single layer.
4. Using your fingers, gently press along the balls to create the cookies.
5. Bake for at least 9 minutes or till golden brown.

Nutrition: Calories: 353 | Fat: 5g | Carbohydrates: 19g | Fiber: 3g | Protein: 25g

10. Sun-Dried Tomato Garlic Bruschetta

Preparation Time: 10 minutes
Cooking Time: 5 minutes
Servings: 6
Ingredients:
- 2 slices sourdough bread, toasted
- 1 tsp. chives, minced
- 1 garlic clove, peeled
- 2 tsp. sun-dried tomatoes in olive oil, minced
- 1 tsp. olive oil

Directions:
1. Vigorously rub garlic clove on 1 side of each of the toasted bread slices
2. Spread equal portions of sun-dried tomatoes on the garlic side of the bread. Sprinkle chives and drizzle olive oil on top.
3. Pop both slices into an oven toaster, and cook until well heated through.
4. Place bruschetta on a plate. Serve warm.

Nutrition: Calories: 149 kcal | Protein: 6.12 g | Fat: 2.99 g | Carbohydrates: 24.39 g

11. Coconut & Banana Cookies

Preparation Time: 15 minutes
Cooking Time: 25 minutes
Servings: 7
Ingredients:
- 2 cups unsweetened coconut, shredded
- 3 medium bananas, peeled
- ½ tsp. ground cinnamon
- ½ tsp. ground turmeric
- Pinch of salt, to taste
- Freshly ground black pepper

Directions:
1. Set the oven to 350°F. Line a cookie sheet a lightly greased parchment paper.
2. In a mixer, put all together ingredients and pulse till a dough-like mixture forms.
3. Form small balls through the mixture and set them onto a prepared cookie sheet in a single layer.
4. Using your fingers, press along the balls to create the cookies.
5. Bake for at least 15-20 minutes or till golden brown.

Nutrition: Calories: 370 | Fat: 4g | Carbohydrates: 28g | Fiber: 11g | Protein: 33g

12. Hash Browns

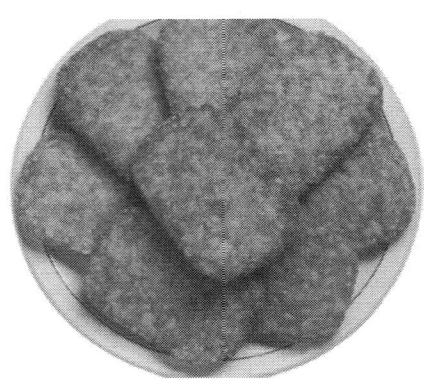

Cooking Time: 15 minutes
Servings: 4
Ingredients:
- 1-pound Russet potatoes, peeled, processed using a grater
- Pinch of sea salt
- Pinch of black pepper, to taste
- 3 Tbsp. olive oil

Directions:
1. Line a microwave safe-dish with paper towels. Spread shredded potatoes on top. Microwave veggies on the highest heat setting for 2 minutes. Remove from heat.
2. Pour 1 tablespoon of oil into a non-stick skillet set over medium heat.
3. Cooking in batches, place a generous pinch of potatoes into the hot oil. Press down using the back of a spatula.
4. Cook for 3 minutes on every side, or until brown and crispy. Drain on paper towels. Repeat step for remaining potatoes. Add more oil as needed.
5. Season with salt and pepper. Serve.

Nutrition: Calories: 200 kcal | Protein: 4.03 g | Fat: 11.73 g | Carbohydrates: 20.49 g

13. Mushroom Crêpes

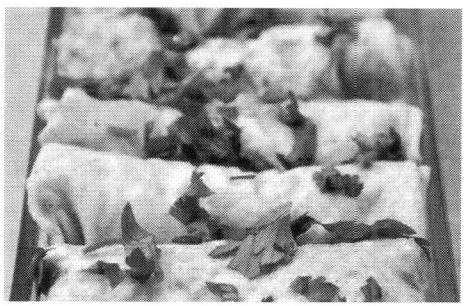

Cooking Time: 30 minutes
Servings: 6
Ingredients:
- 2 eggs
- 3/4 cup milk
- 1/2 cup all-purpose flour
- 1/4 teaspoon salt
- For the filling
- 3 tablespoons all-purpose flour
- 2 cups of cremini mushrooms, sliced
- 3/4 cup chicken broth
- 1/2 cup Parmesan cheese, grated
- 1/8 teaspoon cayenne
- 1/8 teaspoon nutmeg
- ¾ cup milk
- 3 garlic cloves, minced
- 2 tablespoons of parsley (chopped)
- 6 slices of deli-sliced cooked lean ham
- 1/4 teaspoon of salt
- Freshly ground pepper

Directions:
1. Put and combine the salt and flour in a bowl. In another bowl, whisk the eggs and milk. Gradually combine the two mixtures until smooth. Leave for 15 minutes.
2. Spray a skillet using non-stick cooking spray and put it over medium heat. Stir the batter a little. Add 1/4 of the batter into the skillet. Tilt the skillet to form a thin and even crêpe. Cook for 1-2 minutes or until the bottom is golden and the top is set. Flip and cook for 20 seconds. Transfer to a plate.
3. Repeat the steps with the remaining batter. Loosely cover the cooked crêpes with plastic wrap.
4. For the filling. Put all together with the ingredients for filling in a saucepan on medium heat – flour, milk, cayenne, nutmeg, and pepper. Constantly whisk until thick or around 7 minutes. Remove from the stove. Stir in a tablespoon of parsley and cheese. Loosely cover to keep warm.
5. Spray a skillet using non-stick cooking spray and put it over medium heat. Cook the garlic and mushrooms. Season with salt. Cook for 6 minutes or until the mushrooms are soft. Add 2 tablespoons of sherry. Cook for a couple of minutes. Remove from the stove. Add the remaining parsley and stir.
6. Put the crêpes side by side on a flat surface. Spread a tablespoon of the sauce and 2 tablespoons of the cooked mushrooms. Roll up the crêpes and transfer them to a greased baking dish. Put all the sauce on top. Bake in the oven at 450°F for 15 minutes.

Nutrition: Calories: 232 kcal | Protein: 16.51 g | Fat: 10.8 g | Carbohydrates: 16.25 g

14. Bake Apple Turnover

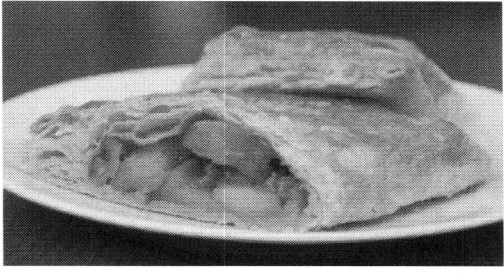

Cooking Time: 25 minutes
Servings: 4
Ingredients:
- For the turnovers
- 4 apples, peeled, cored, diced into bite-sized pieces
- 1 Tbsp. almond flour
- All-purpose flour for rolling out the dough
- 1 frozen puff pastry, thawed
- ½ cup palm sugar, crumbled by hand to loosen granules
- ½ tsp. cinnamon powder
- For the egg wash
- 1 egg white, whisked in

- 2 Tbsp. water

Directions:
1. For the filling: combine almond flour, cinnamon powder, and palm sugar until these resemble coarse meals. Toss in diced apples until well coated. Set aside.
2. On a lightly floured surface, roll the puff pastry until ¼ inch thin. Slice into 8 pieces of 4" x 4" squares.
3. Divide prepared apples into 8 equal portions. Spoon on individual puff pastry squares. Fold in half diagonally. Press edges to seal.
4. Place each filled pastry on a baking tray lined with parchment paper. Make sure there is ample space between pastries.
5. Freeze for at least 20 minutes, or till ready to bake.
6. Preheat oven to 400°F or 205°C for at 10 minutes.
7. Brush frozen pastries with egg wash. Bring in a hot oven, and cook for 12 to 15 minutes, or until these turn golden brown all over.
8. Take off the baking tray in the oven immediately. Cool slightly for easier handling.
9. Place 1 apple turnover on a plate. Serve warm.

Nutrition: Calories: 203 kcal | Protein: 5.29 g | Fat: 4.4 g | Carbohydrates: 38.25 g

15. Almond Pancakes with Coconut Flakes

Preparation: Time: 5 minutes
Cooking Time: 10 minutes
Servings: 6
Ingredients:
- 1 overripe banana, mashed
- 2 eggs, yolks, and whites separated
- ½ cup unsweetened applesauce
- 1 cup almond flour, finely milled
- ¼ cup of water
- ¼ tsp. coconut oil
- Garnish
- 2 Tbsp. blanched almond flakes
- Dash of cinnamon powder
- ¼ cup coconut flakes, sweetened
- Pinch of sea salt
- Pure maple syrup, used sparingly

Directions:
1. Whisk egg whites until soft peaks form.
2. Except for egg whites and coconut oil, combine the remaining ingredients in another bowl. Mix until batter comes together.
3. Gently fold in egg whites. Be sure not to over mix, or the pancake will become dense and chewy.
4. Pour oil into a nonstick skillet set over medium heat.
5. Wait for the oil to heat up before dropping in approximately ½ cup of batter. Cook until each side is set and bubbles form in the center. Turn on the other side, then cook for another 2 minutes.
6. Transfer flapjacks to a plate. Repeat step until all batter is cooked. Pour in more oil into the skillet only if needed. This recipe should yield between 4 to 6 medium-sized pancakes.
7. Stack pancakes. Pour the desired amount of pure maple syrup on top. Garnish each stack with cinnamon-flavored almond-coconut flakes just before serving.
8. For the garnish, set the oven to 350°F for at least 10 minutes before use. Line a baking sheet with parchment paper. Set aside.
9. In a bowl, mix almond and coconut flakes. Spread mixture evenly on a prepared baking sheet.
10. Bake for 7 to 10 minutes until flakes turn golden brown. Stir almond and coconut flakes once midway through roasting to prevent over-browning.
11. Remove the baking sheet from the oven: cool almond and coconut flakes for at least 10 minutes before sprinkling in cinnamon powder and salt. Toss to combine. Set aside.

Nutrition: Calories: 62 kcal | Protein: 2.24 g | Fat: 4.01 g | Carbohydrates: 4.46 g

16. Breakfast Sausage and Mushroom Casserole

Preparation Time: 20 minutes
Cooking Time: 45 minutes
Servings: 4
Ingredients:

- 450g of Italian sausage, cooked and crumbled
- Three-fourth cup of coconut milk
- 8 ounces of white mushrooms, sliced
- 1 medium onion, finely diced
- 2 Tablespoons of organic ghee
- 6 free-range eggs
- 600g of sweet potatoes
- 1 red bell pepper, roasted
- 3/4 tsp. of ground black pepper, divided
- 1 ½ tsp. of sea salt, divided

Directions:
1. Peel and shred the sweet potatoes.
2. Take a bowl, fill it with ice-cold water, and soak the sweet potatoes in it. Set aside.
3. Peel the roasted bell pepper, remove its seeds and finely dice it.
4. Set the oven to 375°F.
5. Get a casserole baking dish and grease it with organic ghee.
6. Put a skillet over medium flame and cook the mushrooms in it. Cook until the mushrooms are crispy and brown.
7. Take the mushrooms out and mix them with the crumbled sausage.
8. Now sauté the onions in the same skillet. Cook up to the onions are soft and golden. This should take about 4 – 5 minutes.
9. Take the onions out and mix them in the sausage-mushroom mixture.
10. Add the diced bell pepper to the same mixture.
11. Mix well and set aside for a while.
12. Now drain the soaked shredded potatoes, put them on a paper towel, and pat dry.
13. Bring the sweet potatoes to a bowl and add about a teaspoon of salt and half a teaspoon of ground black pepper to it. Mix well and set aside.
14. Now take a large bowl and crack the eggs in it.
15. Break the eggs and then blend in the coconut milk.
16. Stir in the remaining black pepper and salt.
17. Take the greased casserole dish and spread the seasoned sweet potatoes evenly in the base of the dish.
18. Next, spread the sausage mixture evenly in the dish.
19. Finally, spread the egg mixture.
20. Now cover the casserole dish using a piece of aluminum foil.
21. Bake for 20 - 30 minutes. To check if the casserole is baked properly, insert a tester in the middle of the casserole, and it should come out clean.
22. Uncover the casserole dish and bake it again, uncovered for 5 - 10 minutes, until the casserole is a little golden on the top.
23. Allow it to cool for 10 minutes.
24. Enjoy!

Nutrition: Calories: 598 kcal | Protein: 28.65 g | Fat: 36.75 g | Carbohydrates: 48.01 g

17. Maple Oatmeal

Preparation Time: 5 minutes
Cooking Time: 20 minutes
Servings: 4
Ingredients:
- 1 tsp. Maple flavoring
- 1 tsp. Cinnamon
- 3 tbsp. Sunflower seeds
- ½ cup Pecans, chopped
- ¼ cup Coconut flakes, unsweetened
- ½ cup Walnuts, chopped
- ½ cup Milk, almond or coconut
- 4 tbsp. Chia seeds

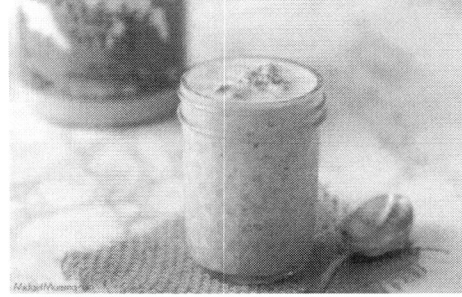

1. Pulse the sunflower seeds, walnuts, and pecans in a food processor to crumble. Or you can just put the nuts in a sturdy plastic bag, wrap the bag with a towel, lay it on a sturdy surface, and beat the towel with a hammer until the nuts are crumbled. Mix the crushed nuts with the rest of the ingredients and pour them into a large pot. Simmer this

mixture over low heat for thirty minutes. Stir often, so the mix does not stick to the bottom. Serve garnished with fresh fruit or a sprinkle of cinnamon if desired.

Nutrition: Calories 374 | 3.2 grams' carbs | 9.25 grams' protein | 4.59 grams' fat

18. Apple, Ginger, and Rhubarb Muffins

Preparation Time: 15 minutes
Cooking Time: 25 minutes
Servings: 4
Ingredients:
- ½ cup finely ground almonds
- ¼ cup brown rice flour
- ½ cup buckwheat flour
- 1/8 cup unrefined raw sugar
- 2 tbsp. arrowroot flour
- 1 tbsp. linseed meal
- 2 tbsp. crystallized ginger, finely chopped
- ½ tsp. ground ginger
- ½ tsp. ground cinnamon
- 2 tsp. gluten-free baking powder
- A pinch of fine sea salt
- 1 small apple, peeled and finely diced
- 1 cup finely chopped rhubarb
- 1/3 cup almond/ rice milk
- 1 large egg
- ¼ cup extra virgin olive oil
- 1 tsp. pure vanilla extract

Directions:
1. Set your oven to 350F grease an eight-cup muffin tin and line with paper cases.
2. Combine the almond four, linseed meal, ginger, and sugar in a mixing bowl. Sieve this mixture over the other flours, spices, and baking powder and use a whisk to combine well.
3. Stir in the apple and rhubarb in the flour mixture until evenly coated.
4. Whisk the milk, vanilla, and egg in a separate bowl, then pour it into the dry mixture. Stir until just combined – don't overwork the batter as this can yield very tough muffins.
5. Scoop the mixture into the arranged muffin tin and top with a few slices of rhubarb. Bake for at least 25 minutes, till they start turning golden or when an inserted toothpick emerges clean.
6. Take off from the oven and let sit for at least 5 minutes before transferring the muffins to a wire rack for further cooling.
7. Serve warm with a glass of squeezed juice.
8. Enjoy!

Nutrition: Calories: 325 kcal | Protein: 6.32 g | Fat: 9.82 g | Carbohydrates: 55.71 g

19. Almond Scones

Preparation Time: 10 minutes
Cooking Time: 20 minutes
Servings: 6
Ingredients:
- 1 cup almonds
- 1 1/3 cups almond flour
- ¼ cup arrowroot flour
- 1 tablespoon coconut flour
- 1 teaspoon ground turmeric
- Salt, to taste
- Freshly ground black pepper, to taste
- 1 egg
- ¼ cup essential olive oil
- 3 tablespoons raw honey

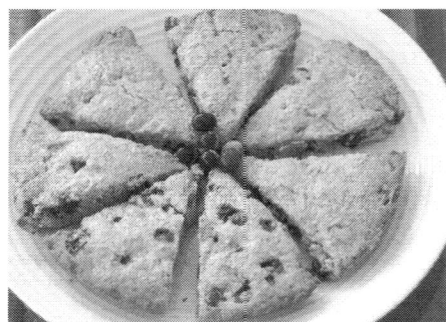

Directions:
1. In a mixer, put almonds, then pulse till chopped roughly
2. Move the chopped almonds to a big bowl.
3. Put flours and spices and mix well.
4. In another bowl, put the remaining ingredients and beat till well combined.
5. Put the flour mixture into the egg mixture, then mix till well combined.
6. Arrange a plastic wrap over the cutting board.

7. Place the dough over the cutting board.
8. Using both of your hands, pat into a 1-inch thick circle.
9. Cut the circle into 6 wedges.
10. Set the scones onto a cookie sheet in a single layer.
11. Bake for at least 15-20 minutes.

Nutrition: Calories: 304 | Fat: 3g | Carbohydrates: 22g | Fiber: 6g | Protein: 20g

20. Cranberry and Raisins Granola

Preparation Time: 15 minutes
Cooking Time: 20 minutes
Servings: 4
Ingredients:
- 4 cups old-fashioned rolled oats
- 1/4 cup sesame seeds
- 1 cup dried cranberries
- 1 cup golden raisins
- 1/8 teaspoon nutmeg
- 2 tablespoons olive oil
- 1/2 cup almonds, slivered
- 2 tablespoons warm water
- 1 teaspoon vanilla extract
- 1 teaspoon cinnamon
- 1/4 teaspoon of salt
- 6 tablespoons maple syrup
- 1/3 cup of honey

Directions:
1. Mix the sesame seeds, nutmeg, almonds, oats, salt, and cinnamon in a bowl.
2. In another bowl, mix the oil, water, vanilla, honey, and syrup. Gradually pour the mixture into the oats mixture. Toss to combine. Spread the mixture into a greased jelly-roll pan. Bake in the oven at 300°F for at least 55 minutes. Stir and break the clumps every 10 minutes.
3. Once you get it from the oven, stir the cranberries and raisins. Allow cooling. This will last for a week when stored in an airtight container and up to a month when stored in the fridge.

Nutrition: Calories: 698 kcal | Protein: 21.34 g | Fat: 20.99 g Carbohydrates: 148.59 g

21. Breakfast Arrozcaldo

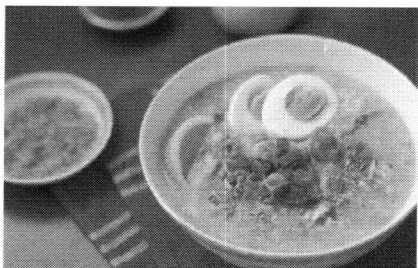

Preparation Time: 20 minutes
Cooking Time: 30 minutes
Servings: 5
Ingredients:
- 6 eggs, white only
- 1½ cups brown rice, cooked
- For the filling
- ¼ cup raisins
- ½ cup frozen peas, thawed
- 1 white onion, minced
- 1 garlic clove, minced
- oil, for greasing

Directions:
1. For the filling, spray a small amount of oil into a skillet set over medium heat. Add in onion and garlic. Stir-fry until the former is limp and transparent.
2. Stir-fry while breaking up clumps, about 2 minutes. Add in remaining ingredients. Stir-fry for another minute.
3. Turn down the heat, and let filling cook for 10 to 15 minutes, or until juices are greatly reduced. Stir often. Turn off heat. Divide into 6 equal portions.
4. For the eggs, spray a small amount of oil into a smaller skillet set over medium heat. Cook eggs. Discard yolk. Transfer to holding the plate.
5. To serve, place 1 portion of rice on a plate, 1 portion of filling, and 1 egg white. Serve warm.

Nutrition: Calories: 53 kcal | Protein: 6.28 g | Fat: 1.35 g | Carbohydrates: 3.59 g

22. Apple Bruschetta with Almonds and Blackberries

Preparation Time: 20 minutes

Cooking Time: 30 minutes
Servings: 5
Ingredients:
- 1 apple, sliced into ¼-inch thick half-moons
- ¼ cup blackberries, thawed, lightly mashed
- ½ tsp. fresh lemon juice
- 1/8 cup almond slivers, toasted
- Sea salt

Directions:
1. Drizzle lemon juice on apple slices. Put these on a tray lined with parchment paper.
2. Spread a small number of mashed berries on top of each slice. Top these off with the desired amount of almond slivers.
3. Sprinkle sea salt on "bruschetta" just before serving.

Nutrition: Calories: 56 kcal | Protein: 1.53 g | Fat: 1.43 g | Carbohydrates: 9.87 g

23. Oat Porridge with Cherry & Coconut

Preparation Time: 10 minutes
Cooking Time: 0 minutes
Servings: 3
Ingredients:
- 1 ½ cups regular oats
- 3 cups coconut milk
- 4 tbsp. chia seed
- 3 tbsp. raw cacao
- Coconut shavings
- Dark chocolate shavings
- Fresh or frozen tart cherries
- A pinch of stevia, optional
- Maple syrup, to taste (optional)

Directions:
1. Combine the oats, milk, stevia, and cacao in a medium saucepan over medium heat and bring to a boil. Lower the heat, then simmer until the oats are cooked to desired doneness.
2. Divide the porridge among 3 serving bowls and top with dark chocolate and coconut shavings, cherries, and a little drizzle of maple syrup.

Nutrition: Calories: 343 kcal | Protein: 15.64 g | Fat: 12.78 g | Carbohydrates: 41.63 g

24. Gingerbread Oatmeal Breakfast

Preparation Time: 10 minutes
Cooking Time: 0 minutes
Servings: 4
Ingredients:
- 1 cup steel-cut oats
- 4 cups drinking water
- Organic Maple syrup, to taste
- 1 tsp ground cloves
- 1 ½ tbsp. ground cinnamon
- 1/8 tsp nutmeg
- ¼ tsp ground ginger
- ¼ tsp ground coriander
- ¼ tsp ground allspice
- ¼ tsp ground cardamom
- Fresh mixed berries

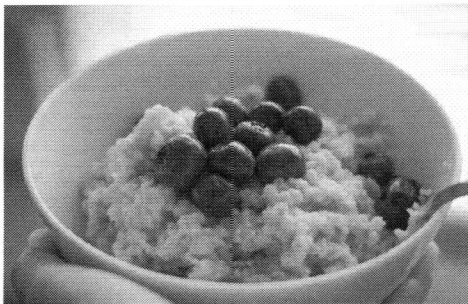

Directions:
1. Cook the oats based on the package instructions. When it comes to a boil, reduce heat and simmer.
2. Stir in all the spices and continue cooking until cooked to desired doneness.
3. Serve in four serving bowls and drizzle with maple syrup and top with fresh berries.
4. Enjoy!

Nutrition: Calories: 87 kcal | Protein: 5.82 g | Fat: 3.26 g

25. Yummy Steak Muffins

Preparation Time: 10 minutes
Cooking Time: 20 minutes
Servings: 4
Ingredients:
- 1 cup red bell pepper, diced
- 2 Tablespoons of water

- 8-ounce thin steak, cooked and finely chopped
- ¼ teaspoon of sea salt
- Dash of freshly ground black pepper
- 8 free-range eggs
- 1 cup of finely diced onion

Directions:
1. Set the oven to 350°F
2. Take 8 muffin tins and line them with parchment paper liners.
3. Get a large bowl and crack all the eggs in it.
4. Beat the eggs well.
5. Blend in all the remaining ingredients.
6. Spoon the batter into the arranged muffin tins. Fill three-fourth of each tin.
7. Put the muffin tins in the preheated oven for about 20 minutes until the muffins are baked and set in the middle.
8. Enjoy!

Nutrition: Calories: 151 kcal | Protein: 17.92 g | Fat: 7.32 g | Carbohydrates: 3.75 g

26. White and Green Quiche

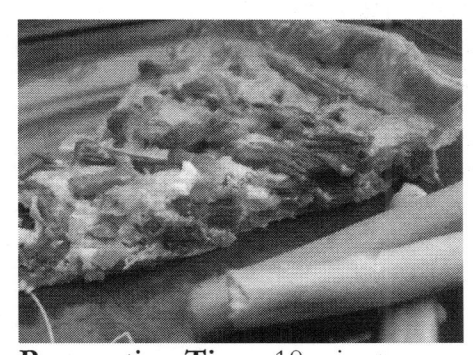

Preparation Time: 10 minutes
Cooking Time: 40 minutes
Servings: 3
Ingredients:
- 3 cups of fresh spinach, chopped
- 15 large free-range eggs
- 3 cloves of garlic, minced
- 5 white mushrooms, sliced
- 1 small sized onion, finely chopped
- 1 ½ teaspoon of baking powder
- Ground black pepper to taste
- 1 ½ cups of coconut milk
- Ghee, as required to grease the dish
- Sea salt to taste

Directions:
1. Set the oven to 350°F.
2. Get a baking dish, then grease it with the organic ghee.
3. Break all the eggs in a huge bowl, then whisk well.
4. Stir in coconut milk. Beat well
5. While you are whisking the eggs, start adding the remaining ingredients to them.
6. When all the ingredients are thoroughly blended, pour all of it into the prepared baking dish.
7. Bake for at least 40 minutes, up to the quiche is set in the middle.
8. Enjoy!

Nutrition: Calories: 608 kcal | Protein: 20.28 g | Fat: 53.42 g | Carbohydrates: 16.88 g

27. Beef Breakfast Casserole

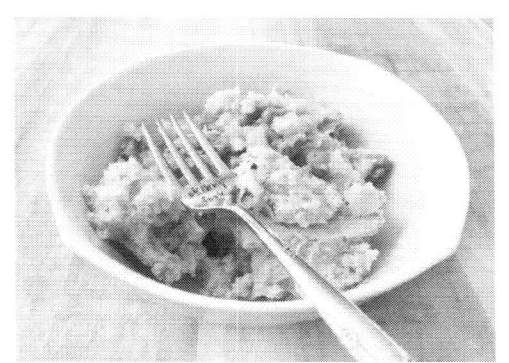

Preparation Time: 10 minutes
Cooking Time: 30 minutes
Servings: 5
Ingredients:
- 1 pound of ground beef, cooked
- 10 eggs
- ½ cup Pico de Gallo
- 1 cup baby spinach
- ¼ cup sliced black olives
- Freshly ground black pepper

Directions:
1. Preheat oven to 350 degrees Fahrenheit. Prepare a 9" glass pie plate with non-stick spray.
2. Whisk the eggs until frothy. Season with salt and pepper.
3. Layer the cooked ground beef, Pico de Gallo, and spinach on the pie plate.
4. Slowly pour the eggs over the top.

5. Top with black olives.
6. Bake for at least 30 minutes until firm in the middle.
7. Slice into 5 pieces and serve.

Nutrition: Calories: 479 kcal | Protein: 43.54 g | Fat: 30.59 g | Carbohydrates: 4.65 g

28. Ham and Veggie Frittata Muffins

Preparation Time: 10 minutes
Cooking Time: 25 minutes
Servings: 12
Ingredients:
- 5 ounces thinly sliced ham
- 8 large eggs
- 4 tablespoons coconut oil
- ½ yellow onion, finely diced
- 8 oz. frozen spinach, thawed and drained
- 8 oz. mushrooms, thinly sliced
- 1 cup cherry tomatoes, halved
- ¼ cup coconut milk (canned)
- 2 tablespoons coconut flour
- Sea salt and pepper to taste

Directions:
1. Preheat oven to 375 degrees Fahrenheit.
2. In a medium skillet, warm the coconut oil on medium heat. Add the onion and cook until softened.
3. Add the mushrooms, spinach, and cherry tomatoes. Season with salt and pepper. Cook until the mushrooms have softened. About 5 minutes. Remove from heat and set aside.
4. In a huge bowl, beat the eggs together with coconut milk and coconut flour. Stir in the cooled veggie mixture.
5. Line each cavity of a 12 cavity muffin tin with the thinly sliced ham. Pour the egg mixture into each one and bake for 20 minutes.
6. Remove from oven and allow to cool for about 5 minutes before transferring to a wire rack.
7. To maximize the benefit of a vegetable-rich diet, it's important to eat a variety of colors, and these veggie-packed frittata muffins do just that. The onion, spinach, mushrooms, and cherry tomatoes provide a wide range of vitamins and nutrients and a healthy dose of fiber.

Nutrition: Calories: 125 kcal | Protein: 5.96 g | Fat: 9.84 g | Carbohydrates: 4.48 g

29. Tomato and Avocado Omelet

Preparation Time: 5 minutes
Cooking Time: 5 minutes
Servings: 1
Ingredients:
- 2 eggs
- ¼ avocado, diced
- 4 cherry tomatoes, halved
- 1 tablespoon cilantro, chopped
- A squeeze of lime juice
- Pinch of salt

Directions:
1. Put together the avocado, tomatoes, cilantro, lime juice, and salt in a small bowl, then mix well and set aside.
2. Warm a medium nonstick skillet on medium heat. Whisk the eggs until frothy and add to the pan. Move the eggs around gently with a rubber spatula until they begin to set.
3. Scatter the avocado mixture over half of the omelet. Remove from heat, and slide the omelet onto a plate as you fold it in half.
4. Serve immediately.

Nutrition Calories: 433 kca | Protein: 25.55 | Fat: 32.75 | Carbohydrates: 10.06 g

BRUNCH

30. Oats with Berries

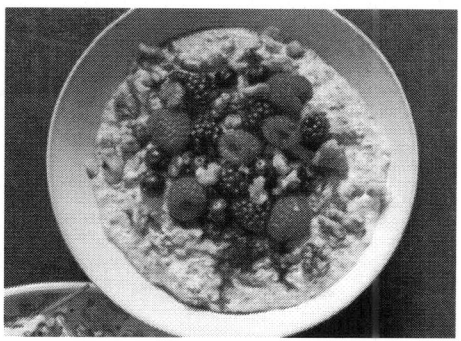

Preparation Time: 10 Minutes

Servings: 4
Ingredients:
- 1 cup Steel Cut Oats
- Dash of Salt
- 3 cups Water
- For toppings:
- ½ cup Berries of your choice
- ¼ cup Nuts or Seeds of your choice like Almonds or Hemp Seeds

Directions:
1. To begin with, place the oats in a small saucepan and heat it over medium-high heat.
2. Now, toast it for 3 minutes while stirring the pan frequently.
3. Next, pour water to the saucepan and mix well.
4. Allow the mixture to boil. Lower the heat.
5. Allow it to cook for 23 to 25 minutes or until the oats are cooked and tender.
6. Once done cooking, transfer the mixture to the serving bowl and top it with the berries and seeds.
7. Serve it warm or cold.

Tip: If you desire, you can add sweeteners like maple syrup or coconut sugar or stevia to it.
Nutrition: Calories: 118Kcal Proteins: 4.1g Carbohydrates: 16.5g Fat: 4.4g

31. Spinach Avocado Smoothie

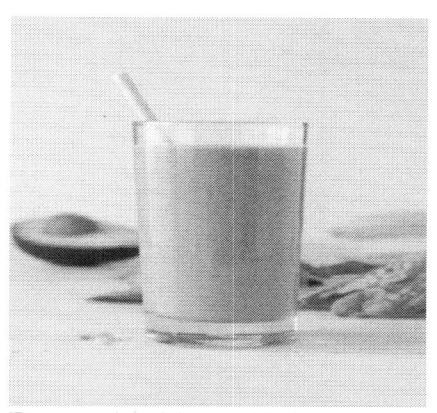

Preparation Time: 5 Minutes

Servings: 1
Ingredients:
- ¼ of 1 Avocado
- 1 cup Plain Yoghurt, non-fat
- 2 tbsp. Water
- 1 cup Spinach, fresh
- 1 tsp. Honey
- 1 Banana, frozen

Directions:
1. Start by blending all the ingredients needed to make the smoothie in a high-speed blender for 2 to 3 minutes or until you get a smooth and creamy mixture.
2. Next, transfer the mixture to a serving glass.
3. Serve and enjoy.

Tip: If you don't prefer to use yogurt, you can use unsweetened almond milk.
Nutrition: Calories: 357Kcal Proteins: 17.7g Carbohydrates: 57.8g Fat: 8.2g

32. Golden Milk

Preparation Time: 5 Minutes
Cooking Time: 5 Minutes
Servings: 2
Ingredients:
- 1 tbsp. Coconut Oil

- 1 ½ cups Coconut Milk, light
- Pinch of Pepper
- 1 ½ cups Almond Milk, unsweetened
- ¼ tsp. Ginger, grated
- 1 ½ tsp. Turmeric, grounded
- ¼ tsp. Cinnamon, grounded
- Sweetener of your choice, as needed

Directions:
1. To make this healthy beverage, you need to place all the ingredients in a medium-sized saucepan and mix it well.
2. After that, heat it over medium heat for 3 to 4 minutes or until it is hot but not boiling. Stir continuously.
3. Taste for seasoning. Add more sweetener or spice as required by you.
4. Finally, transfer the milk to the serving glass and enjoy it.

Tip: Instead of cinnamon powder, you can also use the cinnamon stick, which can be discarded at the end if you prefer a much more intense flavor.
Nutrition: Calories: 205Kcal Proteins: 3.2g Carbohydrates: 8.9g Fat: 19.5g

33. Granola

Preparation Time: 10 Minutes
Cooking Time: 60 Minutes
Servings: 2
Ingredients:
- ½ cup Flax Seeds, grounded
- 1 cup Almonds, whole & raw
- ½ cup Ginger, grated
- 1 cup Pumpkin Seeds, raw
- ½ tsp. Salt
- 1 cup Shredded Coconut, unsweetened
- ¾ cup Water
- 1 cup Oat Bran
- ½ cup Coconut Oil, melted
- 1 cup Dried Cherries, pitted
- 4 tsp. Turmeric Powder

Directions:
1. First, preheat the oven to 300 degrees F.
2. Next, combine dried cherries, almonds, grounded flax, pumpkin seeds, coconut, salt, and turmeric in a large mixing bowl until mixed well.
3. After that, mix ginger, coconut oil, and water in the blender and blend for 30 to 40 seconds or until well incorporated.
4. Now, spoon in the coconut oil mixture to the nut mixture. Mix well.
5. Then, transfer the mixture to a parchment paper-lined baking sheet and spread it across evenly.
6. Bake for 50 to 60 minutes while checking on it once or twice.
7. Allow it to cool completely and enjoy it.

Tip: Substitute dried cherries with raisins if preferred.
Nutrition: Calories: 225Kcal Proteins: 6g Carbohydrates: 18g Fat: 16g

34. Overnight Coconut Chia Oats

Preparation Time: 10 Minutes
Cooking Time: 60 Minutes
Servings: 1 to 2
Ingredients:
- ½ cup Coconut Milk, unsweetened
- 2 tsp. Chia Seeds
- 1 ½ cups Old Fashioned Oats, whole grain
- ½ tsp. Cinnamon, grounded
- 1 cup Almond Milk, unsweetened
- ½ tsp. Cinnamon, grounded
- 2 tsp. Date Syrup
- ½ tsp. Black Pepper, grounded
- 1 tsp. Turmeric, grounded

Directions:
1. To start with, keep the oats in the mason jar.
2. After that, mix the rest of the ingredients in a medium bowl until combined well.
3. Then, pour the mixture to the jars and stir well.
4. Now, close the jar and place it in the refrigerator overnight.
5. In the morning, stir the mixture and then enjoy it.

Tip: You can top it with toasted nuts or berries.
Nutrition: Calories: 335Kcal Proteins: 8g Carbohydrates: 34.1g Fat: 19.9g

35. Blueberry Hemp Seed Smoothie

Preparation Time: 10 Minutes
Cooking Time: 5 Minutes
Servings: 1
Ingredients:
- 1 ¼ cup Blueberries, frozen
- 1 ¼ cup Plant-Based Milk of your choice
- 2 tbsp. Hemp Seeds
- 1 tsp. Spirulina
- 1 scoop of Protein Powder

Directions:
1. First, place all the ingredients needed to make the smoothie in a high-speed blender and blend them for 2 minutes or until smooth.
2. Transfer the mixture to a serving glass and enjoy it.

Tip: Instead of blueberries, you can use any berries of your choice.
Nutrition: Calories: 493Kcal Proteins: 37.8g Carbohydrates: 46.3g Fat: 19.6g

36. Spiced Morning Chia Pudding

Preparation Time: 10 Minutes
Cooking Time: 5 Minutes
Servings: 1
Ingredients:
- ½ tsp. Cinnamon
- 1 ½ cups Cashew Milk
- 1/8 tsp. Cardamom, grounded
- 1/3 cup Chia Seeds
- 1/8 tsp. Cloves, grounded
- 2 tbsp. Maple Syrup
- 1 tsp. Turmeric

Directions:
1. To begin with, combine all the ingredients in a medium bowl until well mixed.
2. Next, spoon the mixture into a container and allow it to sit overnight.
3. In the morning, transfer to a cup and serve with toppings of your choice.

Tip: You can top it with toppings of your choice like coconut flakes or seeds etc.
Nutrition: Calories: 237Kcal Proteins: 8.1g Carbohydrates: 28.9g Fat: 8.1g

37. Green Smoothie

Preparation Time: 10 Minutes
Cooking Time: 10 Minutes
Servings: 1
Ingredients:
- 2 cups Kale
- 1 tbsp. Chia Seeds
- ½ of 1 Banana, medium
- 1 cup Pineapple Chunks, frozen
- ¼ tsp. Turmeric
- 1 cup Green Tea, brewed & cooled
- 1 scoop of Protein Powder
- 2/3 cup Cucumber, cut into chunks
- 3 Mint Leaves
- ½ cup Mango, cut into chunks
- ½-inch Ginger, sliced
- Ice Cubes, if needed

Directions:
1. To start with, place all the ingredients in a high-speed blender, excluding the chia seeds and blend them for 2 to 3 minutes or until smooth.
2. Next, put in the chia seeds and blend them for a further 1 minute.
3. Finally, transfer to a serving glass and enjoy it.

Tip: You can substitute kale with spinach if desired.
Nutrition: Calories: 445Kcal Proteins: 31.9g Carbohydrates: 73.7g Fat: 7.2g

38. Oatmeal Pancakes

Preparation Time: 10 Minutes
Cooking Time: 25 Minutes
Servings: 2
Ingredients:
- 1 ½ cups Rolled Oats, whole-grain
- 2 Eggs, large & pastured
- 2 tsp. Baking Powder
- 1 Banana, ripe
- 2 tbsp. Water
- ¼ cup Maple Syrup

- 1 tsp. Vanilla Extract
- 2 tbsp. Extra Virgin Olive Oil

Directions:
1. To make this delicious breakfast dish, you need to first blend all the ingredients in a high-speed blender for a minute or two or until you get a smooth batter. Tip: To blend easily, pour egg, banana, and all other liquid ingredients first and finally add oats at the end.
2. Now, take a large skillet and heat it over medium-low heat.
3. Once the skillet is hot, ¼ cup of the batter into it and cook it for 3 to 4 minutes per side or until bubbles start appearing in the middle portion.
4. Turn the pancake and cook the other side also.
5. Serve warm.

Tip: You can pair it with maple syrup and fruits.
Nutrition: Calories: 201Kcal Proteins: 5g Carbohydrates: 28g Fat: 8g

39. Anti-inflammatory Porridge

Preparation Time: 10 Minutes
Cooking Time: 25 Minutes
Servings: 2
Ingredients:
- ¾ cup Almond Milk, unsweetened
- 2 tbsp. Hemp Seeds
- 2 tbsp. Chia Seeds, whole
- ¼ cup Walnuts, halved
- ¼ cup Almond Butter
- ¼ cup Coconut Flakes, unsweetened & toasted
- ¼ cup Coconut Milk
- ½ tsp. Turmeric Powder
- Dash of Black Pepper, grounded, as needed
- ½ tsp. Cinnamon
- 1 tbsp. Extra Virgin Olive Oil

Directions:
1. To start with, heat a large saucepan over medium heat.
2. To this, put in the hemp seeds, flaked coconut, and chopped walnuts.
3. Roast for 2 minutes or until toasted.
4. Once the coconut-seed mixture is roasted, transfer to a bowl and set it aside.
5. Then, heat almond milk and coconut milk in a wide saucepan over medium heat.
6. Once it becomes hot but not boiling, remove from the heat. Stir in almond butter and coconut oil to it. Mix.
7. Now, add chia seeds, pepper powder, turmeric powder, and salt to the milk. Combine.
8. Keep it aside for 5 minutes and then add half of the roasted coconut mixture. Mix.
9. Finally, transfer to a serving bowl and top with the remaining coconut mixture.
10. Serve immediately.

Tip: If possible, try adding bee pollen for enhanced taste.
Nutrition: Calories: 575Kcal Proteins: 14.8g Carbohydrates: 6g Fat: 50.2g

40. Cherry Smoothie

Preparation Time: 5 Minutes
Cooking Time: 2 Minutes
Servings: 1
Ingredients:
- ½ cup Cherries, pitted & frozen
- ½ of 1 Banana, frozen
- 10 oz. Almond Milk, unsweetened
- 1 tbsp. Almonds
- 1 Beet, small & quartered

Directions:
1. To make this delightful smoothie, you need to blend all the ingredients in a high-speed blender for 3 minutes or until smooth.
2. Pour to a serving glass and enjoy it.

Tip: If you wish, you can add one more beet to it.
Nutrition: Calories: 208Kcal Proteins: 5.2g Carbohydrates: 34.4g Fat: 7.1g

41. Gingerbread Oatmeal

Preparation Time: 10 Minutes
Cooking Time: 30 Minutes
Servings: 4
Ingredients:
- ¼ tsp. Cardamom, grounded

- 4 cups Water
- ¼ tsp. Allspice
- 1 cup Steel Cut Oats
- 1/8 tsp. Nutmeg
- 1 ½ tbsp. Cinnamon, grounded
- ¼ tsp. Ginger, grounded
- ¼ tsp. Coriander, grounded
- Maple Syrup, if desired
- ¼ tsp. Cloves

Directions:
1. First, place all the ingredients in a large saucepan over medium-high heat and stir well.
2. Next, cook them for 6 to 7 minutes or until cooked.
3. Once finished, add the maple syrup.
4. Top it with dried fruits of your choice if desired.
5. Serve it hot or cold.

Tip: Avoid those spices which you don't prefer.
Nutrition: Calories: 175Kcal Proteins: 6g Carbohydrates: 32g Fat: 32g

42. Roasted Almonds

Preparation Time: 5 minutes
Cooking Time: 10 minutes
Servings: 32
Ingredients:
- 2 cups whole almonds
- 1 tablespoon chili powder
- ½ teaspoon ground cinnamon
- ½ teaspoon ground cumin
- ½ teaspoon ground coriander
- Salt and freshly ground black pepper, to taste
- 1 tablespoon extra-virgin organic olive oil

Directions:
1. Preheat the oven to 350 degrees F. Line a baking dish with a parchment paper.
2. In a bowl, add all ingredients and toss to coat well.
3. Transfer the almond mixture into prepared baking dish in a single layer.
4. Roast for around 10 minutes, flipping twice inside the middle way.
5. Remove from oven and make aside to cool down the completely before serving.
6. You can preserve these roasted almonds in airtight jar.

Nutrition: Calories: 62, Fat: 5g, Carbohydrates: 12g, Protein: 2g, Fiber 6g

43. Roasted Pumpkin Seeds

Preparation Time: 10 minutes
Cooking Time: 20 minutes
Servings: 4
Ingredients:
- 1 cup pumpkin seeds, washed and dried
- 2 teaspoons garam masala
- 1/3 teaspoon red chili powder
- ¼ teaspoon ground turmeric
- Salt, to taste
- 3 tablespoons coconut oil, meted
- ½ tablespoon fresh lemon juice

Directions:
1. Preheat the oven to 350 degrees F.
2. In a bowl, add all ingredients except lemon juice and toss to coat well.
3. Transfer the almond mixture right into a baking sheet.
4. Roast approximately twenty or so minutes, flipping occasionally.
5. Remove from oven and make aside to cool completely before serving.
6. Drizzle with freshly squeezed lemon juice and serve.

Nutrition: Calories: 136 Fat: 4g, Carbohydrates: 15g, Fiber: 9g, Protein: 25g

44. Roasted Chickpeas

Preparation Time: 10 minutes
Cooking Time: one hour
Servings: 8-10
Ingredients:
- 3 cups canned chickpeas, rinsed and dried
- 2 tablespoons nutritional yeast
- 1 tablespoon ground turmeric
- ½ teaspoon garlic powder
- Pinch of cayenne pepper.
- Salt and freshly ground black pepper, to taste

- 2 tablespoons extra-virgin organic olive oil

Directions:
1. Preheat the oven to 400 degrees F.
2. In a bowl, add all ingredients except freshly squeezed lemon juice and toss to coat well.
3. Transfer the almond mixture right into a baking sheet.
4. Roast for around 1 hour, flipping after every 15 minutes.
5. Remove from oven and keep aside for cooling completely before serving.
6. Drizzle with freshly squeezed lemon juice and serve.

Nutrition: Calories: 190 Fat: 5g, Carbohydrates: 16g, Fiber: 7g, Protein: 12g

45. Spiced Popcorn

Preparation Time: 5 minutes
Cooking Time: 2 minutes
Servings: 2-3

Ingredients:
- 3 tablespoons coconut oil
- ½ cup popping corn
- 1 tbsp. olive oil
- 1 teaspoon ground turmeric
- ¼ teaspoon garlic powder
- Salt, to taste

Directions:
1. In a pan, melt coconut oil on medium-high heat.
2. Add popping corn and cover the pan tightly.
3. Cook, shaking the pan occasionally for around 1-2 minutes or till corn kernels begin to pop.
4. Remove from heat and transfer right into a large heatproof bowl.
5. Add essential olive oil and spices and mix well.
6. Serve immediately

Nutrition: Calories: 200, Fat: 4g, Carbohydrates: 12g, Fiber: 1g, Protein: 6g

46. Cucumber Bites

Preparation Time: 15 minutes
Cooking Time: 0 minutes
Servings: 4

Ingredients:
- ½ cup prepared hummus
- 2 teaspoons nutritional yeast
- ¼-½ teaspoon ground turmeric
- Pinch of red pepper cayenne
- Pinch of salt
- 1 cucumber, cut diagonally into ¼-½-inch thick slices
- 1 teaspoon black sesame seeds
- Fresh mint leaves, for garnishing

Directions:
1. In a bowl, mix together hummus, turmeric, cayenne and salt.
2. Transfer the hummus mixture in the pastry bag and pipe on each cucumber slice.
3. Serve while using garnishing of sesame seeds and mint leaves.

Nutrition: Calories: 203 Fat: 4g, Carbohydrates: 20g, Fiber: 3g, Protein: 8g

47. Spinach Fritters

Preparation Time: 15 minutes
Cooking Time: 5 minutes
Servings: 2-3

Ingredients:
- 2 cups chickpea flour
- ¾ teaspoons white sesame seeds
- ½ teaspoon garam masala powder
- ½ teaspoon red chili powder
- ¼ teaspoon ground cumin
- 2 pinches of baking soda
- Salt, to taste
- 1 cup water
- 12-14 fresh spinach leaves
- Olive oil, for frying

Directions:
1. In a sizable bowl, add all ingredients except spinach and oil and mix till an easy mixture forms.
2. In a sizable skillet, heat oil on medium heat.
3. Dip each spinach leaf in chickpea flour mixture evenly and place in the hot oil in batches.
4. Cook, flipping occasionally for about 3-5 minutes or till golden brown from each side.

5. Transfer the fritters onto paper towel lined plate.

Nutrition: Calories: 211 Fat: 2g, Carbohydrates: 13g, Fiber: 11g, Protein: 9g

48. Crispy Chicken Fingers

Preparation Time: 15 minutes
Cooking Time: 18 minutes
Servings: 4-6
Ingredients:
- 2/3 cup almond meal
- ½ teaspoon ground turmeric
- ½ teaspoon red pepper cayenne
- ½ teaspoon paprika
- ½ teaspoon garlic powder
- Salt and freshly ground black pepper, to taste
- 1 egg
- 1-pound skinless, boneless chicken breasts, cut into strips

Directions:
1. Preheat the oven to 375 degrees F. Line a substantial baking sheet with parchment paper.
2. In a shallow dish, beat the egg.
3. In another shallow dish, mix together almond meal and spices.
4. Coat each chicken strip with egg after which roll into spice mixture evenly.
5. Arrange the chicken strips onto prepared baking sheet in the single layer.
6. Bake for approximately 16-18 minutes.

Nutrition: Calories: 236 Fat: 10g, Carbohydrates: 26g, Fiber: 5g, Protein: 37g

49. Quinoa & Veggie Croquettes

Preparation Time: 15 minutes
Cooking Time: 9 minutes
Servings: 12-15
Ingredients:
- 1 tbsp. essential olive oil
- ½ cup frozen peas, thawed
- 2 minced garlic cloves
- 1 cup cooked quinoa
- 2 large boiled potatoes, peeled and mashed
- ¼ cup fresh cilantro leaves, chopped
- 2 teaspoons ground cumin
- 1 teaspoon garam masala
- ¼ teaspoon ground turmeric
- Salt and freshly ground black pepper, to taste
- Olive oil, for frying

Directions:
1. In a frying pan, heat oil on medium heat.
2. Add peas and garlic and sauté for about 1 minute.
3. Transfer the pea mixture into a large bowl.
4. Add remaining ingredients and mix till well combined.
5. Make equal sized oblong shaped patties from your mixture.
6. In a large skillet, heat oil on medium-high heat.
7. Add croquettes and fry for about 4 minutes per side.

Nutrition: Calories: 367 Fat: 6g, Carbohydrates: 17g, Fiber: 5g, Protein: 22g

50. Sweet Potato Cranberry Breakfast bars

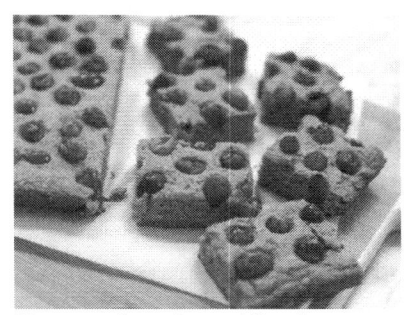

Preparation time: 10 minutes

Servings: 8
Ingredients:
- 1 ½ cups sweet potato puree
- 2 tablespoons coconut oil, melted
- 2 tablespoons maple syrup
- 2 eggs, pasture-raised
- 1 cup almond meal
- 1/3 cup coconut flour
- 1 ½ teaspoon baking soda
- 1 cup fresh cranberry, pitted and chopped

- ¼ cup water

Directions:
1. Preheat the oven to 3500F.
2. Grease a 9-inch baking pan with coconut oil. Set aside.
3. In a mixing bowl. Combine the sweet potato puree, water, coconut oil, maple syrup, and eggs.
4. In another bowl, sift the almond flour, coconut flour, and baking soda.
5. Gradually add the dry ingredients to the wet ingredients. Use a spatula to fold and mix all ingredients.
6. Pour into the prepared baking pan and press the cranberries on top.
7. Place in the oven and bake for 40 minutes or until a toothpick inserted in the middle comes out clean.
8. Allow to rest or cool before removing from the pan.

Nutrition: Calories 98, Total Fat 6g, Saturated Fat 1g, Total Carbs 9g, Net Carbs 8.5g, Protein 3g, Sugar: 7g, Fiber: 0.5g, Sodium:113 mg, Potassium 274mg

51. Savory Breakfast Pancakes

Preparation time: 5 minutes
Cooking time: 6 minutes
Servings: 4
Ingredients:
- ½ cup almond flour
- ½ cup tapioca flour
- 1 cup coconut milk
- ½ teaspoon chili powder
- ¼ teaspoon turmeric powder
- ½ red onion, chopped
- 1 handful cilantro leaves, chopped
- ½ inch ginger, grated
- 1 teaspoon salt
- ¼ teaspoon ground black pepper

Directions:
1. In a mixing bowl, mix all ingredients until well-combined.
2. Heat a pan on low medium heat and grease with oil.
3. Pour ¼ cup of batter onto the pan and spread the mixture to create a pancake.
4. Fry for 3 minutes per side.
5. Repeat until the batter is done.

Nutrition: Calories 108, Total Fat 2g, Saturated Fat 1g, Total Carbs 20g, Net Carbs 19.5g, Protein 2g, Sugar: 4g, Fiber: 0.5g, Sodium: 37mg, Potassium 95mg

52. Scrambled Eggs with Smoked Salmon

Preparation time: 10 minutes
Cooking time: 10 minutes
Servings: 2
Ingredients:
- 4 eggs
- 2 tablespoons coconut ilk
- Fresh chives, chopped
- 4 slices of wild-caught smoked salmon, chopped
- salt to taste

Directions:
1. In a bowl, whisk the egg, coconut milk, and chives.
2. Grease the skillet with oil and heat over medium low heat.
3. Pour the egg mixture and scramble the eggs while cooking.
4. When the eggs start to settle, add in the smoked salmon and cook for 2 more minutes.

Nutrition: Calories 349, Total Fat 23g, Saturated Fat 4g, Total Carbs 3g, Net Carbs 1g, Protein 29g, Sugar: 2g, Fiber: 2g, Sodium: 466mg, Potassium 536mg

53. Raspberry Grapefruit Smoothie

Preparation time: 5 minutes
Cooking time: 0 minutes
Servings: 1
Ingredients:
- Juice from 1 grapefruit, freshly squeezed
- 1 banana, peeled and sliced
- 1 cup raspberries

Directions:
1. Place all ingredients in a blender and pulse until smooth.
2. Chill before serving.

Nutrition: Calories 381, Total Fat 0.8g, Saturated Fat 0.1g, Total Carbs 96g, Net Carbs 85g, Protein 4g, Sugar: 61g, Fiber: 11g, Sodium: 11mg, Potassium 848mg

54. Breakfast Burgers with Avocado Buns

Preparation time: 10 minutes
Cooking time: 5 minutes
Servings: 1
Ingredients:
- 1 ripe avocado
- 1 egg, pasture-raised
- 1 red onion slice
- 1 tomato slice
- 1 lettuce leaf
- Sesame seed for garnish
- salt to taste

Directions:
1. Peel the avocado and remove the seed. Slice the avocado into half. This will serve as the bun. Set aside.
2. Grease a skillet over medium flame and fry the egg sunny side up for 5 minutes or until set.
3. Assemble the breakfast burger by placing on top of one avocado half with the egg, red onion, tomato, and lettuce leaf. Top with the remaining avocado bun.
4. Garnish with sesame seeds on top and season with salt to taste.

Nutrition: Calories 458, Total Fat 39g, Saturated Fat 4g, Total Carbs 20g, Net Carbs 6g, Protein 13g, Sugar: 8g, Fiber: 14g, Sodium: 118mg, Potassium 1184mg

55. Spinach Breakfast

Preparation time: 10 minutes
Cooking time: 35minutes
Servings: 4
Ingredients:
- 2 sweet potatoes, peeled and diced
- 2 tablespoons olive oil
- ½ teaspoon onion powder
- ½ teaspoon garlic powder
- ¼ teaspoon paprika
- 4 eggs, pasture-raised
- ½ onion, sliced
- ½ cup mushrooms, sliced
- 2 cups fresh baby spinach
- salt and pepper to taste
- Coconut oil for greasing

Directions:
1. Preheat the oven to 4250F.
2. Place the potatoes in a baking dish and drizzle with olive oil. Season with onion powder, garlic powder, paprika, salt, and pepper to taste. Once cooked, set aside.
3. Bake in the oven for 30 minutes while turning the sweet potatoes halfway through the cooking time.
4. Heat skillet and grease with coconut oil.
5. Sauté the onion for 30 seconds until fragrant.
6. Add in the mushrooms and egg. Season with salt and pepper to taste.
7. Scramble the eggs.
8. Before the eggs have set, stir in the baby spinach until wilted.
9. Plate the potatoes and top with the egg mixture.

Nutrition: Calories 252, Total Fat 17g, Saturated Fat 4g, Total Carbs 15g, Net Carbs 13g, Protein 11g, Sugar: 4g, Fiber: 2g, Sodium: 151mg, Potassium 472mg

56. Healthy Breakfast Chocolate Donuts

Preparation time: 10 minutes
Cooking time: 15 minutes
Servings: 12
Ingredients:
- 1 cup coconut flour
- ¼ cup raw cacao powder
- ½ teaspoon baking soda
- 4 eggs, pasture-raised
- ¼ cup coconut oil, melted
- ¼ cup unsweetened applesauce
- 1 teaspoon vanilla
- ¼ cup honey
- ¼ teaspoon salt

Directions:

1. Preheat the oven to 3500F.
2. In a mixing bowl, mix the coconut flour, cacao, baking soda, and salt. Set aside.
3. In another bowl, mix the eggs, coconut oil, and applesauce. Stir in the vanilla and honey.
4. Fold the dry ingredients gradually into the wet ingredients until well-combined.
5. Grease the donut pan with coconut oil.
6. Press down the dough into the pan.
7. Bake for 15 minutes or until the dough is cooked through.
8. Remove from the oven and allow cooling before removing from the donut pan.

Nutrition: Calories 115, Total Fat 8g, Saturated Fat 4g, Total Carbs 9g, Net Carbs 8.2g, Protein 4g, Sugar: 7g, Fiber: 0.8g, Sodium:108 mg, Potassium 255mg

57. Baked Eggs with Portobello Mushrooms

Preparation time: 10 minutes
Cooking time: 20 minutes
Servings: 4
Ingredients:
- 4 portobello mushroom caps
- 1 cup arugula
- 1 medium tomato, chopped
- 4 large eggs, pasture-raised
- salt and pepper to taste

Directions:
1. Preheat the oven to 3500F and line a baking sheet with parchment paper.
2. Scoop out the gills from the mushrooms using a spoon. Discard the gills and set aside.
3. Place the mushrooms on the baking sheet inverted (gill side up) and fill each cap with arugula and tomato.
4. Carefully crack an egg on each mushroom cap.
5. Bake in the oven for 20 minutes or until the eggs have set.

Nutrition: Calories 80, Total Fat 5g, Saturated Fat 2g, Total Carbs 5g, Net Carbs 3g, Protein 5g, Sugar: 3g, Fiber: 2g, Sodium: 19mg, Potassium 416mg

58. Breakfast Spinach Mushroom Tomato Fry Up

Preparation time: 5 minutes
Cooking time: 10 minutes
Servings: 2
Ingredients:
- 1 teaspoon olive oil
- 1 red onion, sliced
- 6 button mushrooms, sliced
- ½ cup cherry tomatoes, halved
- ½ teaspoon diced lemon rind
- 3 large handful baby spinach
- salt and pepper to taste

Directions:
1. Heat oil in a skillet over medium low heat.
2. Sauté the onion until fragrant.
3. Add in the mushrooms and tomatoes. Season with lemon rind, salt and pepper. Cook for another 5 minutes.
4. Stir in the baby spinach until wilted.

Nutrition: Calories 38, Total Fat 3g, Saturated Fat 0g, Total Carbs 3g, Net Carbs 1.5g, Protein 2g, Sugar: 1g, Fiber: 1.5g, Sodium: 37mg, Potassium 321mg

59. Sweet Cherry Almond Chia Pudding

Preparation time: 3 hours
Cooking time: 0 minutes
Servings: 4
Ingredients:
- 2 cups whole sweet cherries, pitted
- 2 cups coconut milk
- ¼ cup maple syrup, organic
- 1 teaspoon vanilla extract
- ¾ cup chia seeds
- ½ cup hemp seeds
- 1/8 teaspoon salt

Directions:
1. In the blender, combine the cherries, coconut milk, maple syrup, and vanilla extract. Season with salt. Pulse until smooth.
2. Distribute the chia seeds and hemp seeds in four glasses and pour in the cherry and milk mixture.

3. Allow to chill in the fridge for 3 hours before serving.

Nutrition: Calories 302, Total Fat 17g, Saturated Fat 4g, Total Carbs 29g, Net Carbs 22g, Protein 10g, Sugar: 20g, Fiber: 7g, Sodium: 59mg, Potassium 384mg

60. Pineapple Ginger Smoothie

Preparation time: 5 minutes
Cooking time: 0 minutes
Servings: 1
Ingredients:
- 1 cup pineapple slice
- ½ inch thick ginger, sliced
- 1 cup coconut milk

Directions:
1. Place all ingredients in a blender.
2. Pulse until smooth.
3. Chill before serving.

Nutrition: Calories 299, Total Fat 8g, Saturated Fat 5g, Total Carbs 51g, Net Carbs 49g, Protein 9g, Sugar: 48g, Fiber: 2g, Sodium: 108mg, Potassium 630mg

61. Beet and Cherry Smoothie

Preparation time: 5 minutes
Cooking time: 0 minutes
Servings: 4
Ingredients:
- 10-ounce almond milk, unsweetened
- 2 small beets, peeled and cut into quarters
- ½ cup frozen cherries, pitted
- ½ teaspoon frozen banana
- 1 tablespoon almond butter

Directions:
1. Add all ingredients in a blender.
2. Blend until smooth.

Nutrition: Calories 470, Total Fat 38g, Saturated Fat 6g, Total Carbs 24g, Net Carbs 14g, Protein 16g, Sugar: 10g, Fiber: 10g, Sodium: 67mg, Potassium 733mg

62. Spicy Pineapple Smoothie

Preparation time: 5 minutes
Cooking time: 0 minutes
Servings: 1
Ingredients:
- 1 tablespoon chia seeds
- 1 teaspoon black pepper powder
- 1 orange, peeled
- 1 ½ cups frozen pineapple chunks
- 1 cup coconut water
- 1 teaspoon ground turmeric

Directions:
1. Place all ingredients in a blender.
2. Pulse until smooth.
3. Serve chilled.

Nutrition: Calories 378, Total Fat 10g, Saturated Fat 2g, Total Carbs 73g, Net Carbs 53g, Protein 9g, Sugar: 42g, Fiber: 20g, Sodium: 261mg, Potassium 1281mg

63. Breakfast Cherry Muffins

Preparation time: 10 minutes
Cooking time: 30 minutes
Servings: 6
Ingredients:
- 1 ½ cup almond flour
- ¼ cup arrowroot flour
- ¼ cup coconut oil
- ¼ cup maple syrup
- 3 whole eggs
- 2 teaspoons vanilla extract
- 1 ½ teaspoons almond extract
- 1 teaspoon baking powder
- 1 cup fresh cherry, pitted and chopped
- ¼ teaspoon salt

Directions:
1. Preheat the oven to 3500F.
2. In a mixing bowl, combine all ingredients except for the cherries. Mix until well-combined.
3. Add the cherries last.
4. Fill muffin liners with the batter and bake for 30 minutes or until a toothpick inserted comes out clean.

Nutrition: Calories 528, Total Fat 39g, Saturated Fat 5g, Total Carbs 36g, Net Carbs 29g, Protein 13g, Sugar: 15g, Fiber: 7g, Sodium: 177mg, Potassium 679mg

64. Breakfast Shakshuka

Preparation time: 5 minutes
Cooking time: 10 minutes
Servings: 6
Ingredients:
- 1 tablespoon olive oil
- ½ onion, chopped
- 1 clove garlic, minced
- 1 red bell pepper, seeded and chopped
- 4 cups tomatoes, diced
- 1 teaspoon chili powder
- 1 teaspoon paprika
- 6 eggs, pasture-raised
- ½ tablespoon fresh parsley, chopped
- salt and pepper to taste

Directions:
1. Heat oil in a skillet over medium flame.
2. Sauté the onion and garlic for 30 seconds or until fragrant.
3. Add in the red bell pepper and tomatoes. Season with salt and pepper to taste. Stir in the chili powder and paprika. Allow to simmer until the tomatoes are soft.
4. Reduce the heat and create 6 wells in the skillet.
5. Crack in one egg in each well and increase the heat.
6. Cover and allow to simmer for 5 minutes.
7. Garnish with parsley last.

Nutrition: Calories 177, Total Fat 12g, Saturated Fat 3g, Total Carbs 7g, Net Carbs 5g, Protein 10g, Sugar: 4g, Fiber: 2g, Sodium:109 mg, Potassium 445mg

65. Anti-Inflammatory Crepes

Preparation time: 5 minutes
Cooking time: 4 minutes
Servings: 4
Ingredients:
- 2 tablespoon coconut flour
- 4 large eggs, pasture-raised
- 1 tablespoon coconut oil
- 1 cup hazelnuts, soaked in water overnight
- 2/3 cup dark chocolates
- ½ teaspoon vanilla extract
- 2 tablespoon maple syrup
- ½ cup water

Directions:
1. Preheat the oven to 3500F.
2. In a bowl, mix the coconut flour, eggs, and water until well-combined.
3. Heat oil in a skillet over medium flame and grease the skillet with coconut oil.
4. Scoop 1/3 cup of the crepe mixture into the skillet and cook for 4 minutes while flipping halfway through the cooking time.
5. Repeat until all batter is made into crepes.
6. Make the hazelnut sauce by combining the hazelnuts, dark chocolates, vanilla extract, and maple syrup in a blender.
7. Pulse until smooth.
8. Spread the Nutella sauce over the crepes before serving.

Nutrition: Calories 465, Total Fat 29g, Saturated Fat 6g, Total Carbs 46g, Net Carbs g, Protein 9g, Sugar: 32g, Fiber: 5g, Sodium: 53mg, Potassium 401mg

66. No-Bake Turmeric Protein Donuts

Preparation time: 50 minutes
Cooking time: 0 minutes
Servings: 8
Ingredients:
- 1 ½ cups raw cashews
- ½ cup medjool dates, pitted
- 1 tablespoon vanilla protein powder
- ½ cup shredded coconut
- 2 tablespoons maple syrup
- ¼ teaspoon vanilla extract
- 1 teaspoon turmeric powder
- ¼ cup dark chocolate

Directions:
1. Combine all ingredients except for the chocolate in a food processor.
2. Pulse until smooth.
3. Roll batter into 8 balls and press into a silicone donut mold.
4. Place in the freezer for 30 minutes to set.
5. Meanwhile, make the chocolate topping by melting the chocolate in a double boiler.
6. Once the donuts have set, remove the donuts from the mold and drizzle with chocolate.

Nutrition: Calories 320, Total Fat 26g, Saturated Fat 5g, Total Carbs 20g, Net Carbs 18g, Protein 7g, Sugar: 9g, Fiber: 2g, Sodium:163 mg, Potassium 297mg

67. Breakfast Stir Fry

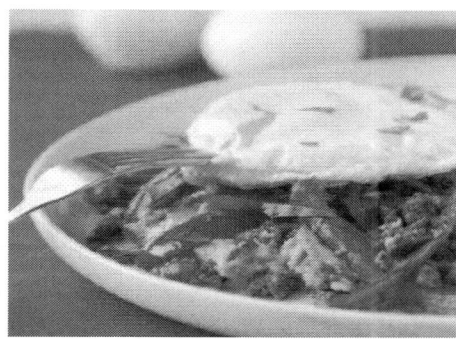

Preparation Time: 20 Minutes

Servings: 2

Ingredients:
- 1/2 pounds beef meat; minced
- 1 tablespoon tamari sauce
- 2 bell peppers; chopped.
- 2 teaspoons red chili flakes
- 1 teaspoon chili powder
- 1 tablespoon coconut oil
- Salt and black pepper to the taste.
- For the bok choy:
- 6 bunches bok choy; trimmed and chopped.
- 1 teaspoon ginger; grated
- 1-tablespoon coconut oil
- Salt to the taste.
- For the eggs:
- 2 eggs
- 1 tablespoon coconut oil

Directions:
1. Heat up a pan with 1 tablespoon coconut oil over medium high heat; add beef and bell peppers; stir and cook for 10 minutes
2. Add salt, pepper, tamari sauce, chili flakes and chili powder; stir, cook for 4 minutes more and take off heat.
3. Heat up another pan with 1 tablespoon oil over medium heat; add bok choy; stir and cook for 3 minutes
4. Add salt and ginger; stir, cook for 2 minutes more and take off heat.
5. Heat up the third pan with 1 tablespoon oil over medium heat; crack eggs and fry them.
6. Divide beef and bell peppers mix into 2 bowls
7. Divide bok choy and top with eggs

Nutrition: Calories: 248 Cal Fat: 14 g Fiber: 4 g Carbs: 10 g Protein: 14 g

LUNCH

68. Strawberries and Cream Trifle

Preparation Time: 10 Minutes
Cooking Time: 45 Minutes
Servings: 12
Ingredients:
- 6 ounces packaged cream cheese, softened
- 1 ½ cups condensed milk
- 12 ounces frozen whipped cream, thawed
- 1 angel food cake, cubed
- 3 pints' fresh strawberries, hulled and sliced

Directions:
1. In a bowl, put together the cream cheese, sweetened condensed milk, and whip in until smooth.
2. In a trifle bowl, put a layer of angel food cake cubes. Add a layer of strawberries and cream on top. Repeat the layers.
3. Bring it in the refrigerator to cool for at least 35 minutes.

Nutrition: Calories: 378 | Fat: 17g | Carbs: 51g | Protein: 7g

69. Maple Toast and Eggs

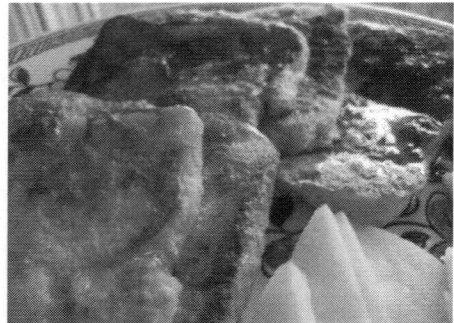

Preparation Time: 20 Minutes
Cooking Time: 20 Minutes
Servings: 6

- 12 bacon strips, diced
- ½ cup maple syrup
- ¼ cup butter
- 12 slices white bread
- 12 large eggs
- Salt and pepper to taste

Directions:
1. Fry the bacon on a skillet on medium heat until the fat has been rendered. Take the bacon out and place it on paper towels to drain excess Fat.
2. Warm the maple syrup and butter until melted in a saucepan. Set aside.
3. Trim the edges of the bread and flatten the slices with a rolling pin. Brush one side with the syrup mixture and press the slices into greased muffin cups.
4. Divide the bacon into the muffin cups.
5. Break one egg into each cup.
6. Sprinkle with salt and pepper to taste
7. Cover using foil, then bake in the oven at 4000F for 20 minutes or until the eggs have set.

Nutrition: Calories: 671 | Fat: 46g | Carbs: 44g | Protein: 21g

70. Sweet Onion and Egg Pie

Preparation Time: 20 Minutes
Cooking Time: 35 Minutes
Servings: 10
Ingredients:
- 2 sweet onions, halved and sliced
- 1 tablespoons butter
- 6 eggs
- 1 cup evaporated milk
- 11 frozen deep-dish pie crust
- Salt and pepper to taste

Directions:
1. Preheat the oven 4000F.
2. Melt the butter in a non-stick skillet. Sauté the onions over medium-low heat until very tender.
3. Place the onions in a bowl. Add in eggs and evaporated milk. Season with salt and pepper to taste.
4. Pour the egg and onion mixture into the commercial pie crust.

5. Bake in the oven for 35 minutes.
Nutrition: Calories: 169 | Fat: 7g | Carbs: 21g

71. Mini Breakfast Pizza

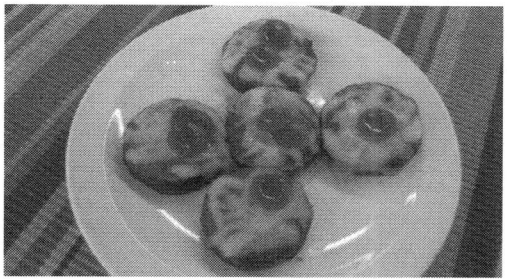

Preparation Time: 5 Minutes
Cooking Time: 10 Minutes
Servings: 4

- 4 eggs, beaten
- 1/3 cup commercial pizza sauce
- 2 English muffins, split and toasted
- ½ cup shredded Italian cheese
- Dried oregano leaves
- Cooking spray
- Salt and pepper to taste

Directions:
1. Preheat the oven to 4000F.
2. Coat a skillet with cooking spray, then heat on medium flame.
3. Season the eggs with salt and pepper to taste and pour into the skillet. As the eggs begin to set, pull the eggs across the pan with an inverted turner. Continue cooking and folding the egg. Set aside.
4. Spread pizza sauce evenly on English muffin halves and top with eggs and cheese.
5. Put on a baking sheet, then bake for 5 minutes.
6. Garnish with oregano last.

Nutrition: Calories: 282 | Fat: 13g | Carbs: 25g | Protein: 17g

72. Chicken Muffins

Preparation Time: 1 hour 10 minutes
Cooking Time: 30 minutes
Servings: 3
Ingredients:
- 3/4-pound chicken breast; boneless
- 1/2 teaspoon garlic powder
- 2 tablespoons green onions; chopped.
- 3 tablespoons hot sauce mixed with 3 tablespoons melted coconut oil
- 6 eggs
- Salt and black pepper to the taste.

Directions:
1. Season chicken breast with pepper, salt, and garlic powder, place on a lined baking sheet, and bake in the oven at 425F for at least 25 minutes.
2. Transfer chicken breast to a bowl, shred with a fork, and mix with half of the hot sauce and melted coconut oil.
3. Toss to coat and leave aside.
4. In a bowl, mix eggs with salt, pepper, green onions, and the rest of the hot sauce mixed with oil and whisk very well.
5. Divide this mix into a muffin tray, top each with shredded chicken, introduce in the oven at 350F, then bake for at least 30 minutes.
6. Serve your muffins hot.

Nutrition: Calories: 140 | Fat: 8 | Fiber: 1 | Carbs: 2 | Protein: 13

73. Pumpkin Pancakes

Preparation Time: 25 minutes
Cooking Time: 10 minutes
Servings: 6
Ingredients:
- 2 ounces' hazelnut flour
- 2 ounces' flax seeds; ground
- 1-ounce egg white Protein:
- 1 teaspoon coconut oil
- 1 tablespoon chai masala
- 1 teaspoon vanilla extract
- 1 teaspoon baking powder
- 1 cup coconut cream
- 1 tablespoon swerve
- 1/2 cup pumpkin puree
- 3 eggs
- 5 drops stevia

Directions:
1. In a bowl, mix flax seeds with hazelnut flour, egg white Protein: baking powder and chai masala and stir.

2. Mix coconut cream with vanilla extract, pumpkin puree, eggs, stevia, and swerve and stir well in another bowl.
3. Combine the 2 mixtures and stir well.
4. Heat a pan with the oil over medium-high heat; pour 1/6 of the batter, spread into a circle, cover, reduce heat to low, cook for 3 minutes on each side and transfer to a plate
5. Repeat the process using the remaining mixture and serve pumpkin pancakes right away.

Nutrition: Calories: 400 | Fat: 23 | Fiber: 4 | Carbs: 5 | Protein: 21

74. Cauliflower and Chorizo

Preparation Time: 55 minutes
Cooking Time: 40 minutes
Servings: 4
Ingredients:
- 1 cauliflower head; florets separated
- 4 eggs; whisked
- 1/2 teaspoon garlic powder
- 2 tablespoons green onions; chopped.
- 1-pound chorizo; chopped.
- 12 ounces canned green chilies; chopped.
- 1 yellow onion; chopped.
- Salt and black pepper to the taste.

Directions:
1. Heat a pan on medium heat; put the chorizo and onion; stir and brown for a few minutes
2. Add green chilies, stir, cook for a few minutes and take off the heat.
3. In your food processor, mix cauliflower with some salt and pepper and blend.
4. Transfer this to a bowl, add eggs, salt, pepper, and garlic powder, and whisk everything.
5. Add chorizo mix as well, whisk again and transfer everything to a greased baking dish.
6. Bake in the oven at 375F, then bake for at least 40 minutes.
7. Leave casserole to cool down for a few minutes, sprinkle green onions on top, slice and serve

Nutrition: Calories: 350 | Fat: 12 | Fiber: 4 | Carbs: 6 | Protein: 20

75. Carrot Bread

Preparation Time: 10 minutes
Cooking Time: 1 hour
Servings: 8
Ingredients:
- 2 cups almond meal
- 1 teaspoon organic baking powder
- 1 tablespoon cumin seeds
- Salt, to taste
- 3 organic eggs
- 2 tablespoons macadamia nut oil
- 1 tablespoon apple cider vinegar
- 3 cups carrot, peeled and grated
- ½-inch piece of fresh ginger, peeled and grated
- ¼ cup sultanas

Directions:
1. Set the oven to 35 F, then line a loaf pan with parchment paper.
2. In a large bowl, put together the almond meal, baking powder, cumin seeds, and salt and mix.
3. In another bowl, add eggs, nut oil, and vinegar and beat till well combined.
4. Put the egg mixture into the flour mixture and mix till well combined.
5. Fold in the remaining ingredients.
6. Place the mixture into the prepared loaf pan equally.
7. Bake for about 1 hour.

Nutrition: Calories: 215 | Total Fat: 17.1g | Total Carbs: 10.8g | Fiber: 4.1g | Sugars: 3.9g | Protein: 7.6g

76. Fruity Muffins

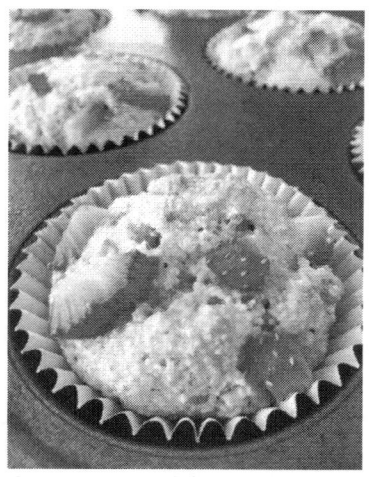

Preparation Time: 10 minutes
Cooking Time: 2-3 minutes
Servings: 8

- ½ cup almond meal
- 1 tablespoon linseed meal
- ¼ cup raw sugar
- 2 tablespoons crystallized ginger, chopped finely
- ½ cup buckwheat flour
- ¼ cup brown rice flour
- 2 tablespoons arrowroot flour
- 2 tablespoons organic baking powder
- ½ teaspoon ground ginger
- 12 teaspoon ground cinnamon
- Pinch of salt
- 1 large organic egg
- 7 tablespoons almond milk
- ¼ cup extra-virgin olive oil
- 1 teaspoon organic vanilla extract
- 1 small apple, peeled, cored, and chopped finely
- 1 cup rhubarb, sliced finely

Directions:
1. Set the oven to 350F. Grease 8 cups of a large muffin tin.
2. In a large bowl, mix together almond meal, linseed meal, sugar, and crystalized ginger.
3. In another bowl, put together flours, baking powder, spices, and salt, and mix.
4. Sift the flour mixture into the bowl of almond meal mixture and mix well.
5. Add egg, milk, oil, and vanilla in a third bowl and beat till well combined.
6. Add egg mixture into the flour mixture and mix till well combined.
7. Fold in apple and rhubarb.
8. Place the mixture into prepared muffin cups equally.
9. Bake for about 20-25 minutes or till a toothpick inserted in the center comes out clean.

Nutrition: Calories: 227 | Total Fat: 4.2g | Total Carbs: 26.9g | Fiber: 4.9g | Sugars: 10.4g | Protein: 4.1g

77. Edamame Omelet

Preparation Time: 5 minutes
Cooking Time: 5 minutes
Servings: 2
Ingredients:

- 3 tbsp. olive oil, divided
- 1 tsp. minced garlic
- 1 bunch scallions, cut into 1-inch pieces
- ½ cup shelled edamame
- 1 tbsp. low-sodium soy sauce, or to taste
- 3 large eggs or ¾ cup egg substitute
- ½ cup shredded regular or soy Cheddar cheese
- Snips of fresh cilantro for garnish

Directions:
1. Warm 2 tablespoons oil in a small skillet over medium heat and sauté the garlic and scallion for about 2 minutes. Add the edamame and soy sauce and sauté 1 minute more. Remove from the skillet and set aside.
2. Warm the other 1 tablespoon oil in the same skillet.
3. Whisk the eggs until mixed and pour into the hot oil. Scatter the shredded cheese on top. Lift up the omelet's edges, tipping the skillet back and forth to cook the uncooked eggs.
4. Once the top looks firm, sprinkle the scallion mixture over one half of the omelet and fold the other half over the top.
5. Lift the omelet out of the skillet. Divide it in half, sprinkle with the cilantro, and serve.

Nutrition: Calories: 416 | Fat: 31 g | Protein: 27 g | Sodium: 640 | Fiber: 3 g | Carbohydrate: 7.5 g

78. Almond Mascarpone Dumplings

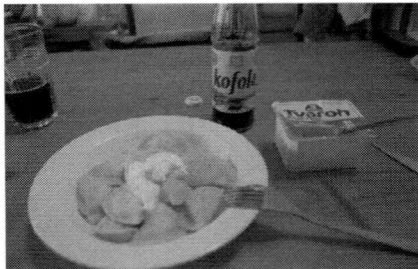

Preparation Time: 10 minutes
Cooking Time: 10 minutes
Servings: 6

- 1 cup whole-wheat flour
- 1 cup all-purpose unbleached flour
- ¼ cup ground almonds
- 4 egg whites
- 3 ounces' mascarpone cheese
- 1 teaspoon extra-virgin olive oil
- 2 teaspoons apple juice
- 1 tablespoon butter
- ¼ cup honey

Directions:
1. Strain together both types of flour in a large bowl. Mix in the almonds.
2. In a separate bowl, whisk together the egg whites, cheese, oil, and juice on medium speed with an electric mixer.
3. Put the flour and egg white mixture with a dough hook on medium speed or by hand until a dough forms.
4. Boil 1-gallon water in a medium-size saucepot. Take a scoop of dough and use a second spoon to push it into the boiling water. Cook up to the dumpling floats to the top, at least 5 to 10 minutes. You can cook several dumplings at once — just take care not to crowd the pot.
5. Take off with a slotted spoon and drain on paper towels.
6. Warm a medium-size sauté pan on medium-high heat.
7. Add the butter, then put the dumplings in the pan and cook until light brown.
8. Set on serving plates and drizzle with honey.

Nutrition: Calories: 254 | Fat: 6.4 g | Protein: 7 g | Sodium: 20 mg | Fiber: 3.5 g | Carbohydrate: 44 g

79. Raisin Bran Muffins

Preparation Time: 15 minutes
Cooking Time: 30 minutes
Servings: 36
Ingredients:

- 1 cup boiling water
- 2½ cups All-Bran cereal
- 2½ cups all-purpose flour
- 2½ teaspoons baking soda
- 1 teaspoon salt
- ½ cup vegetable oil
- 1 cup sugar
- 2 eggs, beaten
- 2 cups buttermilk
- 1½ cups raisins
- 1 cup bran flakes

Directions:
1. Set the oven to 400°F.
2. Grease a muffin tin. Put the boiling water over 1 cup All-Bran, and let sit for 10 minutes.
3. Place the baking soda, flour, and salt in a mixing bowl, then mix, set aside.
4. Stir the oil into the bran and water mixture, then put the remaining bran, sugar, eggs, and buttermilk.
5. Put the flour mixture into the bran mixture and mix to combine. Stir in the raisins, and bran flakes, then fill the muffin cups ¾ full with the batter.
6. Bake muffins for 20 minutes.

Nutrition: Calories: 104 | Fat: 4 g | Protein: 2.5 g | Sodium: 187 mg | Fiber: 2 g | Carbohydrate: 17 g

80. Apple Bread

Preparation Time: 25 minutes
Cooking Time: 1 hour and 10 minutes
Servings: 8
Ingredients:

- 1 packet yeast
- 3 tbsp. sugar
- 11/3 cups warm water

- 3 tbsp. soft butter
- 1 tsp. Salt
- ¼ tsp. baking powder
- 1¾ cups all-purpose flour
- 1¾ cups whole-wheat flour
- 1 cup peeled, chopped apples
- 1 tbsp. cinnamon mixed with 1 tablespoon sugar

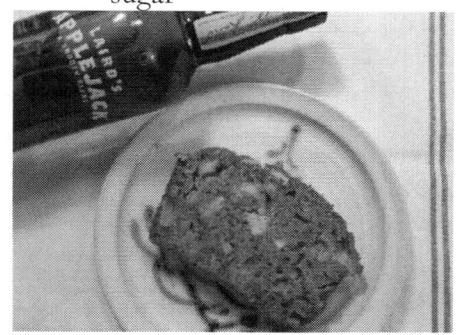

Directions:
1. Combine yeast, ½ teaspoon sugar, and 1/3 cup water in a bowl. Let sit for 5 minutes.
2. Put together remaining water, butter, remaining sugar, salt, and baking powder in a mixing bowl, then mix.
4. Put the dough into an oiled bowl.
5. Cover then rises in a warm place for at least 1 to 2 hours until doubled in bulk.
6. Punch down dough, then form into a rectangle.
7. Scatter the apples on the dough and dust with the cinnamon sugar.
8. Roll into a cylinder and put in an oiled loaf pan. Cover and let it rise in warm for 90 minutes until doubled in size.
9. Preheat oven to 350°F. Uncover bread and bake for 50 minutes.

Nutrition: Calories: 258 |Fat: 5 g|Protein: 7 g |Sodium: 294 mg |Fiber: 4.5 g |Carbohydrate: 48 g

81. Zucchini Bread

Preparation Time: 10 minutes
Cooking Time: 60 minutes
Servings: 16
Ingredients:

- 1½ cups all-purpose flour
- 1½ cups 100% whole-wheat flour
- 1 teaspoon salt
- 1 teaspoon baking soda
- ¼ teaspoon baking powder
- 1 tablespoon cinnamon
- 3 eggs, beaten, or ¾ cup of egg substitute
- 1 cup canola oil
- 2 cups sugar
- 2 cups grated zucchini
- 1 cup chopped pecans
- 1 cup raisins

Directions:
1. Preheat oven to 350°F. Oil 2 loaf pans and set aside.
2. Put the flour, salt, baking soda, baking powder, and cinnamon in a bowl.
3. Mix the eggs, oil, and sugar in another bowl.
4. Add the zucchini and dry ingredients alternately until fully incorporated into a smooth batter. Fold in the pecans and raisins and scrape the batter into the loaf pans.
5. Bake for 60 minutes, cool on a rack and wrap when cool.

Nutrition: Calories: 396|Fat: 20 |Protein: 5 g|Sodium: 237 mg|Fiber: 3 g |Carbohydrate: 52 g

82. Sweetened Brown Rice

Preparation Time: 10 minutes
Cooking Time: 45-60 minutes
Servings: 8
Ingredients:

- 1½ cups soy milk
- 1½ cups water
- 1 cup brown rice
- 1 tablespoon honey
- ¼ teaspoon nutmeg
- Fresh fruit (optional)

Directions:
1. Put all the ingredients, excluding the fresh fruit, in a medium-size saucepan; place the mixture to a slow simmer, then cover using a tight-fitting lid.

2. Simmer for at least 45-60 minutes, up to the rice is tender and done. Serve in bowls, topped with your favorite fresh fruit.

Nutrition: Calories: 155 | Fat: 1.5 g | Protein: 3.5 g | Sodium: 35 mg | Fiber: 1.5 g | Carbohydrate: 13 g

83. Cornmeal Grits

Preparation Time: 5 minutes
Cooking Time: 15 minutes
Servings: 4
Ingredients:
- 4 cups water
- 1 teaspoon salt
- 1 cup polenta meal
- 2 tablespoons butter

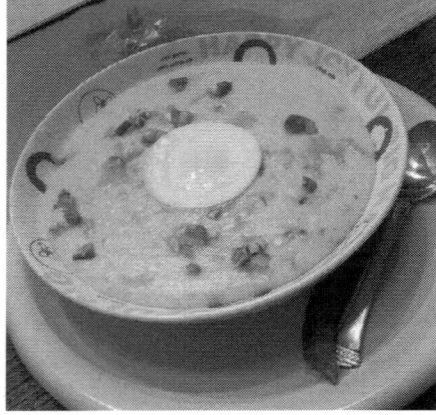

Directions:
1. Put water and salt in a saucepan, then place it to a boil.
2. Gradually add polenta and constantly stir over medium-low heat until it has thickened, about 15 minutes. Stir in butter.
4. Once cool, grits can be sliced and fried, or grilled.

Nutrition: Calories: 177 | Fat: 6 g | Protein: 3 g | Sodium: 641 mg | Fiber: 2.5 g | Carbohydrate: 27 g

84. Grapefruit-Pomegranate Salad

Preparation Time: 10 minutes
Cooking Time: 0 minutes
Servings: 6
Ingredients:
- 2 ruby red grapefruits
- 3 ounces Parmesan cheese
- 1 pomegranate
- 6 cups mesclun leaves
- ¼ cup Basic Vegetable Stock

Directions:
1. Peel the grapefruit using a knife, take off all the pith. (The white layer under the skin).
2. Cut out every section with the knife, ensure that no pith remains. Shave Parmesan using a vegetable peeler to form curls.
3. Peel the pomegranate using a paring knife; take off the berries/seeds.
4. Toss the mesclun greens in the stock.
5. To serve, mound the greens on plates and arrange the grapefruit sections, cheese, and pomegranate on top.

Nutrition: Calories: 84 | Fat: 2 g | Protein: 4 g | Sodium: 102 mg | Fiber: 2 g | Carbohydrate: 14 g

85. Oatmeal-Raisin Scones

Preparation Time: 10 minutes
Cooking Time: 15 minutes
Servings: 6
Ingredients:
- 1½ cups rolled oats
- ½ cup all-purpose flour
- 2 tablespoons wheat germ
- 3 tablespoons sugar
- ½ teaspoon salt
- 11/8 teaspoons baking powder
- 6 tablespoons cold unsalted butter
- 2 eggs or ½ cup egg substitute
- 2/3 cup buttermilk
- ½ teaspoon vanilla
- 1 cup raisins
- 1 egg white
- 2 tablespoons granulated sugar

Directions:
1. Preheat oven to 400°F. Line a baking pan w/ parchment paper or spray lightly with oil. Grind half of the oats into flour in a food processor.
2. Combine remaining oats, oat flour, all-purpose flour, wheat germ, sugar, salt, baking powder, and butter in a food processor with

a metal blade. Process until mixture resembles cornmeal.
3. In a huge bowl, put together eggs, buttermilk, and vanilla, then whisk. Stir in raisins using a spatula or wooden spoon.
4. Put the dry ingredients and fold them in with a spatula. Drop scones into rounds onto the prepared baking sheet.
5. Brush scones with egg white and dust with granulated sugar. Bake for 15 minutes.

Nutrition: Calories: 456 |Fat: 16 g|Protein: 13 g|Sodium: 277 mg|Fiber: 6 g | Carbohydrate: 70 g

86. Yogurt Cheese and Fruit

Preparation Time: 10 minutes
Cooking Time: 0 minutes
Servings: 6
Ingredients:
- 3 cups plain nonfat yogurt
- 1 teaspoon fresh lemon juice
- ½ cup orange juice
- ½ cup water
- 1 fresh Golden Delicious apple
- 1 fresh pear
- ¼ cup honey
- ¼ cup dried cranberries or raisins

Directions:
1. Prepare the yogurt cheese the day before by lining a colander or strainer with cheesecloth. Scoop the yogurt into the cheesecloth, place the strainer over a pot or bowl to catch the whey, and refrigerate for at least 8 hours before serving.
2. In a huge mixing bowl, mix the juices and water. Cut the apple than pear into wedges, place the wedges in the juice mixture, let sit for at least 5 minutes. Strain off the liquid.
3. Please remove the yogurt from the refrigerator, slice, and place it on plates when the yogurt is firm. Arrange the fruit wedges around the yogurt. Drizzle with honey and sprinkle with cranberries or raisins just before serving.

Nutrition: Calories: 177 |Fat: 1 g |Protein: 6.5 g |Sodium: 87 mg | Fiber: 2 g | Carbohydrate: 35 g

87. Chicken & Cabbage Platter

Preparation Time: 9 minutes
Cooking Time: 14 minutes
Servings: 2
Ingredients:
- ½ cup onion, sliced
- 1 tablespoon sesame garlic-flavored oil
- 2 cups Bok-Choy/Spinach, shredded
- 1/2 cup fresh bean sprouts
- 1½ stalks celery, chopped
- 1½ teaspoon garlic, minced
- 1/2 teaspoon stevia
- 1/2 cup chicken broth
- 1 tablespoon coconut aminos
- 1/2 tablespoon freshly minced ginger 2 boneless chicken breast salt, to taste
- pepper, to taste

Directions:
1. Cut chicken breasts into pieces, season with salt and pepper. Fry it in the pan with garlic. Add chicken broth and sauté for a while.
2. Shred the cabbage with a knife.
3. Add onion, bean sprouts, celery, and sauté it until tender. Add stevia, coconut aminos, and ginger. Season with salt and pepper according to your taste.
4. Place the braised cabbage on your platter alongside the rotisserie chicken.
5. Enjoy!

Nutrition: Calories: 368 | Fat: 18g | Net Carbohydrates: 8g | Protein: 42g | Fiber: 3g | Carbohydrates: 11g

88. Balsamic Chicken and Vegetables

Preparation Time: 15 minutes
Cooking Time: 10 minutes
Servings: 4
Ingredients:
- 4 chicken thigh, boneless and skinless
- 5 stalks of asparagus, halved
- 1 bell pepper, cut in chunks
- 1/2 red onion, diced
- 1 garlic cloves, minced

- 2-ounces mushrooms, diced
- ¼ cup balsamic vinegar
- 1 tablespoon olive oil
- ½ teaspoon stevia
- ½ tablespoon oregano
- Salt and pepper, as needed

Directions:
1. Preheat your oven to 425 degrees Fahrenheit. Mix the spices, olive oil, and vinegar. Combine the vegetables and mushrooms in a bowl.
2. Season with spices and sprinkle with oil.
3. Dip the chicken pieces into a spice mix and coat them thoroughly.
4. Place the veggies and chicken onto a pan in a single layer.
5. Cook for 25 minutes.
6. Serve and enjoy!

Nutrition: Calories: 401 | Fat: 17g | Net Carbohydrates: 11g | Protein: 48g | Fiber: 3g | Carbohydrates: 14g

89. Onion Bacon Pork Chops

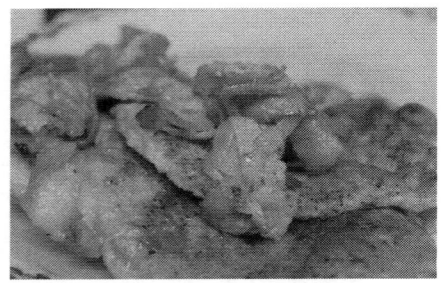

Preparation Time: 10 minutes
Cooking Time: 45 minutes

Ingredients:
- 1 onion, peeled and chopped
- 3 bacon slices, chopped
- 1/4 cup chicken stock
- Salt and pepper to taste
- 2 pork chops

Directions:
1. Heat a pan over medium heat and add bacon. Stir and cook until crispy. Transfer to a bowl. Return pan to medium heat and add onions, season with salt and pepper. Stir and cook for 15 minutes. Transfer to the same bowl with bacon. Return the pan to heat (medium-high) and add pork chops. Season with salt, pepper, and brown for 3 minutes. Flip and lower heat to medium. Cook for 7 minutes more. Add stock and stir cook for 2 minutes. Return the bacon and onions to the pan and stir cook for 1 minute. Serve and enjoy!

Nutrition: Calories: 325 | Fat: 18g | Carbohydrates: 6g | Protein: 36g | Fiber: 2g | Net Carbohydrates: 4g

90. Caramelized Pork Chops

Preparation Time: 5 minutes
Cooking Time: 30 minutes
Servings: 2
Ingredients:
- 2 pounds' chuck roast, sliced
- 2 ounces' green chili, chopped
- 1 tablespoon chili powder
- 1/4 teaspoon dried oregano
- 1/4 teaspoon ground cumin
- 1 garlic cloves, minced
- 2 tablespoons olive oil
- Salt as needed

Directions:
1. Rub up your chop with 1 teaspoon of pepper and 2 teaspoons of seasoning salt. Take a skillet and heat some oil over medium heat. Brown your pork chops on each side. Add some water and chili to the pan. Cover it up and lower down the heat, simmer it for about 20 minutes. Turn your chops over and add the rest of the pepper and salt. Cover it up, cook until the water evaporates, and the chili turns tender.
2. Remove the chops from your pan and serve with some peppers on top.

Nutrition: Calories: 271 | Fat: 19g | Carbohydrates: 4g | Protein: 27g | Fiber: 2g | Net Carbohydrates: 2g

91. Chicken Bacon Quesadilla

Preparation Time: 10 minutes
Cooking Time: 35 minutes
Servings: 2

Ingredients:
- ¼ cup ranch dressing
- ½ cup cheddar cheese, shredded
- 20 slices bacon, center-cut
- 2 cups grilled chicken, sliced

Directions:
1. Re-heat your oven to 400 degrees F.
2. Line baking sheet using parchment paper.
3. Bake bacon slices for 30 minutes.
4. Lay grilled chicken over bacon square, drizzling ranch dressing on top.
5. Sprinkle cheddar cheese and top with another bacon square.
6. Bake for 5 minutes more.
7. Slice and serve. Enjoy!

Nutrition: Calories: 619 | Fat: 35g | Carbohydrates: 2g | Protein: 79g | Fiber: 1g | Net Carbohydrates: 1g

92. Rosemary Roasted Pork with Cauliflower

Preparation Time: 10 minutes
Cooking Time: 20 minutes
Servings: 4
Ingredients:
- 1 ½ pound boneless pork tenderloin
- 1 tablespoon coconut oil
- 1 tablespoon fresh chopped rosemary
- Salt and pepper
- 1 tablespoon olive oil
- 2 cups cauliflower florets

Directions:
1. Rub the coconut oil into the pork, then season with rosemary, salt, and pepper.
2. Heat up the olive oil over medium to high heat in a large skillet.
3. Add the pork on each side and cook until browned for 2 to 3 minutes.
4. Sprinkle the cauliflower over the pork in the skillet.
5. Reduce heat to low, then cover the skillet and cook until the pork is cooked for 8 to 10 minutes.
6. Slice the pork with cauliflower and eat.

Nutrition: Calories: |320 Fats| 37 Protein: 3 |Carbohydrates: 1

93. Grilled Salmon and Zucchini with Mango Sauce

Preparation Time: 5 minutes
Cooking Time: 10 minutes
Servings: 4
Ingredients:
- 4 (6-ounce) boneless salmon fillets
- 1 tablespoon olive oil
- Salt and pepper
- 1 large zucchini, sliced in coins
- 2 tablespoons fresh lemon juice
- ½ cup chopped mango
- ¼ cup fresh chopped cilantro
- 1 teaspoon lemon zest
- ½ cup canned coconut milk

Directions:
1. Preheat a grill pan to heat, and sprinkle with cooking spray liberally.
2. Brush with olive oil to the salmon and season with salt and pepper.
3. Apply lemon juice to the zucchini, and season with salt and pepper.
4. Put the zucchini and salmon fillets on the grill pan.
5. Cook for 5 minutes, then turn all over and cook for another 5 minutes.
6. Combine the remaining ingredients in a blender and combine to create a sauce.
7. Serve the side-drizzled salmon filets with mango sauce and zucchini.

Nutrition: Calories: 350 |Fats: 23 |Protein: 7 |Carbohydrates: 6

94. Beef and Broccoli Stir-Fry

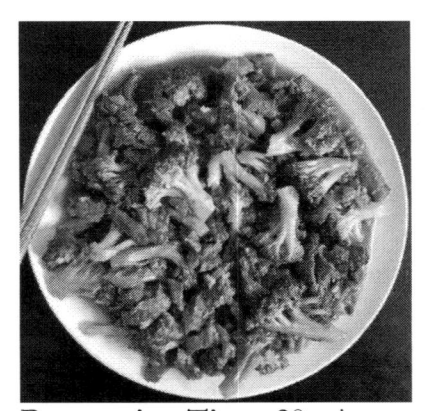

Preparation Time: 20 minutes

Cooking Time: 15 minutes
Servings: 4
Ingredients:
- ¼ cup soy sauce
- 1 tablespoon sesame oil
- 1 teaspoon garlic chili paste
- 1-pound beef sirloin
- 2 tablespoons almond flour
- 2 tablespoons coconut oil
- 2 cups chopped broccoli florets
- 1 tablespoon grated ginger
- 3 cloves garlic, minced

Directions:
1. In a small bowl, whisk the soy sauce, sesame oil, and chili paste together.
2. In a plastic freezer bag, slice the beef and mix with the almond flour.
3. Pour in the sauce and toss to coat for 20 minutes, then let rest.
4. Heat up the oil over medium to high heat in a large skillet.
5. In the pan, add the beef and sauce and cook until the meat is browned.
6. Move the beef to the skillet sides, then add the broccoli, ginger, and garlic.
7. Sauté until tender-crisp broccoli, then throw it all together and serve hot.

Nutrition: Calories: 350 | Fats: 19 | Protein: 37 | Carbohydrates: 6

95. Parmesan-Crusted Halibut with Asparagus

Preparation Time: 10 minutes
Cooking Time: 15 minutes
Servings: 4
Ingredients:
- 2 tablespoons olive oil
- ¼ cup butter softened
- Salt and pepper
- ¼ cup grated Parmesan
- 1-pound asparagus, trimmed
- 2 tablespoons almond flour
- 4 (6-ounce) boneless halibut fillets
- 1 teaspoon garlic powder

Directions:
1. Preheat the oven to 400 F and line a foil-based baking sheet.
2. Throw the asparagus in olive oil and scatter it over the baking sheet.
3. Add the butter, Parmesan cheese, almond flour, garlic powder, salt, and pepper in a blender, and mix until smooth.
4. Place the fillets with the asparagus on the baking sheet, and spoon the Parmesan over the eggs.
5. Bake for 10 to 12 minutes, then broil until browned for 2 to 3 minutes.

Nutrition: Calories: 415 | Fats: 26 | Protein: 42 | Carbohydrates: 3

96. Hearty Beef and Bacon Casserole

Preparation Time: 25 minutes
Cooking Time: 30 minutes
Servings: 8
Ingredients:
- 8 slices uncooked bacon
- 1 medium head cauliflower, chopped
- ¼ cup canned coconut milk
- Salt and pepper
- 2 pounds ground beef (80% lean)
- 8 ounces' mushrooms, sliced
- 1 large yellow onion, chopped
- 2 cloves garlic, minced

Direction:
1. Preheat to 375 F on the oven.
2. Cook the bacon in a skillet until it crispness, then drain and chop on paper towels.
3. Bring to boil a pot of salted water, then add the cauliflower.
4. Boil until tender for 6 to 8 minutes, then drain and add the coconut milk to a food processor.
5. Mix until smooth, then sprinkle with salt and pepper.
6. Cook the beef until browned in a pan, then wash the fat away.
7. Remove the mushrooms, onion, and garlic, then move to a baking platter.
8. Place on top of the cauliflower mixture and bake for 30 minutes.

9. Broil for 5 minutes on high heat, then sprinkle with bacon to serve.

Nutrition: Calories: 410 | Fats: 25 | Protein: 37 | Carbohydrates: 6

97. Sesame Wings with Cauliflower

Preparation Time: 5 minutes
Cooking Time: 30 minutes
Servings: 4
Ingredients:
- 2 ½ tablespoons soy sauce
- 2 tablespoons sesame oil
- 1 ½ teaspoon balsamic vinegar
- 1 teaspoon minced garlic
- 1 teaspoon grated ginger
- Salt
- 1-pound chicken wing, the wings itself
- 2 cups cauliflower florets

Directions:
1. Mix the soy sauce, sesame oil, balsamic vinegar, garlic, ginger, and salt in a freezer bag, then add the chicken wings.
2. Coat flip, then chills for 2 to 3 hours.
3. Preheat the oven to 400 F and line a foil-based baking sheet.
4. Spread the wings along with the cauliflower onto the baking sheet.
5. Bake for 35 minutes, then sprinkle on to serve with sesame seeds.

Nutrition: Calories: 400 | Fats: 15 | Protein: 5 | Carbohydrates: 3

98. Fried Coconut Shrimp with Asparagus

Preparation Time: 15 minutes
Cooking Time: 10 minutes
Servings: 6
Ingredients:
- 1 ½ cups shredded unsweetened coconut
- 2 large eggs
- Salt and pepper
- 1 ½ pound large shrimp, peeled and deveined
- ½ cup canned coconut milk
- 1-pound asparagus, cut into 2-inch pieces

Directions:
1. Pour the coconut onto a shallow platter.
2. Beat the eggs in a bowl with a little salt and pepper.
3. Dip the shrimp into the egg first, then dredge with coconut.
4. Heat up coconut oil over medium-high heat in a large skillet.
5. Add the shrimp and fry over each side for 1 to 2 minutes until browned.
6. Remove the paper towels from the shrimp and heat the skillet again.
7. Remove the asparagus and sauté to tender-crisp with salt and pepper, then serve with the shrimp.

Nutrition: Calories: 535 | Fats: 38 | Protein: 16 | Carbohydrates: 3

99. Coconut Chicken Curry with Cauliflower Rice

Preparation Time: 15 minutes
Cooking Time: 30 minutes
Servings: 6
Ingredients:
- 1 tablespoon olive oil
- 1 medium yellow onion, chopped
- 1 ½ pounds boneless chicken thighs, chopped
- Salt and pepper
- 1 (14-ounce) can coconut milk
- 1 tablespoon curry powder
- 1 ¼ teaspoon ground turmeric
- 3 cups riced cauliflower

Directions:
1. Heat the oil over medium heat in a large skillet.
2. Add the onions, and cook for about 5 minutes, until translucent.
3. Stir in the chicken and season with salt and pepper-cook for 6 to 8 minutes, frequently stirring until all sides are browned.
4. Pour the coconut milk into the pan, then whisk in the curry and turmeric powder.
5. Simmer until hot and bubbling, for 15 to 20 minutes.

6. Meanwhile, steam the cauliflower rice until tender with a few tablespoons of water.
7. Serve the cauliflower rice over the curry.

Nutrition: Calories: 430 | Fats: 29 | Protein: 9 | Carbohydrates: 3

100. Pumpkin Spiced Almonds

Preparation Time: 5 minutes
Cooking Time: 25 minutes
Servings: 4
Ingredients:
- 1 tablespoon olive oil
- 1 ¼ teaspoon pumpkin pie spice
- Pinch salt
- 1 cup whole almonds, raw

Direction:
1. Preheat the oven to 300 ° F, and line a parchment baking sheet.
2. In a mixing bowl, whisk together the olive oil, pumpkin pie spice, and salt.
3. Toss in the almonds until coated evenly, then scatter onto the baking sheet.
4. Bake and place in an airtight container for 25 minutes, then cool down completely.

Nutrition: Calories: 170 | Fats: 15 | Protein: 5 | Carbohydrates: 3

101. Tzatziki Dip with Cauliflower

Preparation Time: 10 minutes
Cooking Time: 0 minutes
Servings: 6
Ingredients:
- ½ (8-ounce) package cream cheese, softened
- 1 cup sour cream
- 1 tablespoon ranch seasoning
- 1 English cucumber, diced
- 2 tablespoons chopped chives
- 2 cups cauliflower florets

Directions:
1. Use an electric mixer to pound the cream cheese until smooth.
2. Stir in the sour cream and ranch seasoning beat until smooth.
3. Fold in the cucumbers and chives, then chill with cauliflower florets for dipping before serving.

Nutrition: Calories: 125 | Fats: 10 | Protein: 5 | Carbohydrates: 3

102. Classic Guacamole Dip

Preparation Time: 15 minutes
Cooking Time: 0 minutes
Servings: 4
Ingredients:
- 2 mediums avocado, pitted
- 1 small yellow onion, diced
- 1 small tomato, diced
- ¼ cup fresh chopped cilantro
- 1 tablespoon fresh lime juice
- 1 jalapeno, seeded and minced
- 1 clove garlic, minced
- Salt
- Sliced veggies to serve

Directions:
1. Mash avocado flesh into a bowl.
2. Stir the onion, tomato, cilantro, lime juice, garlic, and jalapeno in a bowl
3. Season lightly with salt and spoon into a bowl – serve with sliced veggies.

Nutrition: Calories: 225 | Fats: 20 | Protein: 12 | Carbohydrates: 3

103. Creamy Queso Dip

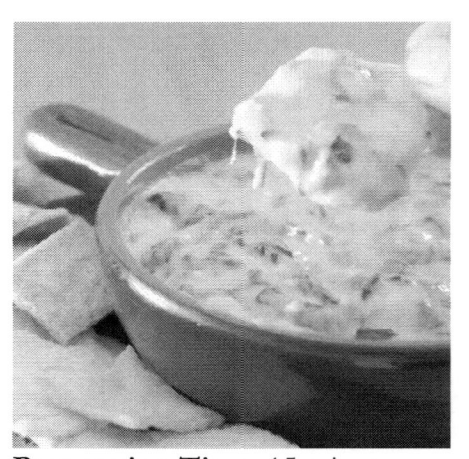

Preparation Time: 15 minutes

Servings: 8
Ingredients:

- 4 ounces' chorizo, crumbled
- 1 clove garlic, minced
- ¼ cup heavy cream
- 6 ounces shredded white cheddar cheese
- 2 ounces shredded pepper jack cheese
- ¼ teaspoon xanthan gum
- Pinch salt
- 1 jalapeno, seeded and minced
- 1 small tomato, diced

Directions:
1. Cook the chorizo in a skillet until browned evenly, then scatter in a dish.
2. At medium-low heat, pressure the skillet and add the garlic–cook for 30 seconds.
3. Stir in the heavy cream, then add the cheese a little at a time, frequently stirring until it melts.
4. Sprinkle with salt and xanthan gum, then mix well, and cook until thickened.
5. Add the tomato and jalapeno, then serve, dipping with vegetables.

Nutrition: Calories: 195 | Fats: 16 | Protein: 12 | Carbohydrates: 1

104. Herb Butter Scallops

Preparation Time: 10 minutes
Cooking Time: 10 minutes
Servings: 3

Ingredients:
- 1-pound sea scallops, cleaned
- Freshly ground black pepper
- 8 tablespoons butter, divided
- 2 teaspoons minced garlic
- Juice of 1 lemon
- 2 teaspoons chopped fresh basil
- 1 teaspoon chopped fresh thyme

Directions:
1. Pat the scallops dry with paper towels and season them lightly with pepper.
2. Place a large skillet over medium heat and add 2 tablespoons of butter.
3. Arrange the scallops in the skillet, evenly spaced but not too close together, and sear each side until they are golden brown, about 2½ minutes per side.
4. Remove the scallops to a plate and set them aside.
5. Add the remaining 6 tablespoons of butter to the skillet and sauté the garlic until translucent, about 3 minutes.
6. Stir in the lemon juice, basil, and thyme and return the scallops to the skillet, turning to coat them in the sauce.
7. Serve immediately.

Nutrition: Calories: 306 | Fat: 24g | Protein: 19g | carbohydrates: 4g | Fiber: 0g

DINNER

105. Pan-Seared Halibut with Citrus Butter Sauce

Preparation Time: 10 minutes
Cooking Time: 15 minutes
Servings: 3
Ingredients:
- 4 (5-ounce) halibut fillets, each about 1 inch thick
- Sea salt
- Freshly ground black pepper
- ¼ cup butter
- 2 teaspoons minced garlic
- 1 shallot, minced
- 1 tablespoon freshly squeezed lemon juice
- 1 tablespoon freshly squeezed orange juice
- 2 teaspoons chopped fresh parsley
- 2 tablespoons olive oil

Directions:
1. Pat the fish dry with paper towels and then lightly season the fillets with salt and pepper. Set aside on a paper towel-lined plate.
2. Place a small saucepan over medium heat and melt the butter.
3. Sauté the garlic and shallot until tender, about 3 minutes.
4. Whisk in the lemon juice and orange juice and bring the sauce to a simmer, cooking until it thickens slightly about 2 minutes.
5. Remove the sauce from the heat and stir in the parsley; set aside.
6. Place a large skillet over medium-high heat and add the olive oil.
7. Panfry the fish until lightly browned and just cooked through, turning them over once, about 10 minutes in total.
8. Serve the fish immediately with a spoonful of sauce for each.

Nutrition: Calories: 319 | Fat: 26g | Protein: 22g | Carbohydrates: 2g | Fiber: 0g

106. Sole Asiago

Preparation Time: 10 minutes
Cooking Time: 8 minutes
Servings: 4
Ingredients:
- 4 (4-ounce) sole fillets
- ¾ cup ground almonds
- ¼ cup Asiago cheese
- 2 eggs, beaten
- 2½ tablespoons melted coconut oil

Directions:
1. Preheat the oven to 350°F. Line a baking sheet with parchment paper and set it aside.
2. Pat the fish dry with paper towels.
3. Stir together the ground almonds and cheese in a small bowl.
4. Place the bowl with the beaten eggs next to the almond mixture.
5. Dredge a sole fillet in the beaten egg and press the fish into the almond mixture to be completely coated. Place on the baking sheet and repeat until all the fillets are breaded.
6. Brush both sides of each piece of fish with coconut oil.
7. Bake the sole until it is cooked through, about 8 minutes in total.
8. Serve immediately.

Nutrition: Calories: 406 | Fat: 31g | Protein: 29g | carbohydrates: 6g | Fiber: 3g

107. Cheesy Garlic Salmon

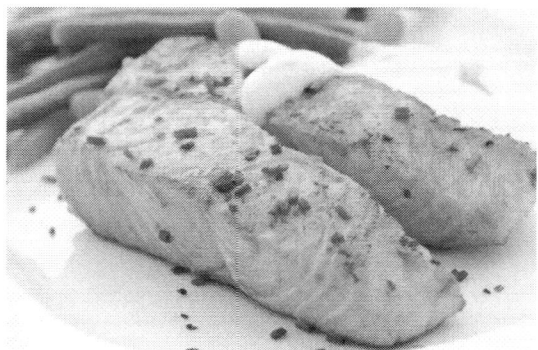

Preparation Time: 15 minutes
Cooking Time: 12 minutes
Servings: 4

- ½ cup Asiago cheese

- 2 tablespoons freshly squeezed lemon juice
- 2 tablespoons butter, at room temperature
- 2 teaspoons minced garlic
- 1 teaspoon chopped fresh basil
- 1 teaspoon chopped fresh oregano
- 4 (5-ounce) salmon fillets
- 1 tablespoon olive oil

Directions:
1. Preheat the oven to 350°F. Line a baking sheet with parchment paper and set it aside.
2. Stir together the Asiago cheese, lemon juice, butter, basil, and oregano in a small bowl.
3. Pat the salmon dry with paper towels and place the fillets on the baking sheet skin-side down. Divide the topping evenly between the fillets and spread it across the fish using a knife or the back of a spoon.
4. Drizzle the fish with the olive oil and bake until the topping is golden and the fish is just cooked through, about 12 minutes.
5. Serve.

Nutrition: Calories: 357 | Fat: 28g | Protein: 24g | Carbohydrates: 2g | Fiber: 0g

108. Stuffed Chicken Breasts

Preparation Time: 30 minutes
Cooking Time: 30 minutes
Servings: 4
Ingredients:
- 1 tablespoon butter
- ¼ cup chopped sweet onion
- ½ cup goat cheese, at room temperature
- ¼ cup Kalamata olives, chopped
- ¼ cup chopped roasted red pepper
- 2 tablespoons chopped fresh basil
- 4 (5-ounce) chicken breasts, skin-on
- 2 tablespoons extra-virgin olive oil

Directions:
1. Preheat the oven to 400°F.
2. In a small skillet over medium heat, melt the butter and add the onion. Sauté until tender, about 3 minutes.
3. Transfer the onion to a medium bowl and add the cheese, olives, red pepper, and basil. Stir until well blended, then refrigerate for about 30 minutes.
4. Cut horizontal pockets into each chicken breast, and stuff them evenly with the filling. Secure the two sides of each breast with toothpicks.
5. Place a large ovenproof skillet over medium-high heat and add the olive oil.
6. Brown the chicken on both sides, about 10 minutes in total.
7. Place the skillet in the oven and roast until the chicken is just cooked through, about 15 minutes. Remove the toothpicks and serve.

Nutrition: Calories: 389 | Fat: 30g | Protein: 25g | Carbohydrates: 3g | Fiber: 0g

109. Spicy Pork Chops

Preparation Time: 4 hours and 10 minutes
Cooking Time: 15 minutes
Servings: 2
Ingredients:
- ¼ cup lime juice 2 pork rib chops
- 1/2 tablespoon coconut oil, melted
- 1/2 garlic cloves, peeled and minced
- 1/2 tablespoon chili powder
- 1/2 teaspoon ground cinnamon
- 1 teaspoon cumin
- Salt and pepper to taste
- 1/4 teaspoon hot pepper sauce
- Mango, sliced

Directions:
1. Take a bowl and mix in lime juice, oil, garlic, cumin, cinnamon, chili powder, salt, pepper, hot pepper sauce. Whisk well.
2. Add pork chops and toss. Keep it on the side, and let it refrigerate for 4 hours.
3. Preheat your grill to medium and transfer pork chops to the preheated grill. Grill for 7 minutes, flip and cook for 7 minutes more.
4. Divide between serving platters and serve with mango slices. Enjoy!

Nutrition: Calories: 200 | Fat: 8g | Carbohydrates: 3g | Protein: 26g | Fiber: 1g | Net Carbohydrates: 2g

110. Almond Breaded Chicken Goodness

Preparation Time: 15 minutes

Cooking Time: 15 minutes
Servings: 2
Ingredients:
- 2 large chicken breasts, boneless and skinless
- 1/3 cup lemon juice
- 1½ cups seasoned almond meal
- 2 tablespoons coconut oil
- Lemon pepper, to taste
- Parsley for decoration

Directions:
1. Slice Hicken breast in half.
2. Pound out each half until a ¼ inch thick.
3. Put a pan over medium heat, add oil, and heat it.
4. Dip each chicken breast slice into lemon juice and let it sit for 2 minutes.
5. Turn over and let the other side sit for 2 minutes as well.
6. Transfer to almond meal and coat both sides.
7. Add coated chicken to the oil and fry for 4 minutes per side, making sure to sprinkle lemon pepper liberally.
8. Transfer to a paper-lined sheet and repeat until all chicken is fried.
9. Garnish with parsley and enjoy.

Nutrition: Calories: 325 | Fat: 24g | Carbohydrates: 3g | Protein: 16g | Fiber: 1g | Net Carbohydrates: 1g

111. Garlic Lamb Chops

Preparation Time: 35 minutes
Cooking Time: 5 minutes
Servings: 2
Ingredients:
- ¼ cup olive oil
- ¼ cup mint, fresh and chopped
- 8 lamb rib chops
- 1 tablespoon garlic, minced
- 1 tablespoon rosemary, fresh and chopped

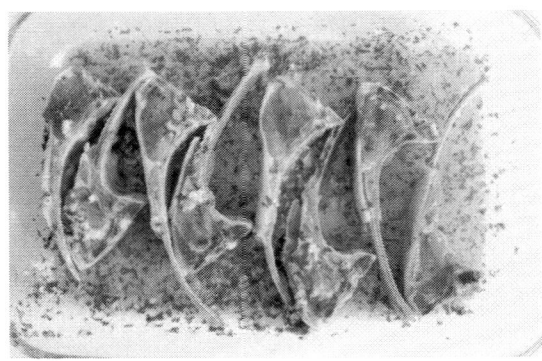

Directions:
1. Add rosemary, garlic, mint, olive oil into a bowl and mix well.
2. Keep a tablespoon of the mixture on the side for later use.
4. Preheat the cast-iron skillet over medium-high heat.
5. Add lamb and cook for 2 minutes per side for medium-rare.
6. Let the lamb rest for a few minutes and drizzle the remaining marinade.
7. Serve and enjoy!

Nutrition: Calories: 566 | Fat: 40g | Carbohydrates: 2g | Protein: 47g | Fiber: 1g | Net Carbohydrates: 1g

112. Mushroom Pork Chops

Preparation Time: 10 minutes
Cooking Time: 40 minutes
Servings: 2
Ingredients:
- 8 ounces' mushrooms, sliced
- 1 teaspoon garlic
- 1 onion, peeled and chopped
- 1 cup keto-friendly mayonnaise
- 3 pork chops, boneless
- 1 teaspoon ground nutmeg
- 1 tablespoon balsamic vinegar
- ½ cup of coconut oil

Directions:
1. Take a pan and place it over medium heat. Add oil and let it heat up. Add mushrooms, onions, and stir. Cook for 4 minutes.
2. Add pork chops, season with nutmeg, garlic powder, and brown both sides. Transfer the

pan to the oven and bake for 30 minutes at 350 degrees F. Transfer pork chops to plates and keep it warm.
3. Take a pan and place it over medium heat. Add vinegar, mayonnaise over the mushroom mixture, and stir for a few minutes.
4. Drizzle sauce over pork chops
5. Enjoy!

Nutrition: Calories: 600 | Fat: 10g | Carbohydrates: 8g | Protein: 30g | Fiber: 2g | Net Carbohydrates: 5g

113. Mediterranean Pork

Preparation Time: 10 minutes
Cooking Time: 35 minutes
Servings: 2
Ingredients:
- 2 pork chops, bone-in
- Salt and pepper, to taste
- 1/2 teaspoon dried rosemary
- 1 garlic clove, peeled and minced

Directions:
1. Season pork chops with salt and pepper. Place in a roasting pan. Add rosemary, garlic in the pan.
2. Preheat your oven to 425 degrees F. Bake for 10 minutes. Lower heat to 350 degrees F. Roast for 25 minutes more. Slice pork and divide on plates.
3. Drizzle pan juice all over. Serve and enjoy!

Nutrition: Calories: 165 | Fat: 2g | Carbohydrates: 2g | Protein: 26g | Fiber: 1g | Net Carbohydrates: 1g

114. Brie-Packed Smoked Salmon

Preparation Time: 4 minutes
Cooking Time: 0 minutes
Servings: 4
Ingredients:
- 4-ounce Brie round
- 1 tablespoon fresh dill
- 1 tablespoon lemon juice
- 2-ounce smoked salmon

Directions:
1. Slice Brie in half lengthwise.
2. Spread salmon, dill, and lemon juice over the Brie cheese.
3. Place the other half on top.
4. Serve with Celery sticks/ cauliflower bites.
5. Enjoy!

Nutrition: Calories: 241 | Fat: 19g | Net Carbohydrates: 0g | Protein: 18g | Fiber: 2g | Carbohydrates: 3g

115. Blackened Tilapia

Preparation Time: 9 minutes
Cooking Time: 9 minutes
Servings: 2
Ingredients:
- 1 cup cauliflower, chopped
- 1 teaspoon red pepper flakes
- 1 tablespoon Italian seasoning
- 1 tablespoon garlic, minced
- 6-ounce tilapia
- 1 cup English cucumber, chopped with peel
- 2 tablespoons olive oil
- 1 sprig dill, chopped
- 1 teaspoon stevia
- 3 tablespoon lime juice
- 2 tablespoon Cajun blackened seasoning

Directions:
1. Take a bowl and add the seasoning ingredients (except Cajun). Add a tablespoon of oil and whip. Pour dressing over cauliflower and cucumber. Brush the fish with olive oil on both sides.
2. Take a skillet and grease it well with 1 tablespoon of olive oil. Press Cajun seasoning on both sides of the fish.
3. Cook fish for 3 minutes per side. Serve with vegetables and enjoy!

Nutrition: Calories: 530 | Fat: 33g | Net Carbohydrates: 4g | Protein: 32g | Fiber: 2g | Carbohydrates: 2g

116. Salsa Chicken Bites

Preparation Time: 4 minutes
Cooking Time: 14 minutes
Servings: 2
Ingredients:

- 2 chicken rest
- 1 cup of salsa
- 1 taco seasoning mix
- 1 cup plain Greek yogurt
- ½ cup cheddar cheese, cubed

Directions:
1. Take a skillet and place it over medium heat.
2. Add chicken breast, a ½ cup of salsa, and taco seasoning.
3. Mix well and cook for 12-15 minutes until the chicken is done.
4. Take the chicken out and cube them.
5. Place the cubes on a toothpick and top with cheddar.
6. Place yogurt and remaining salsa in cups and use them as dips.
7. Serve and Enjoy!

Nutrition: Calories: 359 | Fat: 14g | Net Carbohydrates: 14g | Protein: 43g | Fiber: 3g | Carbohydrates: 17g

117. Tomato & Tuna Balls

Preparation Time: 25 minutes
Cooking Time: 0
Servings: 2
Ingredients:
- 8 tomatoes, medium
- 1 tablespoon of capers
- 2 – 3-ounce cans tuna, drained
- 10 Kalamata olives, pitted and minced
- 2 tablespoon parsley
- 1 tablespoon olive oil
- ½ teaspoon thyme
- Salt, to taste
- pepper, as needed

Directions:
1. Line a cookie pan with a paper towel and scoop guts out from the tomatoes.
2. Keep the tomato shells on the side.
3. Take a bowl and mix olives, tuna, thyme, parsley, pepper in a bowl and mix.
4. Add oil and mix.
5. Fill the tomato shells with tuna mix.
6. Enjoy!

Nutrition: Calories: 169 | Fat: 10g | Net Carbohydrates: 5g | Protein: 13g | Fiber: 5g | Carbohydrates: 10g

118. Fennel & Figs Lamb

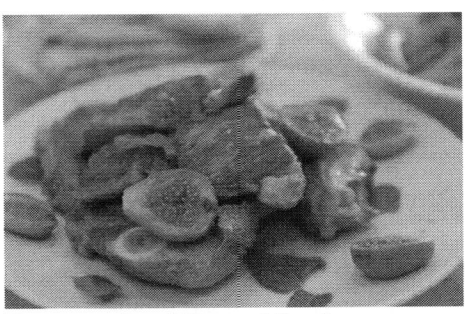

Preparation Time: 10 minutes
Cooking Time: 40 minutes

Ingredients:
- 6 ounces' lamb racks
- 1 fennel bulb, sliced
- Salt
- pepper, to taste
- 1 tablespoon olive oil
- 2 figs, cut in half
- 1/8 cup apple cider vinegar
- 1/2 tablespoon swerve

Directions:
1. Take a bowl and add fennel, figs, vinegar, swerve, oil, and toss. Transfer to baking dish. Season with salt and pepper.
2. Bake it for 15 minutes at 400 degrees F.
3. Season lamb with salt, pepper, and transfer to a heated pan over medium-high heat. Cook for a few minutes. Add lamb to the baking dish with fennel and bake for 20 minutes. Divide between plates and serve. Enjoy!

Nutrition: Calories: 230 | Fat: 3g | Carbohydrates: 5g | Protein: 10g | Fiber: 2g | Net Carbohydrates: 3g

119. Tamari Steak Salad

Preparation Time: 15 minutes
Cooking Time: 10 minutes
Servings: 2
Ingredients:
- 1 large bunches salad greens
- 4 ounces' beef steak
- ½ red bell pepper, diced
- 4 cherry tomatoes, cut into halves

- 2 radishes, sliced
- 2 tablespoons olive oil
- ¼ tablespoon fresh lemon juice
- 1-ounce gluten-free tamari sauce
- Salt as needed

Directions:
1. Marinate steak in tamari sauce.
2. Make the salad by adding bell pepper, tomatoes, radishes, salad green, oil, salt, and lemon juice to a bowl and toss them well.
3. Grill the steak to your desired doneness and transfer the steak on top of the salad platter.
4. Let it sit for 1 minute and cut it crosswise.
5. Serve and enjoy!

Nutrition: Calories: 500 | Fat: 37g | Carbohydrates: 4g | Protein: 33g | Fiber: 2g | Net Carbohydrates: 2g

120. Blackened Chicken

Preparation Time: 10 minutes
Cooking Time: 10 minutes
Servings: 2
Ingredients:
- 1/4 teaspoon paprika
- 1/8 teaspoon salt
- ¼ teaspoon cayenne pepper
- ¼ teaspoon ground cumin
- ¼ teaspoon dried thyme
- 1/8 teaspoon ground white pepper
- 1/8 teaspoon onion powder
- 1 chicken breast, boneless and skinless

Directions:
1. Preheat your oven to 350 degrees Fahrenheit. Grease baking sheet. Take a cast-iron skillet and place it over high heat.
2. Add oil and heat it for 5 minutes until smoking hot.
3. Take a small bowl and mix salt, paprika, cumin, white pepper, cayenne, thyme, onion powder. Oil the chicken breast on both sides and coat the breast with the spice mix.
4. Transfer to your hot pan and cook for 1 minute per side.
5. Transfer to your prepared baking sheet and bake for 5 minutes.
6. Serve and enjoy!

Nutrition: Calories: 136 | Fat: 3g | Carbohydrates: 2g | Protein: 24g | Fiber: 1g | Net Carbohydrates: 1g

121. Mediterranean Mushroom Olive Steak

Preparation Time: 10 minutes
Cooking Time: 14 minutes
Servings: 2
Ingredients:
- 1/2-pound boneless beef sirloin steak, ¾ inch thick, cut into 4 pieces
- 1/2 large red onion, chopped
- 1/2 cup mushrooms
- 2 garlic cloves, thinly sliced
- 2 tablespoons olive oil
- 1/4 cup green olives, coarsely chopped
- 1/2 cup parsley leaves, finely cut

Directions:
1. Take a large-sized skillet and place it over medium-high heat.
2. Add oil and let it heat up. Add beef and cook until both sides are browned, remove beef and drain fat. Add the rest of the oil to the skillet and heat it.
3. Add onions, garlic, and cook for 2-3 minutes. Stir well.
4. Add mushrooms olives and cook until mushrooms are thoroughly done. Return beef to skillet and lower heat to medium.
5. Cook for 3-4 minutes (covered). Stir in parsley.
6. Serve and enjoy!

Nutrition: Calories: 386 | Fat: 30g | Carbohydrates: 11g | Protein: 21g | Fiber: 5g | Net Carbohydrates: 6g

122. Buttery Scallops

Preparation Time: 10 minutes
Cooking Time: 10 minutes
Servings: 6
Ingredients:
- 2 pounds' sea scallops
- 3 tablespoons butter, melted
- 2 tablespoons fresh thyme, minced
- Salt and pepper, to taste

Directions:
1. Preheat your air fryer to 390 degrees F. Grease the air fryer cooking basket with butter.
2. Take a bowl, mix in all remaining ingredients, and toss well to coat the scallops.
3. Transfer scallops to air fryer-cooking basket and cook for 5 minutes.
4. Repeat if any ingredients are left, serve, and enjoy!

Nutrition: Calories: 186, |Total Fat: 24g, |Total Carbs: 4g, |Fiber: 1g, |Net Carbs: 2g, |Protein: 20g

123. Brussels sprouts and Garlic Aioli

Preparation Time: 15 minutes
Cooking Time: 10 minutes
Servings: 4
Ingredients:
- 1 pound Brussels sprouts, trimmed and excess leaves removed
- Salt and pepper, to taste
- 1½ tablespoons olive oil
- 2 teaspoons lemon juice
- 1 teaspoon powdered chili
- 3 garlic cloves
- ¾ cup whole egg, keto-friendly mayonnaise
- 2 cups of water

Directions:
1. Take a skillet and place it over medium heat.
2. Add garlic cloves (with peel) and roast until brown and fragrant.
3. Remove the skillet with garlic and put a pot with water over medium heat. Bring the water to a boil.
4. Take a knife and cut Brussels sprouts in halves lengthwise, add them to the boiling water, blanch for minutes.
5. Drain them through a sieve and keep them on the side.
6. Preheat your air fryer to 350 degrees F.
7. Remove garlic from the skillet and peel, crush them, and keep them on the side.
8. Add olive oil to skillet and place it over medium heat, stir in Brussels and season with salt and pepper,
9. cook for 2 minutes.
10. Remove heat and transfer sprouts to your air fryer cooking basket. Cook for 5 minutes. Make aioli by taking a small bowl and adding mayonnaise, crushed garlic, lemon juice, powdered chili, pepper, salt, mix.
11. Serve Brussels with the aioli, enjoy!

Nutrition: Calories: 42, |Total Fat: 2g, |Total Carbs: 3g, |Fiber: 1g, |Net Carbs: 2g, |Protein: 5g

124. Broccoli Bites

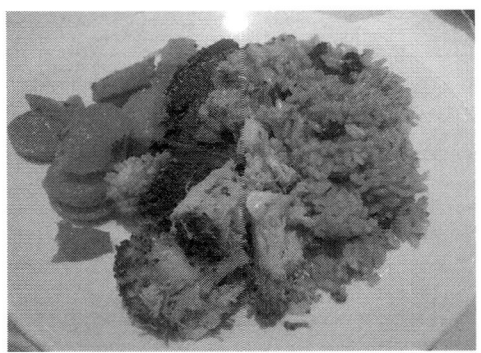

Preparation Time: 15 minutes
Cooking Time: 12 minutes

Ingredients:
- 2 eggs, beaten
- ¼ cup parmesan cheese, grated
- 2 cups broccoli florets
- 1½ cups cheddar cheese, grated
- Salt and pepper, to taste

Directions:
1. Add broccoli to the food processor and pulse until crumbly.
2. Mix broccoli and the remaining ingredients in a large bowl.
3. Make small balls from the mixture and arrange them on a baking sheet.
4. Let it refrigerate for 30 minutes.
5. Preheat your Air Fryer to 360 degrees F.
6. Transfer balls to air fryer cooking basket and cook for 12 minutes.
7. Serve and enjoy!

Nutrition: Calories: 234, |Total Fat: 17g, |Total Carbs: 4g, |Fiber: 1g, |Net Carbs: 2g, |Protein: 16g

125. Bacon Burger Cabbage Stir Fry

Preparation Time: 10 minutes

Cooking Time: 20 minutes
Servings: 10
Ingredients:
- Ground beef (1 lb.)
- Bacon (1 lb.) Small onion (1)
- Minced cloves of garlic (3)
- Cabbage (1 lb./1 small head)

Directions:
1. Dice the bacon and onion. Combine the beef and bacon in a wok or large skillet.
2. Prepare it until done and store it in a bowl to keep warm. Mince the onion and garlic.
3. Toss both into the hot grease. Slice and toss in the cabbage and stir-fry until wilted.
4. Blend in the meat and combine. Sprinkle with pepper and salt as desired.

Nutrition: Net Carbohydrates: 4.5 grams | Protein Counts: 32 grams | Total Fats: 22 grams | Calories: 357

126. Bacon Cheeseburger

Preparation Time: 15 minutes
Cooking Time: 30 minutes
Servings: 12
Ingredients:
- Low-sodium bacon (16 oz. pkg.)
- Ground beef (3 lb.)
- Eggs (2)
- Medium chopped onion (half of 1)
- Shredded cheddar cheese (8 oz.)

Directions:
1. Fry the bacon and chop it to bits. Shred the cheese and dice the onion.
2. Combine the mixture with the beef and blend in the whisked eggs.
3. Prepare 24 burgers and grill them the way you like them.
4. You can make a double-decker since they are small.
5. If you like a bigger burger, you can make 12 burgers as a single-decker.

Nutrition: Net Carbohydrates: 0.8 grams | Protein Counts: 27 grams | Total Fats: 41 grams | Calories: 489

127. Cauliflower Mac & Cheese

Preparation Time: 15 minutes
Cooking Time: 20 minutes
Servings: 4
Ingredients:
- Cauliflower (1 head)
- Butter (3 tbsp.)
- Unsweetened almond milk (.25 cup)
- Heavy cream (.25 cup)
- Cheddar cheese (1 cup)

Directions:
1. Use a sharp knife to slice the cauliflower into small florets. Shred the cheese. Prepare the oven to reach 450º Fahrenheit. Cover a baking pan with a layer of parchment baking paper or foil.
2. Add two tablespoons of the butter to a pan and melt. Add the florets, butter, salt, and pepper together. Place the cauliflower on the baking pan and roast 10 to 15 minutes.
3. Warm up the rest of the butter, milk, heavy cream, and cheese in the microwave or double boiler. Pour the cheese over the cauliflower and serve.

Nutrition: Net Carbohydrates: 7 grams | Protein Counts: 11 grams | Total Fats: 23 grams | Calories: 294 grams

128. Mushroom & Cauliflower Risotto

Preparation Time: 5 minutes
Cooking Time: 10 minutes
Servings: 4
Ingredients:
- Grated head of cauliflower (1)
- Vegetable stock (1 cup)
- Chopped mushrooms (9 oz.)
- Butter (2 tbsp.)
- Coconut cream (1 cup)

Directions:
1. Pour the stock in a saucepan. Boil and set aside. Prepare a skillet with butter and saute the mushrooms until golden.
2. Grate and stir in the cauliflower and stock. Simmer and add the cream, cooking until the cauliflower is al dente. Serve.

Nutrition: Net Carbohydrates: 4 grams | Protein Counts: 1 gram | Total Fats: 17 grams | Calories: 186

129. Pita Pizza

Preparation Time: 15 minutes
Cooking Time: 10 minutes
Servings: 2
Ingredients:
- Marinara sauce (.5 cup)
- Low-carb pita (1)
- Cheddar cheese (2 oz.)
- Pepperoni (14 slices)
- Roasted red peppers (1 oz.)

Directions:
1. Program the oven temperature setting to 450° Fahrenheit.
2. Slice the pita in half and place it onto a foil-lined baking tray. Rub with a bit of oil and toast for one to two minutes.
3. Pour the sauce over the bread. Sprinkle using the cheese and other toppings. Bake until the cheese melts (5 min.). Cool thoroughly.

Nutrition: Net Carbohydrates: 4 grams | Protein Counts: 13 grams | Total Fats: 19 grams | Calories: 250

130. Skillet Cabbage Tacos

Preparation Time: 10 minutes
Cooking Time: 15 minutes
Servings: 4
Ingredients:
- Ground beef (1 lb.)
- Salsa - ex. Pace Organic (.5 cup)
- Shredded cabbage (2 cups)
- Chili powder (2 tsp.)
- Shredded cheese (.75 cup)

Directions:
1. Brown the beef and drain the fat. Pour in the salsa, cabbage, and seasoning.
2. Cover and lower the heat. Simmer for 10 to 12 minutes using the medium heat temperature setting.
3. When the cabbage has softened, remove it from the heat and mix in the cheese.
4. Top it off using your favorite toppings, such as green onions or sour cream, and serve.

Nutrition: Net Carbohydrates: 4 grams | Protein Counts: 30 grams | Total Fats: 21 grams | Calories: 325

131. Taco Casserole

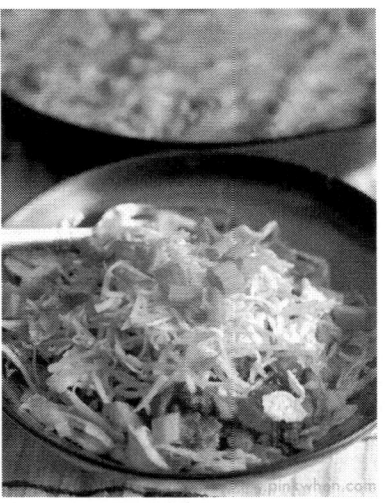

Preparation Time: 10 minutes
Cooking Time: 20 minutes

Ingredients:
- Ground turkey or beef (1.5 to 2 lb.)
- Taco seasoning (2 tbsp.) Shredded cheddar cheese (8 oz.)
- Salsa (1 cup) Cottage cheese (16 oz.)

Directions:
1. Heat the oven to reach 400° Fahrenheit.
2. Combine the taco seasoning and ground meat in a casserole dish. Bake it for 20 minutes.
3. Combine the salsa and both kinds of cheese. Set aside for now.
4. Carefully transfer the casserole dish from the oven. Drain away the cooking juices from the meat.
5. Break the meat into small pieces and mash with a potato masher or fork.
6. Sprinkle with cheese. Bake in the oven for 15 to 20 more minutes until the top is browned.

Nutrition: Net Carbohydrates: 6 grams | Protein Counts: 45 grams | Total Fats: 18 grams | Calories: 367

132. Creamy Chicken Salad

Preparation Time: 10 minutes
Cooking Time: 30 minutes
Servings: 4
Ingredients:
- Chicken Breast - 1 Lb.
- Avocado - 2
- Garlic Cloves - 2,
- Minced Lime Juice - 3 T.
- Onion - .33 C.,
- Minced Jalapeno Pepper - 1,
- Minced Salt - Dash Cilantro - 1 T.
- Pepper - Dash

Directions:
1. You will want to start this recipe off by prepping the stove to 400. As this warms up, get out your cooking sheet and line it with paper or foil.
2. Next, it is time to get out the chicken.
3. Go ahead and layer the chicken breast up with some olive oil before seasoning to your liking.
4. When the chicken is all set, you will want to line them along the surface of your cooking sheet and pop it into the oven for about twenty minutes.
5. By the end of twenty minutes, the chicken should be cooked through and taken out of the oven for chilling.
6. Once cool enough to handle, you will want to either dice or shred your chicken, dependent upon how you like your chicken salad.
7. Now that your chicken is all cooked, it is time to assemble your salad!
8. You can begin this process by adding everything into a bowl and mashing down the avocado.
9. Once your ingredients are mended to your liking, sprinkle some salt over the top and serve immediately.

Nutrition: Fats: 20g | Carbs: 4g | Proteins: 25g

133. Spicy Keto Chicken Wings

Preparation Time: 20 minutes
Cooking Time: 30 minutes
Servings: 4
Ingredients:
- Chicken Wings - 2 Lbs.
- Cajun Spice - 1 t.
- Smoked Paprika - 2 t.
- Turmeric - .50 t.
- Salt - Dash
- Baking Powder - 2 t.
- Pepper - Dash

Directions:
1. When you first begin the Ketogenic Diet, you may find that you won't be eating the traditional foods that may have made up a majority of your diet in the past.
2. While this is a good thing for your health, you may feel you are missing out! The good news is that there are delicious alternatives that aren't lacking in flavor! To start this recipe, you'll want to prep the stove to 400.
3. As this heats up, you will want to take some time to dry your chicken wings with a paper towel. This will help remove any excess moisture and get you some nice, crispy wings!
4. When you are all set, take out a mixing bowl and place all of the seasonings along with the baking powder. If you feel like it, you can adjust the seasoning levels however you would like.
5. Once these are set, go ahead and throw the chicken wings in and coat evenly. If you have one, you'll want to place the wings on a wire rack that is placed over your baking tray. If not, you can just lay them across the baking sheet.
6. Now that your chicken wings are set, you are going to pop them into the stove for thirty minutes. By the end of this time, the tops of the wings should be crispy.
7. If they are, take them out from the oven and flip them so that you can bake the other side. You will want to cook these for an additional thirty minutes.
8. Finally, take the tray from the oven and allow it to cool slightly before serving up your spiced keto wings. For additional flavor, serve with any of your favorite keto-friendly dipping sauces.

Nutrition: Fats: 7g |Carbs: 1g |Proteins: 60g

134. Cheesy Ham Quiche

Preparation Time: 10 minutes
Cooking Time: 30 minutes
Servings: 6
Ingredients:
- Eggs - 8
- Zucchini - 1 C.,
- Shredded heavy Cream - .50 C.
- Ham - 1 C., Diced
- Mustard - 1 t.
- Salt – Dash

Directions:
1. For this recipe, you can start off by prepping your stove to 375 and getting out a pie plate for your quiche.
2. Next, it is time to prep the zucchini. First, you will want to go ahead and shred it into small pieces.
3. Once this is complete, take a paper towel and gently squeeze out the excess moisture. This will help avoid a soggy quiche.
4. When the step from above is complete, you will want to place the zucchini into your pie plate along with the cooked ham pieces and your cheese.
5. Once these items are in place, you will want to whisk the seasonings, cream, and eggs together before pouring it over the top.
6. Now that your quiche is set, you are going to pop the dish into your stove for about forty minutes.
7. By the end of this time, the egg should be cooked through, and you will be able to insert a knife into the center and have it come out clean.
8. If the quiche is cooked to your liking, take the dish from the oven and allow it to chill slightly before slicing and serving.

Nutrition: Fats: 25g |Carbs: 2g |Proteins: 20g

135. Feta and Cauliflower Rice Stuffed Bell Peppers

Preparation Time: 10 minutes
Cooking Time: 20 minutes
Servings: 3
Ingredients:
- 1 green Bell Pepper
- 1 red Bell Pepper
- 1 yellow Bell Pepper
- ½ cup Cauliflower rice
- 1 cup Feta cheese
- 1 Onion, sliced
- 2 Tomatoes, chopped
- 1 tbsp. Black Pepper
- 2-3 Garlic clove, minced
- 3 tbsp. Lemon juice
- 3-4 green Olives, chopped
- 3-4 tbsp. Olive oil
- Yogurt Sauce:
- 1 clove Garlic, pressed
- 1 cup Greek Yogurt
- kosher Salt, to taste
- juice from 1 Lemon
- 1 tbsp. fresh Dill

Directions:
1. Grease the Instant Pot with olive oil. Cut at the top of the bell peppers near the stem. Place feta cheese, onion, olives, tomatoes, cauliflower rice, salt, black pepper, garlic powder, and lemon juice into a bowl; mix well.
2. Please fill up the bell peppers with the feta mixture and insert them in the Instant Pot. Set on Manual and cook on High pressure for 20 minutes. When the timer beeps, allow the pressure to release naturally for 5 minutes, then do a quick pressure release.
3. To prepare the yogurt sauce, combine garlic, yogurt, lemon juice, salt, and fresh dill.

Nutrition: Calories 388, |Protein 13.5g, |Net Carbs 7.9g, |Fat 32.4g

136. Shrimp with Linguine

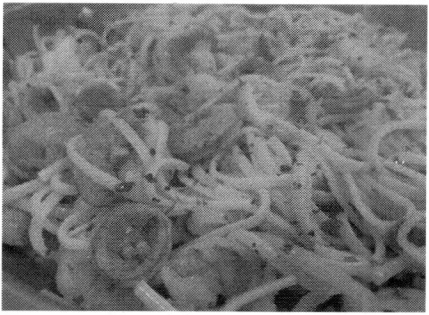

Preparation Time: 10 minutes
Cooking Time: 10 minutes

Ingredients:
- 1 lb. Shrimp, cleaned
- 1 lb. Linguine
- 1 tbsp. Butter
- ½ cup Parmesan cheese, shredded
- 2 Garlic cloves, minced
- 1 cup Parsley, chopped
- Salt and Pepper, to taste
- ½ cup Coconut Cream, for garnish
- ½ Avocado, diced, for garnish
- 2 tbsp. fresh Dill, for garnish

Directions:
1. Melt the butter on Sauté. Stir in linguine, garlic cloves, and parsley. Cook for 4 minutes until aromatic. Add shrimp; season with salt and pepper, seal the lid.
2. Select Manual and cook for 5 minutes on High pressure. When ready, quickly release the pressure. Unseal and remove the lid. Press Sauté, add the cheese, and stir well until combined, for 30-40 seconds. Serve topped with coconut cream, avocado, and dill.

Nutrition: Calories 412, |Protein 48g, |Net Carbs 5.6g, |Fat 21g

137. Mexican Cod Fillets

Preparation Time: 10 minutes
Cooking Time: 10 minutes
Servings: 3

Ingredients:
- 3 Cod fillets
- 1 Onion, sliced
- 2 cups Cabbage
- Juice from 1 Lemon
- 1 Jalapeno Pepper
- ½ tsp Oregano
- ½ tsp Cumin powder
- ½ tsp Cayenne Pepper
- 2 tbsp. Olive oil
- Salt and Black Pepper to taste

Directions:
1. Heat the oil on Sauté, add onion, cabbage, lemon juice, jalapeño pepper, cayenne pepper, cumin powder, and oregano, and stir to combine. Cook for 8-10 minutes.
2. Season with salt and black pepper. Arrange the cod fillets in the sauce, using a spoon to cover each piece with some sauce. Seal the lid and press Manual. Cook for 5 minutes on High pressure. When ready, do a quick release and serve.

Nutrition: Calories 306, |Protein 21g, |Net Carbs 6.8g, | Fat 19.4g

138. Simple Mushroom Chicken Mix

Preparation Time: 5 minutes
Cooking Time: 18 minutes
Servings: 2

Ingredients:
- 2 Tomatoes, chopped
- ½ lb. Chicken, cooked and mashed
- 1 cup Broccoli, chopped
- 1 tbsp. Butter
- 2 tbsp. Mayonnaise
- ½ cup Mushroom soup
- Salt and Pepper, to taste
- 1 Onion, sliced

Directions:
1. Once cooked, put the chicken into a bowl. Mix the mayo, mushroom soup, tomatoes, onion, broccoli, and salt and pepper in a separate bowl. Add the chicken.
2. Grease a round baking tray with butter. Put the mixture in a tray. Add 2 cups of water into the Instant Pot and place the trivet inside. Place the tray on top. Seal the lid, press Manual, and cook for 14 minutes on

High pressure. When ready, do a quick release.
Nutrition: Calories 561, |Protein 28.5g, | Net Carbs 6.3g, |Fat 49.5g

139. Squash Spaghetti with Bolognese Sauce

Preparation Time: 5 minutes
Cooking Time: 10 minutes
Servings: 3
Ingredients:
- 1 large Squash, cut into 2, and seed pulp removed
- 2 cups Water
- Bolognese Sauce to serve

Directions:
1. Place the trivet and add the water. Add in the squash, seal the lid, select Manual and cook on High Pressure for 8 minutes. Once ready, quickly release the pressure. Carefully remove the squash; use two forks to shred the inner skin. Serve with Bolognese sauce.

Nutrition: Calories 37, |Protein 0.9g, |Net Carbs 7.8g, |Fat 0.4g

140. Healthy Halibut Fillets

Preparation Time: 5 minutes
Cooking Time: 10 minutes
Servings: 2
Ingredients:
- 2 Halibut fillets
- 1 tbsp. Dill
- 1 tbsp. Onion powder
- 1 cup Parsley, chopped
- 2 tbsp. Paprika
- 1 tbsp. Garlic powder
- 1 tbsp. Lemon Pepper
- 2 tbsp. Lemon juice

Directions:
1. Mix lemon juice, lemon pepper, and garlic powder, and paprika, parsley, and dill and onion powder in a bowl. Pour the mixture into the Instant pot and place the halibut fish over it.
2. Seal the lid, press Manual mode, and cook for 10 minutes on High pressure. When ready, do a quick pressure release by setting the valve to venting.

Nutrition: Calories 283, |Protein 22.5g, |Net Carbs 6.2g, |Fat 16.4g

141. Clean Salmon with Soy Sauce

Preparation Time: 10 minutes
Cooking Time: 30 minutes
Servings: 2
Ingredients:
- 2 Salmon fillets
- 2 tbsp. Avocado oil
- 2 tbsp. Soy sauce
- 1 tbsp. Garlic powder
- 1 tbsp. fresh Dill to garnish
- Salt and Pepper, to taste

Directions:
1. To make the marinade, thoroughly mix the soy sauce, avocado oil, salt, pepper, and garlic powder into a bowl. Dip salmon in the mixture and place in the refrigerator for 20 minutes.
2. Transfer the contents to the Instant pot. Seal, set on Manual, and cook for 10 minutes on high pressure. When ready, do a quick release. Serve topped with the fresh dill.

Nutrition: Calories 512, |Protein 65g, |Net Carbs 3.2g, |Fat 21g

142. Simple Salmon with Eggs

Preparation Time: 2 minutes
Cooking Time: 5 minutes
Servings: 3
Ingredients:
- 1 lb. Salmon, cooked, mashed
- 2 Eggs, whisked
- 2 Onions, chopped
- 2 stalks celery, chopped
- 1 cup Parsley, chopped
- 1 tbsp. Olive oil
- Salt and Pepper, to taste

Directions:
1. Mix salmon, onion, celery, parsley, and salt and pepper, in a bowl. Form into 6 patties

about 1-inch-thick and dip them in the whisked eggs. Heat oil in the Instant pot on Sauté mode.
2. Add the patties to the pot, cook on both sides for about 5 minutes and transfer to the plate. Allow to cool and serve.

Nutrition: Calories 331, |Protein 38g, |Net Carbs 5.3g, | Fat 16g

143. Easy Shrimp

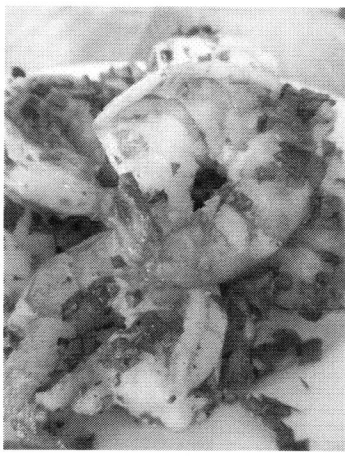

Preparation Time: 4 minutes
Cooking Time: 5 minutes
Servings: 2
Ingredients:
- 1 lb. Shrimp, peeled and deveined
- 2 Garlic cloves, crushed
- 1 tbsp. Butter.
- A pinch of red Pepper
- Salt and Pepper, to taste
- 1 cup Parsley, chopped

Directions:
1. Melt butter on Sauté mode. Add shrimp, garlic, red pepper, salt, and pepper. Cook for 5 minutes, occasionally stirring the shrimp until pink. Serve topped with parsley.

Nutrition: Calories 245, |Protein 45g, |Net Carbs 4.8g, | Fat 4g

144. Scallops with Mushroom Special

Preparation Time: 15 minutes
Cooking Time: 20 minutes
Servings: 2
Ingredients:
- 1 lb. Scallops
- 2 Onions, chopped
- 1 tbsp. Butter
- 2 tbsp. Olive oil
- 1 cup Mushrooms
- Salt and Pepper, to taste
- 1 tbsp. Lemon juice
- ½ cup Whipping Cream
- 1 tbsp. chopped fresh Parsley

Directions:
1. Heat the oil on Sauté. Add onions, butter, mushrooms, salt, and pepper. Cook for 3 to 5 minutes. Add the lemon juice and scallops. Lock the lid and set it to Manual mode.
2. Cook for 15 minutes on High pressure. When ready, do a quick pressure release and carefully open the lid. Top with a drizzle of cream and fresh parsley.

Nutrition: Calories 312, |Protein 31g, |Net Carbs 7.3g, | Fat 10.4g

145. Delicious Creamy Crab Meat

Preparation Time: 5 minutes
Cooking Time: 10 minutes
Servings: 3
Ingredients:
- 1 lb. Crab meat
- ½ cup Cream cheese
- 2 tbsp. Mayonnaise
- Salt and Pepper, to taste
- 1 tbsp. Lemon juice
- 1 cup Cheddar cheese, shredded

Directions:
1. Mix mayo, cream cheese, salt and pepper, and lemon juice in a bowl. Add in crab meat and make small balls. Place the balls inside the pot. Seal the lid and press Manual.
2. Cook for 10 minutes on High pressure. When done, allow the pressure to release naturally for 10 minutes. Sprinkle the cheese over and serve!

Nutrition: Calories 443, |Protein 41g, |Net Carbs2.5g,|Fa30.4g

SNACKS AND APPETIZERS

146. Candied Dates

Preparation Time: 5 minutes
Cooking Time: 0 minutes
Servings: 2
Ingredients:
- 4 pitted Medjool dates
- 2 tablespoons of peanut butter
- 2 tablespoons of dark cocoa nibs

Directions:
1. Slice the pitted dates in half, and spread half a tablespoon of peanut butter on each date.
2. Top each date with half a tablespoon of dark cocoa nibs.
3. Divide the candied dates between two plates, and enjoy!

Nutrition: Total Carbohydrates: 20g | Dietary Fiber: 3g | Net Carbs: | Protein: 5g | Total Fat: 12g | Calories: 187

147. Berry Delight

Preparation Time: 15 minutes
Cooking Time: 0 minutes
Servings: 6
Ingredients:
- 1 cup of fresh organic blueberries
- 1 cup of fresh organic raspberries
- 1 cup of fresh organic blackberries
- ¼ cup of raw honey
- 1 tablespoon of cinnamon

Directions:
1. Mix all the berries in a large bowl, add in the honey, and gently stir.
2. Sprinkle with cinnamon.

Nutrition: Total Carbohydrates: 20g | Dietary Fiber: 3g | Net Carbs: | Protein: 1g | Total Fat: 0g | Calories: 78

148. Blueberry & Chia Flax Seed Pudding

Preparation Time: 10 minutes
Cooking Time: 15 minutes
Servings: 4
Ingredients:
- 2 cups of almond milk
- 3 tablespoons of chia seeds
- 3 tablespoons of ground flaxseed
- ¼ cup of blueberries

Directions:
1. Warm a pan on medium heat, then put all together of the ingredients except the blueberries.
2. Stir all the ingredients until the pudding is thick; this will take around 3 minutes.
3. Put the pudding into a bowl, then top with blueberries.

Nutrition: Total Carbohydrates: 23g | Dietary Fiber: 12g | Net Carbs: | Protein: 7g | Total Fat: 15g | Calories: 243

149. Spicy Roasted chickpeas

Preparation Time: 10 minutes
Cooking Time: 40 minutes
Servings: 6
Ingredients:
- 2 (15 ounces) cans of chickpeas, drained and rinsed
- 1 teaspoon of paprika
- 1 teaspoon of turmeric
- ¼ teaspoon of cayenne pepper
- 2 teaspoons of coconut oil, melted

Directions:
1. Set the oven to 425°F.
2. Line a baking sheet using a paper towel, then place the chickpeas on them and use more paper towels to take off the excess water in the chickpeas. Remove all of the paper towels.
3. Put the oil and spices into the chickpeas and mix well.
4. Roast your chickpeas for 40 minutes, stirring every 10 minutes.
5. Once the chickpeas are done, take them off from the oven and let them completely cool.

Nutrition: Total Carbohydrates: 19g|Dietary Fiber: 3g|Net Carbs: |Protein: 5g|Total Fat: 12g|Calories: 177

150. Berry Energy bites

Preparation Time: 10 minutes
Cooking Time: 0 minutes
Servings: 6
Ingredients:
- ½ cup of coconut flour
- 1 teaspoon of cinnamon
- 1 tablespoon of coconut sugar
- ¼ cup of dried blueberries
- ½ - 1 cup of almond milk

Directions:
1. Put together the coconut flour, cinnamon, coconut sugar, and blueberries in a huge mixing bowl, and mix well.
2. Add the almond milk slowly until a firm dough is formed.
3. Form into bite-sized balls and refrigerate for 30 minutes so they can harden up.
4. Store leftovers in the refrigerator.

Nutrition: Total Carbohydrates: 18g|Dietary Fiber: 1g|Net Carbs: |Protein: 5g|Total Fat: 12g|Calories: 87

151. Roasted Beets

Preparation Time: 10 minutes
Cooking Time: 35-45 minutes
Servings: 6
Ingredients:
- 2 and a ½ pounds of beets, peeled and diced
- 1 tablespoon of coconut oil, melted
- 1 teaspoon of salt

Directions:
1. Preheat the oven to 400°F.
2. Spread the beets onto a baking sheet and drizzle with melted coconut oil.
3. Add salt and mix well.
4. Roast the beets in the oven for 35-45 minutes until the beets are soft.

Nutrition: Total Carbohydrates: 7g|Dietary Fiber: 2g|Net Carbs: |Protein: 5g|Total Fat: 12g|Calories: 57

152. 473.Bruschetta

Preparation Time: 60 minutes
Cooking Time: 0 minutes
Servings: 4
Ingredients:
- 4 medium tomatoes, diced
- 1 red onion, diced
- ¼ cup of extra virgin olive oil
- 2 tablespoons of balsamic vinegar
- 2 cloves of garlic, minced
- 1 teaspoon of sea salt
- ¼ teaspoon of ground black pepper

Directions:
1. Place the ingredients into a large bowl, and stir gently.
2. Refrigerate for 1 hour before serving on gluten-free toast (toast is not included in nutritional information)

Nutrition: Total Carbohydrates: 8g|Dietary Fiber: 2g|Net Carbs: |Protein: 5g|Total Fat: 12g|Calories: 185

153. Cashew Cheese

Preparation Time: 2 hours
Cooking Time: 0 minutes
Servings: 6
Ingredients:
- 1 cup of raw cashews
- Juice of ½ lemon
- 1 tablespoon of nutritional yeast
- Salt and pepper to taste
- ¼ cup of fresh basil

Directions:
1. In a1 cup of water, soak the cashew for at least 2 hours. Drain.
2. Place the cashews, lemon juice, nutritional yeast, and fresh basil into a food processor and blend until smooth. Put in 1 tablespoon of water at a time to make it creamy but not runny.
3. Season with pepper and salt, then spread it on gluten-free bread or toast.
4. Store in an airtight jar in the refrigerator.

Nutrition: Total Carbohydrates: 10g | Dietary Fiber: 1g | Net Carbs: | Protein: 5g | Total Fat: 12g | Calories: 127

154. Low Cholesterol-Low Calorie Blueberry Muffin

Preparation Time: 10 minutes
Cooking Time: 25 minutes
Servings: 12
Ingredients:
- 1 cup blueberries, fresh
- 2 tablespoons melted margarine
- 2 teaspoons baking powder
- 1 and ½ cup of flour, all-purpose
- 1 egg white
- ½ cup skim milk or non-fat milk
- 1 tablespoon coconut oil
- ½ cup white sugar
- Pinch of salt

Directions:
1. Set the oven to 205C.
2. Grease a 12-cup muffin pan using oil.
3. In a small bowl, place the blueberries. Add ¼ cup of the flour and mix it. Set aside.
4. In another bowl, whisk the egg white and the coconut oil. Add the melted margarine.
5. In a separate bowl, mix the dry ingredients and sift. Sift again over the egg white mixture. Mix to moisten the flour. The flour should look lumpy, so do not overmix.
6. Fold in the blueberries. Separate the blueberries so that each scoop will have blueberries. Scoop the mixture into the muffin pans. Fill only up to two-thirds of the pan.
7. Bake for 25 minutes or until the muffin turns golden brown.

Nutrition: Calories: 114 kcal | Protein: 2.66 gFat: 5.34 g | Carbohydrates: 14.25 g

155. Carrot Sticks with Avocado Dip

Preparation Time: 10 minutes
Cooking Time: 0 minutes
Servings: 6
Ingredients:
- 1 large avocado, pitted
- 6 ounces shelled edamame
- ½ cup cilantro, tightly packed
- ½ onion
- Juice of one lemon
- 2 tablespoons olive oil
- 1 tablespoon of chili-garlic sauce or chili sauce
- Salt and pepper

Directions:
1. Place the edamame, cilantro, onion, and chili sauce in a blender or food processor. Pulse it to chop and mix the ingredients. Add the avocado and lemon juice. Gradually add the olive oil as you blend. Transfer to a jar.
2. Scoop 2 spoons and serve with carrot sticks.

Nutrition: Calories: 154 kcal | Protein: 5.16 g | Fat: 11.96 g | Carbohydrates: 8.44 g

156. Boiled Okra and Squash

Preparation Time: 5 minutes
Cooking Time: 5 minutes
Servings: 1
Ingredients:
- ½ cup of okra, cut in 1" cubes
- ½ cup of squash, cut in 1" cubes
- 1 clove garlic, minced
- 2/3 cup Vegetable stock or fish stock, plain water may be used as well
- Salt to taste

Directions:
1. Boil the liquid in high heat.
2. Add the okra and squash. Bring to a boil. Add the garlic. Reduce the heat and simmer for at least 5 minutes or until the squash is tender.
3. Add salt to taste and serve hot.

Nutrition: Calories: 117 kcal | Protein: 8.2 g | Fat: 6.25 g | Carbohydrates: 7.82 g

157. Oven Crisp Sweet Potato

Preparation Time: 10 minutes
Cooking Time: 20 minutes
Servings: 2
Ingredients:
- 1 medium-sized sweet potato, raw

- 1 teaspoon sugar
- 1 teaspoon coconut oil

Directions:
1. Preheat the oven to 160C.
2. Using a mandolin slicer or a peeler, slice the sweet potato into thin chips or strips. Wash and pat dry.
3. Drizzle the coconut oil over the potatoes. Toss until all chips are coated.
4. Arrange in an oven baking sheet. Bake for 10 minutes. Check the crispiness. If it is not that crispy enough, bake for another 5 or 1o minutes or until the chips attain the crispiness desired.
5. Take out the crispy sweet potatoes. Sprinkle with sugar and serve.

Nutrition: Calories: 123 kcal|Protein: 4.23 g|Fat: 5.39 g |Carbohydrates: 14.63 g

158. Olive and Tomato Balls

Preparation Time: 10 minutes
Cooking Time: 35 minutes
Servings: 5
Ingredients:
- 5 tbsp. Parmesan cheese, grated
- .25 tsp. Salt
- Black pepper (as desired)
- 2 cloves Garlic, crushed
- 4 Kalamata olives, pitted
- 4 pcs. Sun-dried tomatoes, drained
- 2 tbsp. Oregano, chopped
- 2 tbsp. Thyme, chopped
- 2 tbsp. Basil, chopped
- .25 cup Coconut oil
- .5 cup Cream cheese

Directions:
1. Chop the coconut oil, add it to a small mixing bowl with the cream cheese, and leave them to soften for about 30 minutes. Mash together and mix well to combine.
2. Add in the Kalamata olives and sun-dried tomatoes and mix well before adding in the herbs and seasonings. Combine thoroughly before placing the mixing bowl in the refrigerator to allow the results to solidify.
3. Once it has solidified, form the mixture into a total of 5 balls using an ice cream scoop. Roll each of the finished balls into the parmesan cheese before plating.
4. Stored the extras in the fridge in an air-tight container for up to 7 days.

Nutrition: Calories: 212 kcal|Protein: 4.77 g|Fat: 20.75 g|Carbohydrates: 3.13 g

159. Mini Pepper Nachos

Preparation Time: 5 minutes
Cooking Time: 10 minutes
Servings: 8
Ingredients:
- .5 cup Tomato, chopped
- 1 tbsp. Chili powder
- cup Cheddar cheese, shredded
- 1 tsp. Cumin, ground
- 16 oz. Mini peppers, seeded, halved
- 1 tsp. Garlic powder
- 16 oz. Ground beef
- 1 tsp. Paprika
- .25 tsp. Red pepper flakes
- 5 tsp. Salt
- .5 tsp. Oregano
- 5 tsp. Pepper

Directions:
1. Mix seasonings together in a bowl.
2. On medium heat, brown the meat, be sure all the clumps are broken up.
3. Mix in the spices and continue to sauté until the seasoning has gone through all of the meat.
4. Heat the oven to 400F.
5. Place the peppers in a single line. They can touch.
6. Coat with the beef mix.
7. Sprinkle with cheese.
8. Bake for at least 10 minutes or until cheese has melted.
9. Pull out of the oven and top with the toppings.

Nutrition: Calories: 240 kcal|Protein: 11.01 g|Fat: 18.2 g |Carbohydrates: 9.49 g

160. Avocado Hummus

Preparation Time: 15 minutes
Cooking Time: 0 minutes

Servings: 4
Ingredients:
- .25 tsp. Pepper
- .5 tsp. Salt
- 5 tsp. Cumin
- 1 clove pressed garlic
- .5 Lemon juice
- .25 cup Tahini
- .25 cup Sunflower seeds
- .5 cup Coconut oil
- .5 cup Cilantro
- 3 Avocados

Directions:
1. Halve the avocados, take off the pits, and then spoon out the flesh.
2. Put all together ingredients in a blender and mix until completely smooth.
3. Add water, lemon juice, or oil if you need to loosen the mixture bit.

Nutrition: Calories: 651 kcal | Protein: 9.62 g | Fat: 64.05 g | Carbohydrates: 19.95 g

161. Flavorsome Almonds

Preparation Time: 10 minutes
Cooking Time: 15 minutes
Servings: 8
Ingredients:
- 2 cups of whole almonds
- 3 tbsp. of raw honey
- 1 tsp. of extra-virgin olive oil
- 1 tbsp. of filtered water
- ½ tsp. of chili powder
- ½ tsp. of ground cinnamon
- ¼ tsp. of ground cumin
- ¼ tsp. of cayenne pepper
- Salt, to taste

Directions:
1. Preheat the oven to 350 degrees F.
2. Arrange the almonds onto a large rimmed baking sheet in a single layer.
3. Roast for about 10 minutes.
4. Meanwhile, in a microwave-safe bowl, add honey and microwave on Hugh for about 30 seconds.
5. Remove from microwave and stir in oil and water.
6. In a small bowl, mix all spices.
7. Remove the almonds from the oven, add it into the bowl of honey mixture, and stir to combine well.
8. Transfer the almond mixture onto the baking sheet in a single layer.
9. Sprinkle with spice mixture evenly.
10. Roast for about 3-4 minutes.
11. Take off from the oven and keep aside to cool completely before serving.
12. You can preserve these roasted almonds in an airtight jar.

Nutrition: Calories: 168 | Fat: 12.5g | Carbs: 11.8g | Protein: 5.1g | Fiber: 3.1g

162. Chewy Blackberry Leather

Preparation Time: 15 minutes
Cooking Time: 5-6 hours
Servings: 8
Ingredients:
- 2 cups of fresh blackberries
- 1 tbsp. of fresh mint leaves
- 1 tsp. of ground cinnamon
- 1/8 tsp. of fresh lemon juice
- ¼ cup of raw honey

Directions:
1. Set the oven to 170F. Line baking sheet with parchment paper.
2. In a food processor, put all ingredients and pulse till smooth.
3. Take the mixture onto the prepared baking sheet and smooth the top with the back of a spoon.
4. Bake for about 5-6 hours.
5. Cut the leather into equal-sized strips.
6. Now, roll each rectangle to make fruit rolls.

Nutrition: Calories: 48 | Fat: 12.5g | Carbs: 11.8g | Protein: 5.1g | Fiber: 2.1g

163. Party-Time Chicken Nuggets

Preparation Time: 10 minutes
Cooking Time: 25 minutes
Servings: 6
Ingredients:

- 2 (6-ounce) grass-fed skinless, boneless chicken breasts
- 2 large organic eggs
- 1½ cups of blanched almond flour
- ½ cup tapioca flour
- ½ tsp. of paprika
- ½ tsp. of onion powder
- ½ tsp. of garlic powder
- Salt, to taste
- Freshly ground black pepper, to taste

Directions:
1. Set the oven to 400F, then grease a large baking sheet.
2. With a rolling pin, roll the chicken breasts to an even thickness.
3. Cut each breast into bite-sized pieces.
4. In a shallow dish, crack the eggs and beat well.
5. In another shallow dish, mix flours and spices.
6. Dip the chicken nuggets in beaten eggs.
7. Then roll in flour mixture completely.
8. Arrange the nuggets onto the prepared baking sheet in a single layer.
9. Bake for about 10-12 minutes, flipping once after 5 minutes.

Nutrition: Calories: 238 | Fat: 12.5g | Carbs: 11.8g | Protein: 4.1g | Fiber: 2.1g

164. Protein-Packed Croquettes

Preparation Time: 10 minutes
Cooking Time: 5 minutes
Servings: 12
Ingredients:
- ¼ cup plus 1 tbsp. of olive oil, divided
- ½ cup of thawed frozen peas
- 2 minced garlic cloves
- 1 cup of cooked quinoa
- 2 large peeled and mashed boiled potatoes
- ¼ cup of chopped fresh cilantro leaves
- 2 tsp. of ground cumin
- ½ tsp. of paprika
- ¼ tsp. of ground turmeric
- Salt, to taste
- Freshly ground black pepper, to taste

Directions:
1. In a frying pan, heat 1 tbsp. of oil on medium heat.
2. Add peas and garlic and sauté for about 1 minute.
3. Transfer the peas mixture into a large bowl.
4. Put remaining ingredients, then mix till well combined.
5. Make equal sized oblong shaped patties from the mixture.
6. In a huge skillet, warm the remaining oil on medium-high heat.
7. Add croquettes in batches and fry for about 4 minutes per side.

Nutrition: Calories: 165 | Fat: 12.5g | Carbs: 10.8g | Protein: 5.1g | Fiber: 3.1g

165. Energy Dates Balls

Preparation Time: 10 minutes
Cooking Time: 25 minutes
Servings: 7
Ingredients:
- 1 cup of toasted almonds
- 1 cup of pitted and chopped dates
- ¼ cup of fresh lemon juice
- ½ cup of shredded sweetened coconut

Directions:
1. Line a large baking sheet using parchment paper. Keep aside.
2. In a food processor, add almonds and pulse till chopped coarsely.
3. Add dates and lemon juice and pulse till a soft dough forms.
4. Make equal-sized balls from the mixture.
5. In a shallow, dish place shredded coconut.
6. Roll the balls in shredded coconut evenly.
7. Put the balls onto the baking sheet in a single layer.
8. Refrigerate to set completely before serving.

Nutrition: Calories: 148 | Fat: 14.5g | Carbs: 11.8g | Protein: 5.1g | Fiber: 2.1g

166. Energetic Oat Bars

Preparation Time: 10 minutes
Cooking Time: 25 minutes
Servings: 6
Ingredients:
- ½ cup of gluten-free rolled oats

- 2 tbsp. of flax seeds
- 1 tbsp. of sunflower seeds
- 1 tbsp. of chopped walnuts
- 2 tbsp. of raisins
- ¾ cup fresh blueberries
- 1 peeled and mashed banana
- 2 tbsp. of pitted and chopped finely dates
- 1 tbsp. of fresh pomegranate juice

Directions:
1. Set the oven to 350F. Lightly oil an 8-inch baking dish.
2. In a huge mixing bowl, put all ingredients and mix till well combined.
3. Place the mixture into the prepared baking dish evenly.
4. Bake for about 25 minutes. Take off from the oven, then cool.
5. Using a knife, divide the bars into the size of your desired pieces, then serve.

Nutrition: Calories: 88 | Fat: 12.5g | Carbs: 11.8g | Protein: 5.1g | Fiber: 2.8g

167. Soft Flourless Cookies

Preparation Time: 10 minutes
Cooking Time: 25 minutes
Servings: 4
Ingredients:
- ¾ cup of shredded unsweetened coconut
- 1 peeled large banana
- Pinch of ground cinnamon
- ¼ teaspoon of organic vanilla extract

Directions:
1. Set the oven to 350F. Line a cookie sheet with a large greased parchment paper.
2. In a large food processor, put all ingredients and pulse till well combined.
3. Spoon the mixture onto the prepared cookie sheet. With your hands, flatten the cookies slightly.
4. Bake for at least 25 minutes or till golden brown.

Nutrition: Calories: 68 | Fat: 9.5g | Carbs: 11.8g | Protein: 5.1g | Fiber: 2.1g

168. Delectable Cookies

Preparation Time: 20 minutes
Cooking Time: 15-20 minutes
Servings: 6
Ingredients:
- 1 cup of almonds
- 1 1/3 cups of almond flour
- ¼ cup of arrowroot flour
- 1 tbsp. of coconut flour
- 1 tsp. ground turmeric
- Salt, to taste
- Freshly ground black pepper, to taste
- 1 organic egg
- ¼ cup of olive oil
- 3 tbsp. of raw honey
- 1 tsp. of organic vanilla extract

Directions:
1. In a food processor, put the almonds and pulse till chopped roughly
2. Transfer the chopped almonds to a large bowl.
3. Put the flours and spices and mix well.
4. In another bowl, put the remaining ingredients, then beat till well combined.
5. Place the flour mixture into the egg mixture and mix till well combined.
6. Arrange a plastic wrap over the cutting board.
7. Place the dough over the cutting board.
8. Using your hands, pat into about a 1-inch thick circle.
9. Gently cut the circle into 6 wedges.
10. Set the scones onto a cookie sheet in a single layer.
11. Bake for about 15-20 minutes.

Nutrition: Calories: 335 | Fat: 27.7g | Carbs: 17.6g | Protein: 9g | Fiber: 4.8g

169. Turmeric Chickpea Cakes

Preparation Time: 20 minutes
Cooking Time: 30 minutes
Servings: 8
Ingredients:
- 2 small onions, minced
- 2 cans (15oz.) chickpeas, rinsed, drained
- Freshly ground pepper to taste
- 1 teaspoon cayenne pepper, to taste (optional)

- 4 cloves garlic, minced
- 4 tablespoons cornstarch
- 1 teaspoon salt or to taste
- 2 teaspoons turmeric powder
- 8-10 tablespoons chickpea flour
- Avocado dipping sauce to serve
- ½ cup fresh parsley, minced
- Grapeseed oil to fry

Directions:
1. Place a skillet over medium heat. Add a little oil. When the oil is heated, put onion and garlic and sauté until translucent. Turn off the heat and cool completely.
2. Add chickpeas into the food processor bowl and process until very finely chopped.
3. Add the onion mixture, salt, pepper, cayenne pepper, and turmeric powder and pulse again until well combined.
4. Transfer into a bowl. Add parsley and mix well.
5. Make small balls of the mixture (of about 1-inch diameter) and shape them into patties. Place chickpea flour on a plate.
6. Place a nonstick pan over medium heat. Add a little oil and swirl the pan so that the oil spreads.
7. Dredge the patties in the chickpea flour and place a few on the pan. Cook in batches.
8. Cook until the underside is golden brown. Flip, then cook the other side till it's golden brown.
9. Repeat steps 6-8 to fry the remaining patties.
10. Serve with avocado dipping sauce.

Nutrition: Calories: 154 kcal|Protein: 7.32 g|Fat: 2.85 g|Carbohydrates: 25.43 g

170. Almonds and Blueberries Yogurt Snack

Preparation Time: 10 minutes
Cooking Time: 0 minutes
Servings: 2
Ingredients:
- 1 ½ cups nonfat Greek yogurt
- 20 almonds, chopped
- 1 cup blueberries

Directions:
1. Take 2 bowls and add ¾ cup yogurt into each bowl.
2. Divide the blueberries among the bowls and stir.
3. Sprinkle half the almonds in each bowl and serve.

Nutrition: Calories: 223 kcal|Protein: 6.57 g|Fat: 9.45 g|Carbohydrates: 30.82 g

171. Cottage Cheese with Apple Sauce

Preparation Time: 5 minutes
Cooking Time: 0 minutes
Servings: 2
Ingredients:
- 5-6 tablespoons cottage cheese
- ½ teaspoon cinnamon powder
- 2-3 tablespoons applesauce or more if required

Directions:
1. Divide the cottage cheese into 2 bowls.
2. Spread applesauce over the cottage cheese.
3. Sprinkle ¼ teaspoon cinnamon powder on each and serve.

Nutrition: Calories: 79 kcal|Protein: 8.09 g|Fat: 3.45 g |Carbohydrates: 3.92 g

172. Cucumber Rolls Hors D'oeuvres

Preparation Time: 20 minutes
Cooking Time: 0 minutes
Servings: 8-10
Ingredients:
- 2 large organic English cucumbers or 4 normal cucumbers
- For the avocado spread:
- ½ cup capers
- 1 teaspoon Himalayan pink salt
- ¼ cup fresh dill, finely chopped
- ½ cup fresh parsley + extra to garnish, finely chopped
- 5-6 ripe avocadoes, peeled, pitted, mashed
- Freshly cracked pepper to taste

Directions:
1. Peel the cucumbers and cut thin slices along the length on a mandolin slicer.

2. Place the cucumber slices on your countertop.
3. To make the avocado spread: Add all the ingredients of avocado spread into a bowl and mix until well combined.
4. Spread the avocado mixture evenly and thinly on the cucumber slices.
5. Start rolling from one of the shorter ends to the other end and place on a serving platter with its seam side facing down.
6. Repeat the above step with the remaining cucumber slices.
7. Serve immediately as the cucumbers tend to get soggy after a while.

Nutrition: Calories: 227 kcal | Protein: 3.77 g | Fat: 19.88 g | Carbohydrates: 12.99 g

173. Ginger Turmeric Protein Bars

Preparation Time: 10 minutes + 20 cooling time
Cooking Time: 25 minutes
Servings: 7
Ingredients:
- ½ cup coconut
- 1 Tbsp. ginger
- 1 scoop turmeric protein bone broth
- 2 Tbsp. maple syrup
- 1/3 cup sunflower butter
- 1 cup cashews

Directions:
1. Add coconut pieces and cashews to a blender or food processor. Use the pulse option to obtain a coarse mixture.
2. Add butter, broth, maple syrup, and ginger and pulse the mixture to form a coarse yet even and somewhat sticky mass.
3. Evenly place the mixture in a baking pan (8x8 inches) with your hands or a spoon. Push firmly to the baking pan.
4. Please bring it to a refrigerator and let it cool for 20 minutes.
5. Cut the mixture into even squares.
6. You can consume it immediately or store it in a glass container in your fridge (up to 7 days).

Nutrition: 107 kcal | Protein: 1.15 g | Fat: 9.59 g | Carbohydrates: 4.63 g

174. Avocado with Tomatoes and Cucumber

Preparation Time: 10 minutes
Cooking Time: 0 minutes
Servings: 2
Ingredients:
- 2 avocados
- 1 cucumber
- 4 Roma tomatoes
- ½ red onion
- 1/8 cup parsley
- ¼ cup cilantro
- ¼ cup olives – to your choice
- 1 lemon
- 1 Tbsp. turmeric
- Salt and pepper – to your taste

Directions:
1. Dice the tomatoes, cucumber, avocado, and olives.
2. Slice the cilantro, parsley, and onion.
3. Add the above ingredients into a bowl.
4. Squeeze the lemon juice, then add to the vegetables.
5. Add olive oil, turmeric, salt, and pepper.
6. Toss well.
7. Consume immediately after adding lemon juice and olive oil.
8. If you prefer to consume the salad later, add the dressing immediately before consuming it.

Nutrition: Calories: 480 kcal | Protein: 11.57 g | Fat: 35.27 g | Carbohydrates: 39.77 g

175. Salmon & Avocado Toast

Preparation Time: 10 minutes
Cooking Time: 5 minutes
Servings: 1
Ingredients:
- oz. pink salmon (wild)
- 2 slices of gluten-free bread
- ½ avocado
- ¼ tsp red pepper
- 1 tsp lemon juice
- salt and pepper - to taste

Directions:

1. Slice the avocado.
2. Toast the bread to your taste.
3. Mix the salmon and lemon juice.
4. When the toast is ready, lay avocado slices onto it.
5. Cover with salmon.
6. Add some red pepper, salt, and pepper to your taste.
7. Feel free to put the other ingredients you like (tomatoes, onions)
8. Enjoy your salmon snack!

Nutrition: Calories: 481 kcal | Protein: 28.08 g | Fat: 27.52 g | Carbohydrates: 33 g

176. Avocado and Egg Sandwich

Preparation Time: 10 minutes
Cooking Time: 0 minutes
Servings: 2
Ingredients:
- 1 avocado (ripe)
- 1 egg, organic
- ½ lime juice
- 2 slices of who wheat, seed bread
- 2 radishes
- Black pepper – to your taste
- A pinch of salt (sea or Himalayan)
- 1 scallion
- Mixed seeds – to your choice

Directions:
1. Peel the avocado.
2. Boil the egg (soft boiled).
3. Cut the radishes into thin slices.
4. Dice the scallion (finely).
5. Mix avocado, salt, and lime juice in a bowl. Mash the mixture thoroughly.
6. Spread the mixture onto the bread.
7. Add some radish.
8. Put soft-boiled eggs on top.
9. Add some scallion, seeds, and pepper.

Nutrition: Calories: 342 kcal | Protein: 12.36 g | Fat: 22.99 g | Carbohydrates: 26.54 g

177. Coconut Porridge

Preparation Time: 20 minutes
Cooking Time: 10 minutes
Servings: 2
Ingredients:
- 2 cups oats
- 1 tbsp. coconut oil
- Coconut milk
- Fresh, shredded coconut (for serving)
- 750 ml of water
- 2 tsp turmeric
- 330ml evaporated coconut milk
- 1 vanilla bean
- 2 tbsp. maple syrup
- 2 tsp ginger
- 1 tsp cinnamon

Directions:
1. Mix 750 ml water and turmeric in a bowl. Let it sit for 10 minutes.
2. Mix all ingredients except coconut milk and shredded coconut in a saucepan.
3. Heat it on medium heat, stirring constantly, and cook for 8 minutes.
4. Let it cool for 10 minutes.
5. Divide into serving bowls.
6. Add coconut milk and shredded coconut on top.
7. Add some extra cinnamon to your taste.
8. Eat warm.

Nutrition: Calories: 417 kcal | Protein: 20.63 g | Fat: 16.8 g | Carbohydrates: 83.03 g

178. Almond and Honey Homemade Bar

Preparation Time: 15 minutes + 30 minutes' fridge time
Cooking Time: 15 minutes
Servings: 8
Ingredients:
- A ¼ cup of almonds
- 1 cup oats
- ¼ cup sunflower seeds
- 1/3 cup currants
- 1 tbsp. flaxseeds
- 1/3 cup apricots (dried and chopped)
- 1/3 cup raisins (chopped)
- 1 tbsp. sesame seeds
- 1 cup whole-grain puffed cereal (unsweetened)

- ¼ cup almond butter
- ¼ cup honey
- 1/8 tsp salt
- ¼ cup sugar (or another sweetener to your taste in adjusted amount)
- ½ teaspoon vanilla extract

Directions:
1. Preheat the oven to 350 degrees Fahrenheit.
2. Put a baking paper to an 8-inch pan or coat it with cooking spray/oil.
3. Mix the almonds, oats, and seeds and spread the mixture on a rimmed baking sheet.
4. Bake the mixture until you notice that the oats are lightly toasted (for about 10 minutes).
5. Transfer the mixture to a bowl.
6. Add cereal, raisins, currants, and apricots to the bowl.
7. Toss well to combine.
8. Mix honey, almond butter, vanilla, salt, and sugar in a saucepan.
9. Heat over medium heat. Stir frequently for 2-5 minutes until you see light bubbles.
10. As soon as you notice the bubbles, pour the mixture over the dry mixture with apricots and oats you prepared previously.
11. Mix well with a spatula. There mustn't be any dry spots.
12. Transfer the new mixture to the previously prepared pan.
13. Press it to the pan to make a firm and flat layer.
14. Refrigerate for 30 minutes.
15. Cut the layer into eight equal bars or squares, to your taste.
16. Consume immediately or refrigerate for up to seven days.
17. You can store these energy bars in the freezer as well (for long-term storage). Wrap them in stretch plastic folium and store them at −16 to −18 degrees.

Nutrition: Calories: 213 kcal Protein: 6.92 g Fat: 9.59 g Carbohydrates: 32.33 g

SIDE DISHES

179. Simply Vanilla Frozen Greek Yogurt

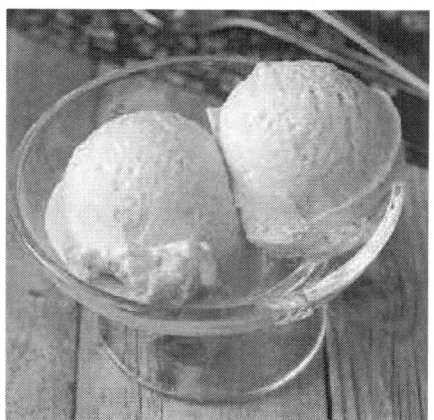

Preparation Time: 5 minutes + 8 hours to freeze
Cooking Time: 0 minutes

Ingredients:
- 4 cups nonfat plain Greek yogurt
- 4 tablespoons vanilla whey protein powder
- 4 tablespoons vanilla extract
- 4 teaspoons stevia or no-calorie sweetener

Directions:
1. 1.In a large bowl or loaf pan, combine the yogurt, protein powder, vanilla extract, and stevia.
2. 2.Cover and freeze overnight or for at least 8 hours.
3. 3.About an hour before serving, set in the refrigerator to thaw slightly. Serve and enjoy.

Nutrition: PER SERVING (1 CUP): Calories: 183; Protein: 28g; Fat: 1g; Carbohydrates: 12g; Fiber: 1g; Sugar: 8g; Sodium: 96mg

180. Salad Bites

Preparation Time: 10 minutes
Cooking Time: 8 minutes
Servings: 2-3

Ingredients:
- For the Bites
- 24 cherry tomatoes
- 12 mozzarella balls
- 12 fresh basil leaves
- For the Balsamic Glaze
- ½ cup balsamic vinegar
- 2 tablespoons extra-virgin olive oil
- 1 garlic clove, minced
- 1 teaspoon Italian seasoning

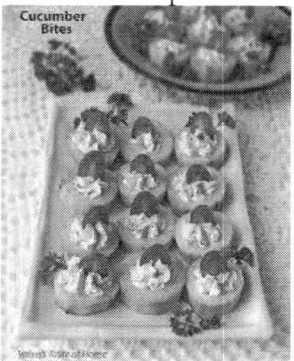

Directions:
1. To make the bites
3. 2.Place on a serving platter or in a large glass storage container that can be sealed.
4. To make the glaze
5. 1.In a small saucepan, bring the balsamic to a simmer. Simmer for 15 minutes, or until syrupy. Set aside to cool and thicken.
6. 2.In a small bowl, whisk olive oil, garlic, Italian seasoning, and cooled vinegar.
7. 3.Drizzle the olive oil and balsamic glaze over the skewers. Serve immediately or keep in the refrigerator for a tasty snack.

Nutrition: Calories: 39; Total fat: 3g; Protein: 1g; Carbohydrates: 3g; Fiber: 0g; Sugar: 0g; Sodium: 11mg.

181. Greek Chop-Chop Salad

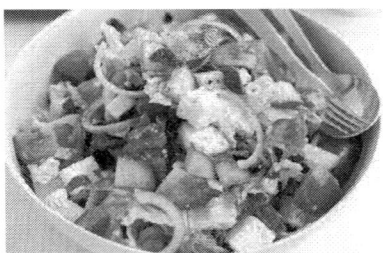

Preparation Time: 15 minutes
Cooking Time: 0 minutes

Ingredients:
- 1 medium English cucumber, chopped (2 cups)
- 1 cup halved cherry tomatoes
- 1 red bell pepper, seeded and diced
- ½ red onion, diced
- ½ cup pitted Kalamata olives, roughly chopped
- 1 cup crumbled feta cheese
- ½ cup balsamic dressing

Directions:
1. 1.In a large bowl, toss the cucumber, tomatoes, bell pepper, onion, olives, and cheese with the dressing, and serve.

Nutrition: Calories: 173; Total fat: 13g; Protein: 4g; Carbohydrates: 10g; Fiber: 1g; Sugar: 4g; Sodium: 883mg.

182. Cauliflower Fried Rice

Preparation Time: 15 minutes
Cooking Time: 8 minutes
Servings: 2-3

Ingredients:
- 1 teaspoon sesame oil, plus 1 tablespoon
- 2 large eggs, beaten
- 4 cups cauliflower rice (or florets of 1 head of cauliflower riced in a food processor)
- 1 cup frozen mixed vegetables
- 2 garlic cloves, minced
- 2 tablespoons low-sodium soy sauce
- 2 scallions, diced

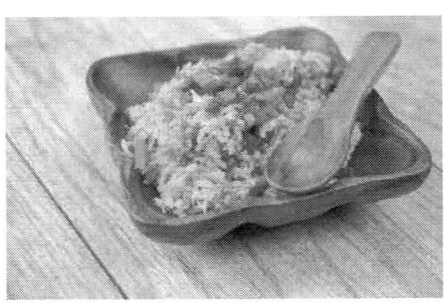

Directions:
1. 1.In a large skillet over medium heat, heat 1 teaspoon of sesame oil. Add the eggs, and stir until they are cooked. Set aside.

Nutrition: Calories: 121; Total fat: 7g; Protein: 6g; Carbohydrates: 9g; Fiber: 3g; Sugar: 3g; Sodium: 357mg.

183. Roasted Garden Vegetables

Preparation Time: 5 minutes
Cooking Time: 15 minutes
Servings: 2-3

Ingredients:
- 1 medium bell pepper, cut into strips
- 1 small onion, halved then sliced
- 1 small zucchini, sliced into rounds
- 1-pint grape tomatoes
- 2 tablespoons extra-virgin olive oil
- Salt
- Freshly ground black pepper

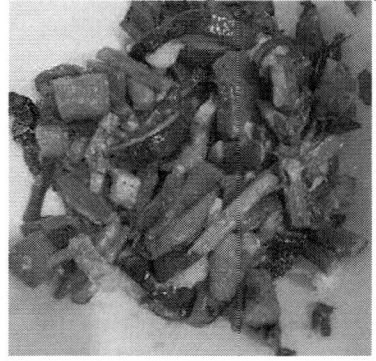

Directions:

1. 1.Preheat the oven to 400°F.
2. 2.Using 1 or 2 large baking sheets, arrange the vegetables so they are lying flat, lightly touching each other.
3. 3.Evenly pour the olive oil over the vegetables, and gently toss to coat, using either a spoon or your hands. Add salt and pepper to taste.
4. 4.Roast for 20 to 30 minutes, or until soft and lightly charred, stirring halfway through, and serve.

Nutrition: Calories: 75; Total fat: 5g; Protein: 0g; Carbohydrates: 8g; Fiber: 1g; Sugar: 4g; Sodium: 2mg.

184. Asian Cabbage Salad

Preparation Time: 10 minutes
Cooking Time: 0 minutes
Servings: 2-3
Ingredients:
- 1 (14-ounce) package coleslaw
- 1 red bell pepper, thinly sliced
- 1 large carrot, grated
- ¼ cup diced scallions
- ¼ cup chopped fresh cilantro
- ¼ cup chopped peanuts
- 1/3 cup Spicy Peanut Dressing, plus more if desired

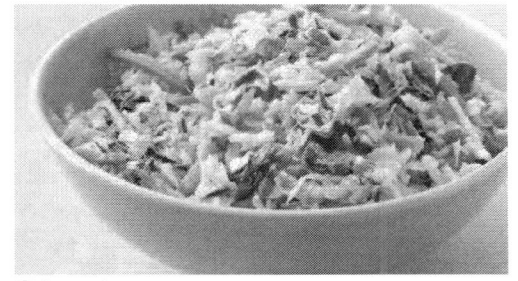

Directions:
1. 1.In a large bowl, combine coleslaw, bell pepper, carrot, scallions, cilantro, and peanuts.

Nutrition: Calories: 123; Total fat: 6g; Protein: 6g; Carbohydrates: 16g; Fiber: 6g; Sugar: 6g; Sodium: 198mg.

185. Southwest Deviled Eggs

Preparation Time: 10 minutes
Cooking Time: 0 minutes
Servings: 2-3
Ingredients:
- 6 large hard-boiled eggs
- 2 tablespoons low-fat, plain Greek yogurt
- ¼ teaspoon spicy mustard
- 1/8 teaspoon salt
- ½ teaspoon Taco Seasoning

Directions:
1. 1.Peel the eggs, and halve them lengthwise.
2. 2.Remove the yolks, and transfer them to a small bowl, setting the whites aside.
3. 3.Add the yogurt, spicy mustard, salt, and taco seasoning to the bowl with the yolks, and mash everything together.
4. 4.Spoon the mixture into the egg white halves, and serve.

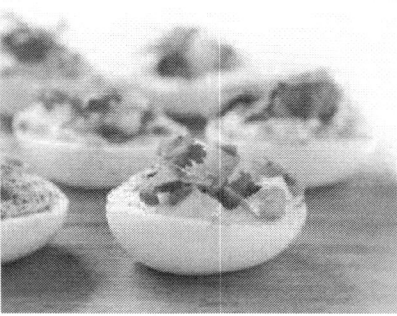

Nutrition: Calories: 83; Total fat: 5g; Protein: 7g; Carbohydrates: 1g; Fiber: 0g; Sugar: 1g; Sodium: 129mg.

186. Rajun' Cajun Roll-Ups

Cooking Time: 0 minutes
Servings: 2-3
Ingredients:
- 4 slices nitrate-free Cajun deli turkey
- 4 teaspoons spicy mustard, divided
- 4 slices pepper Jack cheese
- ½ steak tomato, seeded and diced
- ¼ red onion, thinly sliced
- 2 cups shredded lettuce
- ½ avocado, diced

- ¼ cup chopped banana peppers

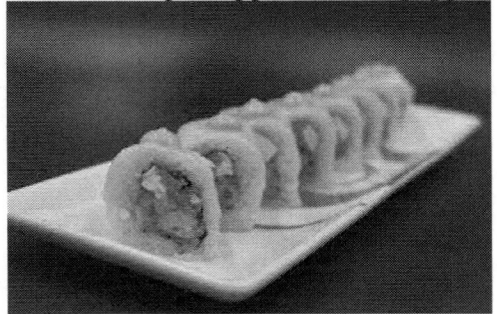

Directions:
1. 1.On a cutting board, lay out 1 slice of deli turkey and spread with 1 teaspoon of mustard.
3. 3.Wrap the deli turkey tightly, but delicately, around the filling, and pin with a toothpick.
4. 4.Repeat the process 3 times with the remaining ingredients, and serve.

Nutrition: Calories: 152; Total fat: 9g; Protein: 10g; Carbohydrates: 6g; Fiber: 2g; Sugar: 1g; Sodium: 498mg.

187. Everything Parmesan Crisps

Preparation Time: 10 minutes
Cooking Time: 5 minutes
Servings: 2-3
Ingredients:
- 1 teaspoon poppy seeds
- 1 teaspoon sesame seeds
- 1 teaspoon garlic flakes
- 1 teaspoon onion flakes
- 12 tablespoons grated Parmesan cheese

Directions:
1. 1.Preheat the oven to 400°F.
2. 2.In a small bowl, mix the poppy seeds, sesame seeds, garlic flakes, and onion flakes together.
3. 3.Line a sheet pan with a silicon baking mat or parchment paper. Pour 1 tablespoon of Parmesan onto the mat, and gently pat down with your fingers to make a 2- to 2½-inch round.
4. 4.Repeat 11 more times, making sure to keep at least 1 inch between each round.
5. 5.Bake for 3 minutes. Remove from the oven, and sprinkle ¼ teaspoon of the seasoning over each Parmesan round.
6. 6.Bake for another 3 to 5 minutes, or until golden and crisp, and serve.

Nutrition: Calories: 23; Total fat: 2g; Protein: 2g; Carbohydrates: 0g; Fiber: 0g; Sugar: 0g; Sodium: 85mg.

188. Edamame Hummus

Preparation Time: 10 minutes
Cooking Time: 5 minutes
Servings: 2-3
Ingredients:
- 1½ cups frozen edamame, thawed, rinsed, and drained
- ¼ cup tahini
- 2 tablespoons extra-virgin olive oil
- 2 garlic cloves, peeled
- ½ teaspoon ground cumin
- 3 to 4 teaspoons freshly squeezed lemon juice (juice of 1 lemon)
- Salt
- Freshly ground black pepper
- 2 to 4 tablespoons water
- Raw veggies, for serving

Directions:
1. 1.In a food processor, combine the edamame, tahini, olive oil, garlic, cumin, and lemon juice. Process until smooth, stopping to scrape down the sides as needed.
2. 2.Add salt and pepper to taste. Process again until combined.
3. 3.To thin, if desired, add 1 tablespoon of water and process. Repeat this step until you reach your desired consistency.
4. 4.Transfer to a serving bowl, and serve with raw veggies.

Nutrition: Calories: 115; Total fat: 9g; Protein: 4g; Carbohydrates: 6g; Fiber: 2g; Sugar: 1g; Sodium: 20mg.

189. Chia Chocolate Pudding

Preparation Time: 5 minutes + 2-8 hours to chill
Cooking Time: 0 minutes
Servings: 2-3

Ingredients:
- ½ cup unsweetened almond milk
- ½ cup nonfat plain Greek yogurt
- 2 tablespoons chia seeds
- 1 tablespoon vanilla whey protein
- 1 teaspoon unsweetened cocoa powder
- ½ teaspoon stevia or no-calorie sweetener

Directions:
1. 1.In a canning jar, combine the almond milk, yogurt, chia seeds, whey protein, cocoa powder, and stevia.
2. 2.Seal with lid and let sit in refrigerator overnight.
3. 3.Enjoy straight from the jar, or in a separate bowl if you are consuming a smaller serving.

Nutrition: Calories: 257; Protein: 25g; Fat: 12g; Carbohydrates: 21g; Fiber: 11g; Sugar: 5g; Sodium: 122mg

190. Mashed Cauliflower

Preparation Time: 10 minutes
Cooking Time: 5 minutes
Servings: 2-3

Ingredients:
- 1 large head cauliflower
- ¼ cup water
- 1/3 cup low-fat buttermilk
- 1 tablespoon minced garlic
- 1 tablespoon extra-virgin olive oil

Directions:
1. 1.Break the cauliflower into small florets. Place in a large microwave-safe bowl with the water. Cover and microwave for about 5 minutes, or until the cauliflower is soft. Drain the water from the bowl.
2. 2.In a blender or food processor, puree the buttermilk, cauliflower, garlic, and olive oil on medium speed until the cauliflower is smooth and creamy.
3. 3.Serve immediately.

Nutrition: Calories: 62; Total fat: 2g; Protein: 3g; Carbs: 8g; Fiber: 3g; Sugar: 3g; Sodium: 54mg

191. Pickle Roll-Ups

Preparation Time: 20 minutes
Cooking Time: 0 minutes
Servings: 2-3

Ingredients:
- ¼ pound deli ham (nitrate-free), thinly sliced (about 8 slices)
- 8 ounces Neufchâtel cheese, at room temperature
- 1 teaspoon dried dill
- 1 teaspoon onion powder
- 8 whole kosher dill pickle spears

Directions:
1. 1.Get a large cutting board or clean counter space to assemble your roll-ups.
2. 2.Lay the ham slices on the work surface and carefully spread on the Neufchâtel cheese.
3. 3.Season each lightly with the dill and onion powder.
4. 4.Place an entire pickle on an end of the ham and carefully roll.
5. 5.Slice each pickle roll-up into mini rounds about ½- to 1-inch wide.
6. 6.Skew each with a toothpick for easier serving.

Nutrition: Calories: 86; Total fat: 7g; Protein: 4g; Carbs: 4g; Fiber: 0 g; Sugar: 2g; Sodium: 540mg

192. Baked Zucchini Fries

Preparation Time: 15 minutes
Cooking Time: 15 minutes
Servings: 2-3

Ingredients:
- 3 large zucchinis
- 2 large eggs
- 1 cup whole-wheat bread crumbs
- ¼ cup shredded Parmigiano-Reggiano cheese
- 1 teaspoon garlic powder
- 1 teaspoon onion powder

Directions:
1. 1.Preheat the oven to 425°F. Line a large rimmed baking sheet with aluminum foil.
2. 2.Halve each zucchini lengthwise and continue slicing each piece into fries about ½ inch in diameter. You will have about 8 strips per zucchini.
3. 3.In a small bowl, crack the eggs and beat lightly.

4. 4.In a medium bowl, combine the bread crumbs, Parmigiano-Reggiano cheese, garlic powder, and onion powder.
5. 5.One by one, dip each zucchini strip into the egg, then roll it in the bread crumb mixture. Place on the prepared baking sheet.
6. 6.Roast for 30 minutes, stirring the fries halfway through. Zucchini fries are done when brown and crispy.
7. 7.Serve immediately.

Nutrition: Calories: 89; Total fat: 3g; Protein: 5g; Carbs: 10g; Fiber: 1g; Sugar: 3g; Sodium: 179mg

193. Italian Eggplant Pizzas

Preparation Time: 15 minutes
Cooking Time: 15 minutes
Servings: 2-3
Ingredients:
- 1 large eggplant, cut into ¼- to ½-inch rounds
- 1 tablespoon salt
- 1 tablespoon extra-virgin olive oil
- 2 teaspoons minced garlic
- ½ teaspoon dried oregano
- 1 cup Marinara Sauce with Italian Herbs
- 1 cup fresh basil leaves
- 1 cup shredded part-skim Mozzarella cheese
- ¼ cup shredded Parmigiano-Reggiano cheese

Directions:
1. 1.Preheat the oven to 425°F. Line a large rimmed baking sheet with aluminum foil.
2. 2.Put the eggplant rounds on paper towels and sprinkle them with the salt. Let them sit for 10 to 15 minutes to help release some of the water in the eggplant. Pat dry afterward. It's okay to wipe off some of the salt before baking.
3. 3.In a small bowl, mix together the olive oil, garlic, and oregano.
4. 4.Place the eggplant rounds 1-inch apart on the baking sheet. Using a pastry brush, coat each side of the eggplant with the olive oil mixture. Bake the eggplant for 15 minutes.
5. 5.Create pizzas by layering 1 to 2 tablespoons of marinara sauce, 2 basil leaves, about 1 tablespoon of mozzarella cheese, and about ½ tablespoon of Parmigiano-Reggiano cheese on each baked eggplant round.
6. 6.Bake the pizzas for an additional 10 minutes or until the cheese is melted and starting to brown.
7. 7.Serve immediately and enjoy!

Nutrition: Calories: 99; Total fat: 6g; Protein: 5g; Carbs: 7g; Fiber: 2g; Sugar: 4g; Sodium: 500mg

194. Tomato, Basil, and Cucumber Salad

Preparation Time: 15 minutes
Cooking Time: 15 minutes
Servings: 2-3
Ingredients:
- 1 large cucumber, seeded and sliced
- 4 medium tomatoes, quartered
- 1 medium red onion, thinly sliced
- ½ cup chopped fresh basil
- 3 tablespoons red wine vinegar
- 1 tablespoon extra-virgin olive oil
- ½ teaspoon Dijon mustard
- ½ teaspoon freshly ground black pepper

Directions:
1. 1.In a medium bowl, mix together the cucumber, tomatoes, red onion, and basil.
2. 2.In a small bowl, whisk together the vinegar, olive oil, mustard, and pepper.
3. 3.Pour the dressing over the vegetables, and gently stir until well combined.
4. 4.Cover and chill for at least 30 minutes prior to serving.

Nutrition: Calories: 72; Total fat: 4g; Protein: 1g; Carbs: 8g; Fiber: 1g; Sugar: 4g; Sodium: 5mg

195. Roasted Root Vegetables

Preparation Time: 15 minutes
Cooking Time: 45 minutes
Servings: 2-3
Ingredients:
- Nonstick cooking spray
- 2 medium red beets, peeled
- 2 large parsnips, peeled
- 2 large carrots, peeled

- 1 medium butternut squash (about 2 pounds), peeled and seeded
- 1 medium red onion
- 2 tablespoons extra-virgin olive oil
- 4 teaspoons minced garlic
- 2 teaspoons dried thyme

Directions:
1. 1.Preheat the oven to 425°F. Spray a large rimmed baking sheet with the cooking spray.
2. 2.Roughly chop the beets, parsnips, carrots, and butternut squash into 1-inch pieces. Cut the onion into half and then each half into 4 large chunks.
3. 3.Arrange the vegetables in a single, even layer on the baking sheet, and sprinkle them with the olive oil, garlic, and thyme. Use a spoon to mix the vegetables to coat them with the oil and seasonings.
4. 4.Roast for 45 minutes, stirring the vegetables every 15 minutes, until all the vegetables are tender.
5. 5.Serve immediately.

Nutrition: Calories: 68; Total fat: 3g; Protein: 1g; Carbs: 11g; Fiber: 1g; Sugar: 5g; Sodium: 30mg

196. Cauliflower Rice

Preparation Time: 5 minutes
Cooking Time: 5 minutes
Servings: 2-3
Ingredients:
- 1 cauliflower head
- 1 teaspoon extra-virgin olive oil

Directions:
1. 1.Prepare the cauliflower head by removing the stems and leaves. Cut it into four large pieces.
2. 2.Put the cauliflower in a food processor and pulse until it breaks down into pieces the size of rice. You may need to remove any leftover pieces of stem. Alternatively, you can use a box grater to shred the cauliflower.
3. 3.Transfer the riced cauliflower to a plate or bowl and pat it dry with a paper towel.
4. 4.Place a small skillet over medium heat and add the olive oil. When the oil is hot, add the cauliflower. Sauté for 5 to 6 minutes, or until tender. Alternatively, steam the cauliflower rice and drain off any excess liquid before serving.

Nutrition: Calories: 12; Total fat: 0g; Protein: 1g; Carbs: 2g; Fiber: 1g; Sugar: 1g; Sodium: 5mg

197. Tomato and Mozzarella Bites

Preparation Time: 30 minutes
Cooking Time: 15 minutes
Servings: 2-3
Ingredients:
- 20 grape tomatoes, halved
- fresh basil leaves (20)
- 20 small balls fresh mozzarella cheese
- salt and pepper as need
- balsamic vinegar (½ cup)
- ¼ cup of extra virgin olive oil
- 20 toothpicks

Directions:
1. 1.Use a toothpick to spear half a tomato, a basil leaf, a ball of mozzarella, and another half a tomato. With the ingredients, repeat.
2. 2.Place and sprinkle with salt and pepper on a serving plate. In a small bowl, mix the vinegar and oil together to act as a dipping sauce.

Nutrition: 225 calories; carbohydrates 5.4g; fat 17.9g; cholesterol 39.3mg; sodium 151.8mg

198. Homemade Potato Chips

Preparation Time: 30 minutes
Cooking Time: 5 min/ batch
Servings: 2-3
Ingredients:
- 7 unpeeled medium potatoes (about 2 pounds)
- ice water (2 quarts)
- Salt (5 tsp.)
- Garlic powder (2 tsp.)
- 1-1/2 tsp. celery salt
- 1-1/2 tsp. pepper
- Oil for deep-fat frying

Directions:
1. 1.Slice the potatoes into very thinly slices, using a vegetable peeler or a metal cheese

slicer. Place it in a wide bowl; add salt and ice water. For 30 minutes, soak.
2. 2.Place the potatoes on paper towels and pat them dry. Combine the garlic powder, celery salt and pepper in a small bowl; set aside.
3. 3.Heat 1-1/2 in. in a cast-iron. Up to 375 ° crude. Fry the potatoes until golden brown in clusters, stirring on a constant basis for 3-4 minutes.
4. 4.With a slotted spoon, remove; drain onto paper towels. Sprinkle with the seasoning mixture immediately. Store it in an air-tight jar.

Nutrition: 3/4 cup of: 176 calories, 8g fat, 0 cholesterol, 703mg sodium, 24g carbohydrate, 3g protein.

199. Brie with Apricot Topping

Preparation Time: 25 minutes
Cooking Time: 0 cooking
Servings: 2-3
Ingredients:
- 1/2 cup of chopped dried apricots
- 2 tbsp. brown sugar
- 2 tbsp. water
- 1 tsp. balsamic vinegar
- Dash salt
- 1/2 to 1 tsp. minced fresh rosemary or 1/4 tsp. dried rosemary, crushed
- 1 round Brie cheese (8 ounces)
- Assorted crackers

Directions:
1. 1.Heat the oven to 400F. Mix the all first five ingredients in a small saucepan; bring it to a boil. Cook and when slightly thickened, stir with medium heat. Remove from heat; add rosemary and stir.
2. 2.From the top of the cheese, cut the rind off. Put the cheese in an ovenproof, non-greased serving dish. Spoon the apricot mix with the cheese. Bake until the cheese is softened, 10-12 minutes, uncovered. Serve soft, crackers included.

Nutrition: 1 Servings: 4-529 calories, 8g fat, 28mg cholesterol, 204mg sodium, 9g carbohydrate, 6g protein.

200. Chocolate Peanut Butter Protein Balls

Preparation Time: 10 minutes
Cooking Time: 5 minutes
Servings: 2-3
Ingredients:
- 1 1/2 cup of old-fashioned rolled oats
- 1 cup of natural peanut butter
- 1/4 cup of honey
- 2 scoops (64 grams) chocolate protein powder
- 2 Tbsp. chocolate chips

Directions:
1. 1.Place the oats, peanut butter, honey, chocolate chips and protein powder in a large bowl and stir to blend.
2. 2.It takes a little arm muscle to get the mixture to blend and it can seem too thick at first but as you keep mixing, it will come together. I used my hands at the end to knead the dough and that seemed to help.
3. 3.Use a cookie scoop to scoop and shape the dough into balls until mixed.
4. 4.Store in the freezer.

Nutrition: Calories: 114; Sugar: 5g; Fat: 6g; Carbohydrates: 8g; Fiber: 1g; Protein: 6g

201. Hummus

Preparation time: 02:20:00
Cooking Time: 0 minutes
Servings: 2-3
Ingredients:
- 1 can chickpeas, drained and rinsed
- 1 tbsp peanut butter
- 1/2 lemon, juice only
- 1 tsp lemon rind, minced
- 1 tsp salt
- 1/4 tsp red pepper flakes, crushed
- 1 tbsp olive oil
- 1 clove garlic
- Option, substitute pesto for peanut butter

Directions:
1. 1.Place everything in the food processor. Start to puree while slowly drizzling in two

tablespoons of water. Puree until exceptionally creamy.
2. 2.Place in a bowl and keep cool in the fridge until ready to enjoy with any chopped, sliced, or whole vegetable of your choice. These could include sweet bell peppers, cherry tomatoes, radishes, fennel, jicama, and snap peas.

Nutrition: Protein: 19 kcal Fat: 77 kcal Carbohydrates: 80 kcal

202. Cheese Chips

Preparation time: 20 min
Cooking time: 30 min
Servings: 2-3
Ingredients:
- 10 tbsp parmesan cheese shredded
- Garlic powder
- 2 tbsp fresh basil finely chopped

Directions:
1. 1.Heat the oven to 350 degrees. Line a baking sheet with parchment paper.
2. 2.Scoop one tablespoon of cheese and drop in a plop on the baking sheet.
3. 3.With your fingers, gently spread the cheese into a thin circle and add a pinch of garlic powder and a pinch of basil.
4. 4.Repeat until all of the cheese is gone.
5. 5.Place sheet in oven until circle edges are golden brown. Give them a minute to cool.

Nutrition: Protein: 26 kcal Fat: 239 kcal Carbohydrates: 231 kcal

203. Caprese Salad Bites

Preparation time: 10 min
Cooking time: 15 min
Servings: 2-3
Ingredients:
- For the bites
- 24 cherry tomatoes
- 12 mozzarella balls
- 12 fresh basil leaves
- For the balsamic glaze
- Preparation time: 30 min
- Cooking time: 20 min
- Ingredients ½ cup balsamic vinegar
- 2 tablespoons extra-virgin olive oil
- 1 garlic clove, minced
- 1 teaspoon Italian seasoning

Directions:
1. To make the bites
2. 1.Using 12 toothpicks or short skewers, assemble each with 1 cherry tomato, 1 mozzarella ball, 1 basil leaf, and another tomato.
3. 2.Place on a Servings: platter or in a large glass storage container that can be sealed.
4. To make the glaze
5. 1.In a small saucepan, bring the balsamic to a simmer. Simmer for 15 min, or until syrupy. Set aside to cool and thicken.
6. 2.In a small bowl, whisk olive oil, garlic, Italian seasoning, and cooled vinegar.
7. 3.Drizzle the olive oil and balsamic glaze over the skewers. Servings: immediately or keep in the refrigerator for a tasty snack.

Ingredient tip: if you do not have mozzarella balls, you can use string cheese—cut each piece into sixths.

Nutrition: calories: 39; total fat: 3g; protein: 1g; carbohydrates: 3g; fiber: 0g; sugar: 0g; sodium: 11mg.

204. Kale, Butternut Squash, and Sausage Pasta

Servings: 2-3
Preparation time: 35 min
Cooking time: 25min
Ingredients
- 6 links Italian sausage (spicy or sweet)
- 4 cups kale (roughly chopped)
- 1 cup butternut squash (diced)
- 3 cloves garlic (grated)
- ¼ cup parsley (minced)
- 1-pound whole wheat pasta (orecchiette)
- ½ cup Parmigiano-Reggiano (grated)
- ¼ cup olive oil (divided)
- Salt and pepper, to taste

Directions
1. 1.Preheat oven to 400 f.
2. 2.Line a baking sheet with foil. Coat butternut squash with olive oil, salt, and pepper. Arrange onto a single layer on the baking sheet. Roast until golden brown,

about 25-30 min. Toss once, halfway through.
3. 3.Preparation timer orecchiette pasta according to package directions. Set aside 1 cup of cooked pasta liquid. Set cooked pasta aside.
4. 4.In a deep pan over medium-high heat, heat 1 tablespoon of olive oil. Remove sausage from casings and add to pan. Begin browning the meat.
5. 5.Add grated garlic when sausage is halfway cooked. Continue cooking time until thoroughly cooked, about 7-9 min. Deglaze pan with cooked pasta liquid.
6. 6.Stir kale, 2 tablespoons of olive oil, salt, and pepper into sausage pan. Wait 2-3 min, until kale is bright green.
7. 7.Toss in cooked pasta, roasted butternut squash, parsley, and Parmigiano-Reggiano.
8. 8.Topped with Parmigiano-Reggiano and parsley as preferred.

Nutrition: Calories: 384kcalcarbohydrates: 53.2gprotein: 24gfat: 12.2gsaturated fat: 3.9gcholesterol:54mg sodium: 820mg fiber: 7.9g

205. Lemon Juice Salmon with Quinoa

Preparation time: 10 min
Cooking time: 15 min
Servings: 2-3
Ingredients: 1 lemon
- 2 8-ounce boneless salmon fillets
- 14 cherry tomatoes (halved)
- 10 white button mushrooms (thinly sliced)
- 8-10 asparagus spears
- 2 tablespoon dill (roughly chopped)
- 2 cloves garlic (minced) 2 teaspoons olive oil
- 2 teaspoons capers (optional)

Directions
1. 1.Preheat oven to 350 f.
2. 2.On a large piece of parchment paper, layer minced garlic.
3. 3.Place layer of asparagus on top of garlic.
4. 4.Arrange a salmon fillet on top of the asparagus.
5. 5.Place the mushrooms and cherry tomatoes around the salmon.
6. 5.Drizzle with lemon juice and olive oil. Season with salt, pepper, dill, and capers.
7. 7.Fold paper up above the ingredients, careful to maintain the layered arrangement.
8. 8.Tightly seal by folding the edges several times.
9. 9.Bake for 20-25 min, or until salmon is flaky. Servings: with rice, pasta, or quinoa.

Nutrition: Calories: 302kcal carbohydrates: 2.2g protein: 30.4g fat: 18.9g saturated fat: 3g cholesterol: 88mg sodium: 634mg

206. Asian Peanut Cabbage Slaw

Servings: 2-3
Preparation time: 10 min
Cooking time: 10 min
Ingredients
- 1 (14-ounce) package coleslaw
- 1 red bell pepper, thinly sliced
- 1 large carrot, grated
- ¼ cup diced scallions
- ¼ cup chopped fresh cilantro
- ¼ cup chopped peanuts
- 1/3 cup spicy peanut dressing, plus more if desired

Directions:
1. 1.In a large bowl, combine coleslaw, bell pepper, carrot, scallions, cilantro, and peanuts. Toss with the dressing, add more as desired, and servings.
2. 2.Ingredient tip: powdered peanut butter is made by dehydrating peanuts and grinding them into a powder. This reduces fat content but Preserving: protein and flavor. Use powdered peanut butter in any recipe that calls for traditional peanut butter, and you'll achieve the same great flavor. You can find powdered peanut butter in your local grocery store with the nut butters.

Nutrition: calories: 123; total fat: 6g; protein: 6g; carbohydrates: 16g; fiber: 6g; sugar: 6g; sodium: 198mg.

207. Cinnamon Fried Bananas

Preparation time: 7 minutes
Cooking Time: 5 minutes

Servings: 2-3
Ingredients:
- 1 cup panko breadcrumbs
- tbsp. cinnamon
- ½ cups almond flour
- egg whites
- ripe bananas
- tbsp. coconut oil

Directions:
1. 1.Heat coconut oil and add breadcrumbs, then mix around 3 minutes until golden and pour into a bowl.
2. 2.Peel and cut bananas in half.
3. 3.Roll the half of each banana into flour, eggs, and crumb mixture.
4. 4.Place into the Smart Air Fryer Oven. Cook 10 minutes at 280 °F.

Nutrition: Calories 221 Fat9g Carbs5g Protein 4g

208. Melting Tuna and Cheese Toasties

Preparation Time: 10 minutes
Cooking Time: 8 minutes
Servings: 2-3
Ingredients:
- 6oz. canned line caught tuna in water
- tsp. lemon juice
- 1/2 tbsp. olive oil
- A pinch of sea salt and black pepper
- 1/4 cooked yellow corn
- 4 slices of whole meal bread
- ½ cup low fat cheddar

Directions:
1. 1.Preheat your broiler/grill on its highest setting.
2. 2.Drain the tuna and flake into a bowl.
3. 3.Mix in the lemon juice and olive oil.
4. 4.Season with salt and freshly ground black pepper.
5. 5.Add in the corn.
6. 6.Toast the bread under the grill until it's nicely browned on both sides, then spread the tuna mixture on top, right up to the edges of the toast.
7. 7.Grate over the cheese and grill until the cheese is bubbling.
8. 8.Slice in half, grab a plate, and enjoy.

Nutrition: Calories: 170 Protein: 15g Carbs: 14g Fiber: 2g Sugar: 2g Fat: 4g

209. Spinach and Artichoke Dip

Preparation Time: 10 minutes
Cooking Time: 5 minutes
Servings: 2-3
Ingredients:
- 10 ounces – Baby spinach
- 14 ounces – Artichokes, frozen
- 8 ounces – Light cream cheese
- ½ cup – Onion, finely chopped
- ½ cup – Parmesan cheese
- Ingredients from the kitchen store:
- 1 tablespoon – Lemon juice
- 3 cloves – Garlic, finely grated
- ½ teaspoon – Red pepper flakes
- ½ teaspoon – Oregano
- ½ teaspoon – Pepper ground
- ¼ teaspoon – Salt

Directions:
1. 1.Wash, dry, and steam baby spinach.
2. 2.In a medium-size nonstick saucepan, pour cooking oil and sauté onion and garlic for 5 minutes on low-medium heat for about 5 minutes.
3. 3.In a food processor, put the spinach and chop.
4. 4.Now add artichokes and blend it a few moments.
5. 5.Transfer the blended artichokes and spinach into a medium-size bowl.
6. 6.Add oregano, lemon juice, red pepper, and cream cheese and stir well.
7. 7.Cook it on low-medium temperature until it starts bubbling.
8. 8.Now add salt, parmesan cheese, and pepper.
9. 9.Serve fresh

Nutrition: Calories 122, Fat 4, Carbs 18, Protein 12, Sodium 280

210. Slow Cooker Boston Beans

Preparation Time: 5 minutes
Cooking Time: 15 minutes

Servings: 2-3
Ingredients:
- 1 pound – White Northern beans, dry.
- 1 cup – Onion, finely chopped
- 2 slices – turkey bacon, chopped
- 1 cup – Dark molasses
- 2 tablespoons – Ketchup
- ¼ cup – Brown sugar
- 1 tablespoon – Mustard
- ½ teaspoon – Salt
- ½ teaspoon – Black pepper
- 3 cups – Water

Directions:
1. 1.In a medium bowl, soak the beans. Drain the beans and keep aside.
2. Put all the ingredients in a slow cooker. Set the timer for 30 minutes and start cooking. Serve hot.

Nutrition: Calories 134, Fat 6, Carbs 12, Protein 8, Sodium 234

211. Low Cholesterol Scalloped Potatoes

Preparation Time: 10 minutes
Cooking Time: 35 minutes
Servings: 2-3
Ingredients:
- 4 cups - Potatoes
- ½ cup – Onion, coarsely chopped
- 1 tablespoon – Parsley chopped
- 1½ cup – Skim milk
- 3 tablespoons – Low cholesterol margarine
- ¼ teaspoon – Ground pepper
- ½ teaspoon – Salt
- 3 tablespoons – Whole grain flour

Directions:
1. 1.Wash, clean potatoes and finely slice the potatoes.
2. 2.Stack the potatoes and onion layer by layer in a casserole.
3. 3.Drizzle flour between onion and potatoes.
4. 4.Pour milk in a medium bowl and add parsley, pepper, and salt and bring to low-medium heat. Once the milk becomes hot, pour it over the potato-onion layer.
5. 5.Cover the casserole and bake it for one hour at 350°F. Remove the cover and bake it for another 3 minutes.

Nutrition: Calories 184, Fat 6, Carbs 32, Protein 6, Sodium 324

212. Green Beans Greek Style

Preparation Time: 5 minutes
Cooking Time: 8 minutes
Servings: 2-3
Ingredients:
- 1 cup - Tomato Bouillon Soup
- 2 cups - Green beans
- 8 ounces - Water
- 1 teaspoon - Onion powder
- 1 teaspoon - Oregano
- 1 teaspoon - Garlic powder
- Parsley dash

Directions:
1. 1.In a large saucepan, pour water.
2. 2.Add tomato soup into the water.
3. 3.Now add all the ingredients into the saucepan.
4. 4.Cover the pan and cook for about 15 minutes until the beans become tender.
5. 5.Serve hot as a side dish.

Nutrition: Calories 134, Fat 2, Carbs 32, Protein 12, Sodium 309

213. Marinated Mushrooms

Preparation Time: 10 minutes
Cooking Time: 15 minutes
Servings: 2-3
Ingredients:
- 1 cup - Beef soup
- 1 teaspoon - Parsley flakes
- 1 pound - Mushrooms
- Ingredients from kitchen store:
- 1 teaspoon – Onion powder
- 8 ounces – Water
- 1 teaspoon – Garlic powder
- ¼ teaspoon – Salt

Directions:
1. 1.In a medium bowl, dissolve the beef soup in water

2. 2.Put all the remaining ingredients in the soup and water mix. Cover it and boil in low-medium heat at least for 2 hours.

Nutrition: Calories 186, Fat 2, Carbs 31, Protein 8, Sodium 155

214. Moch Mashed Potatoes

Preparation Time: 5 minutes
Cooking Time: 18 minutes
Servings: 2-3
Ingredients:
- 1 cup - Tomato chicken soup
- 4 ounces – Frozen cauliflower
- ¼ teaspoon - Salt
- 6 cup – Water

Directions:
1. 1.Cook cauliflower for about 15 minutes in a small saucepan by adding the salt until it becomes soft.
2. 2.Drain excess water after cooking.
3. 3.Mash the cooked cauliflower. Add the chicken soup into the masked cauliflower and heat the mix for 2 minutes. Serve hot.

Nutrition: Calories 165, Fat 3, Carbs 33, Protein 12, Sodium 318

215. No Dish Summer Medley

Preparation Time: 10 minutes
Cooking Time: 10 minutes
Servings: 2-3
Ingredients:
- 2 cup - Chicken soup
- ½ cup – Sliced celery
- ½ cup - Yellow summer squash
- ½ cup – Mushrooms, chopped
- ¼ teaspoon – Salt
- ¼ teaspoon – Black pepper powder

Directions:
1. 1.In a medium saucepan mix all the ingredients, except the chicken soup.
2. 2.Now pour the chicken soup over it.
3. 3.Add salt and pepper.
4. 4.Cover and cook for 20 minutes until it starting to boil

Nutrition: Calories 212, Fat 4, Carbs 18, Protein 8, Sodium 234

216. Pureed Classic Egg Salad

Preparation Time: 5 minutes
Cooking Time: 2 minutes
Servings: 2-3
Ingredients:
- 2 - Eggs, hard-boiled
- 1 tablespoon - Low-fat mayonnaise
- 1 tablespoon – Greek yogurt, plain

Directions:
1. 1.Cut the boiled eggs to even portions.
2. 2.Put the slices of eggs into a food-mixer and chop it.
3. 3.Add salt, mayonnaise, and Greek yogurt as the seasonings to the eggs
4. 4.Mix finely as far as the egg salad becomes smooth.

Nutrition: Calories 134, Fat 2, Carbs 12, Protein 6, Sodium 320

217. Maple-Mashed Sweet Potatoes

Preparation Time: 5 minutes
Cooking Time: 5 minutes
Servings: 2-3
Ingredients:
- 1 pound – Sweet potatoes
- 1 cup – Carrots, thinly sliced
- 2 tablespoons – Maple syrup
- ¼ teaspoon – Nutmeg
- ¼ teaspoon – Fresh ground pepper
- 4 cup – Water

Directions:
1. 1.Wash and clean sweet potatoes.
2. 2.Peel and cut into small chunks.
3. 3.In a large bowl, pour water and bring to boil.
4. 4.5.Put carrots and sweet potatoes into it.
5. 6.7.Reduce heat and continue cooking for about 10 minutes until the carrots and sweet potatoes become soft.
6. 8.Drain the vegetables using a colander and put them into a bowl.
7. 9.Mas the vegetables until it becomes smooth.
8. 10.Sprinkle ground pepper and nutmeg into it and stir.

9. 11.Drizzle maple syrup over it, and stir.

Nutrition: Calories 212, Fat 4, Carbs 18, Protein 6, Sodium 176

218. Garlic-Parmesan Cheesy Chips

Preparation Time: 2 minutes + 20 minutes to cool
Cooking Time: 7 minutes
Servings: 2-3
Ingredients:
- ¼ cup shredded Parmesan cheese
- ¼ cup shredded sharp Cheddar cheese
- ¼ teaspoon garlic powder
- Dash salt

Directions:

1. 1.Preheat the oven to 400°F. Line a large baking sheet with parchment paper.
2. 2.In a medium mixing bowl, combine the Parmesan cheese, Cheddar cheese, garlic powder, and salt. Mix well.
3. 3.Place 2 teaspoons of the cheese mixture about an inch or two apart on the baking sheet, making about 12 chips.
4. 4.Bake for 5 to 7 minutes, or until the chips are golden brown around the edges.
5. 5.Remove from the oven and let sit for 15 to 20 minutes, or until the chips start to crisp. Enjoy.

Nutrition: PER SERVING (6 CHIPS): Calories: 98; Protein: 8g; Fat: 7g; Carbohydrate: 1g; Fiber: 0g; Sugar: 0g; Sodium: 333mg

STAPLES, SAUCES, DIPS AND DRESSINGS

219. Roasted Garlic Dip

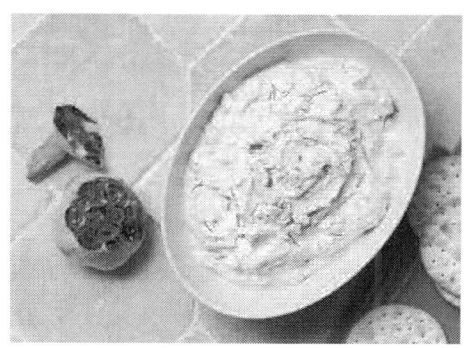

Preparation Time: 10 minutes

Servings: 2-3
Ingredients:
- 1 head garlic
- ½ tablespoon olive oil

Directions:
1. Slice the top off the garlic.
2. Drizzle with the olive oil.
3. Add to the air fryer.
4. Set it to roast.
5. Cook at 390 degrees F for 20 minutes.
6. Peel the garlic.
7. Transfer to a food processor.
8. Pulse until smooth.

Nutrition: Calories: 207cal, Carbs: 17g, Protein: 9g, Fat: 12g.

220. Cashew Yogurt

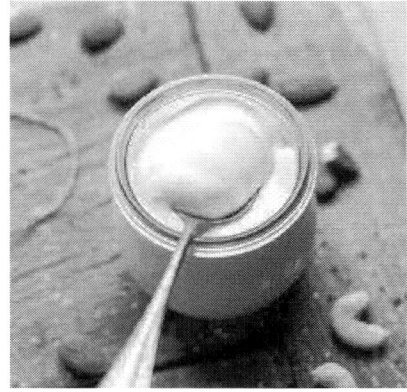

Preparation time: 12 hours and 5 minutes

Servings: 8
Ingredients:
- 3 probiotic supplements
- 2 2/3 cups cashews, unsalted, soaked in warm water for 15 minutes
- 1/4 teaspoon sea salt
- 4 tablespoon lemon juice
- 1 1/2 cup water

Directions:
1. Drain the cashews, add them into the food processor, then add remaining ingredients, except for probiotic supplements, and pulse for 2 minutes until smooth.
2. Tip the mixture in a bowl, add probiotic supplements, stir until mixed, then cover the bowl with a cheesecloth and let it stand for 12 hours in a dark and cool room.
3. Serve straight away.

Nutrition: Calories: 252 Cal Fat: 19.8 g Carbs: 14.1 g Protein: 8.3g Fiber: 1.5g

221. Artichoke Spinach Dip

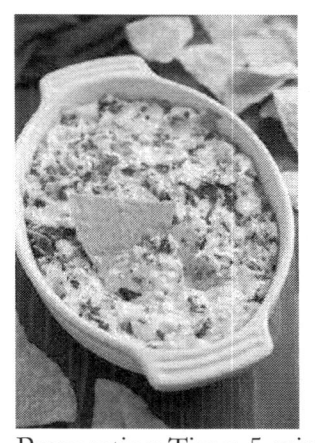

Preparation Time: 5 minutes

Servings: 3 ½ cups
Ingredients:
- 1 (10-ounce package spinach, chopped
- ⅓ cup nutritional yeast
- 2 (8-ounce jars marinated artichoke hearts
- ½ teaspoon Tabasco sauce
- 3 scallions, minced

- 1 tablespoon fresh lemon juice
- 1 cup vegan cream cheese
- ½ teaspoon salt

Directions:
1. Drain the artichoke hearts and chop them finely.
2. Add the scallions, lemon juice, salt, artichoke hearts, sauce, spinach and yeast in an instant pot.
3. Cover and cook for about 3 minutes.
4. Add the cheese and stir well.
5. Serve warm.

Nutrition: Calories 194, Total Fat 10g, Total Carbs 2g, Protein 7g, Cholesterol 54mg, Sugar 1g

222. Chickpea & Artichoke Mushroom Pâté

Preparation Time: 15 minutes
Cooking Time: 1 minutes
Servings: 6-8

Ingredients:
- 2 cups canned artichoke hearts, drained
- 1½ cups cooked chickpeas
- 3 garlic cloves, chopped
- 1 tablespoon fresh lemon juice
- 1 teaspoon dried basil
- ½ cup raw cashews, soaked overnight and drained
- 1 cup chopped mushrooms
- Shredded fresh basil leaves, for garnish
- 1 cup crumbled extra-firm tofu
- Salt and black pepper
- Paprika, for garnish

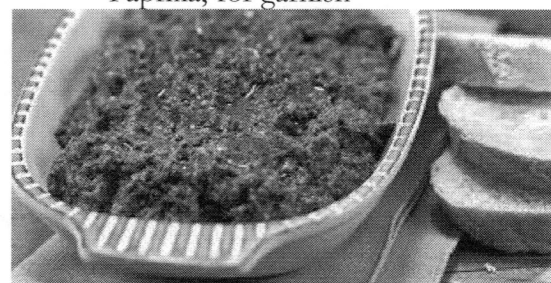

Directions:
2. Drain them to get rid of excess liquid.
3. Add the cashews, tofu in a blender and blend until smooth.
4. Add the artichoke mixture, lemon juice, salt, chickpeas, basil and pepper.
5. Blend again and pour into a loaf pan.
6. Cover with aluminum foil and poke some holes on top.
7. Add to your instant pot and cook for about 3 minutes.
8. Let it cool down and refrigerate until served.
9. Garnish using basil, paprika.

Nutrition: Calories: 260, Fat: 12 g, Carbs: 29 g, Protein: 12 g Fiber: 7 g, Sugar 2 g, Sodium 63 mg.

223. Buffalo Dip

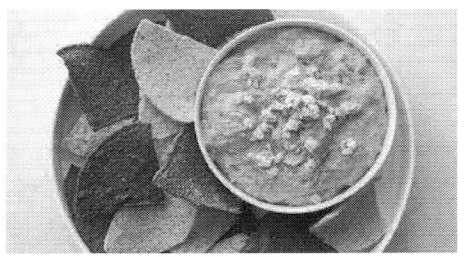

Preparation time: 20 minutes

Servings: 4
Ingredients:
- 2 cups cashews
- 2 teaspoons garlic powder
- 1 1/2 teaspoons salt
- 2 teaspoons onion powder
- 3 tablespoons lemon juice
- 1 cup buffalo sauce
- 1 cup of water
- 14-ounce artichoke hearts, packed in water, drained

Directions:
1. Switch on the oven, then set it to 375 degrees F and let it preheat.
2. Meanwhile, pour 3 cups of boiling water in a bowl, add cashews and let soak for 5 minutes.
3. Then drain the cashew, transfer them into the blender, pour in water, add lemon juice

and all the seasoning and blend until smooth.
4. Add artichokes and buffalo sauce, process until chunky mixture comes together, and then transfer the dip to an ovenproof dish.
5. Bake for 20 minutes and then serve.

Nutrition: Calories: 100 Cal Fat: 100 g Carbs: 100 g Protein: 100 g Fiber: 100g

224. Barbecue Sauce

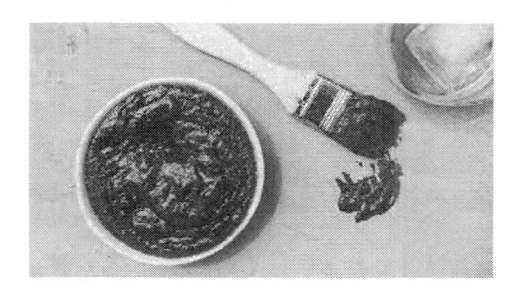

Cooking Time: 0 minutes
Servings: 16
Ingredients:
- 8 ounces tomato sauce
- 1 teaspoon garlic powder
- ¼ teaspoon ground black pepper
- 1/2 teaspoon. sea salt
- 2 Tablespoons Dijon mustard
- 3 packets stevia
- 1 teaspoon molasses
- 1 Tablespoon apple cider vinegar
- 2 Tablespoons tamari
- 1 teaspoon liquid aminos

Directions:
1. Take a medium bowl, place all the ingredients in it, and stir until combined.
2. Serve straight away

Nutrition: Calories: 29 Cal Fat: 0.1 g Carbs: 7 g Protein: 0.1 g Fiber: 0.1 g

225. Barbecue Tahini Sauce

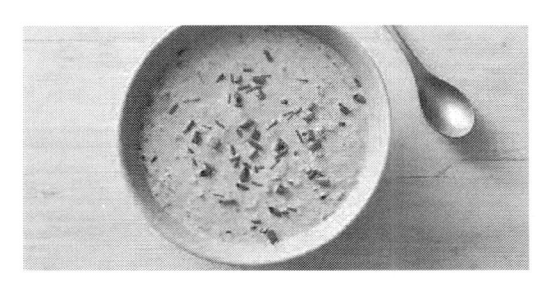

Cooking Time: 0 minutes
Servings: 8
Ingredients:
- 6 tablespoons tahini
- 3/4 teaspoon garlic powder
- 1/8 teaspoon red chili powder
- 2 teaspoons maple syrup
- 1/4 teaspoon salt
- 3 teaspoons molasses
- 3 teaspoons apple cider vinegar
- 1/4 teaspoon liquid smoke
- 10 teaspoons tomato paste
- 1/2 cup water

Directions:
1. Place all the ingredients in the order in a food processor or blender and then pulse for 3 to 5 minutes at high speed until smooth.
2. Tip the sauce in a bowl and then serve.

Nutrition: Calories: 86 Cal Fat: 5 g Carbs: 7 g Protein: 2 g Fiber: 0 g

226. Bolognese Sauce

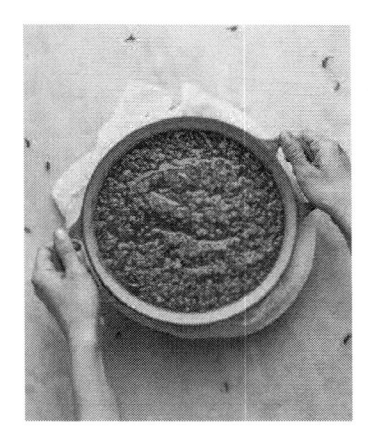

Cooking Time: 0 minutes
Servings: 8
Ingredients:
- ½ of small green bell pepper, chopped
- 1 stalk of celery, chopped
- 1 small carrot, chopped
- 1 medium white onion, peeled, chopped
- 2 teaspoons minced garlic
- 1/2 teaspoon crushed red pepper flakes
- 3 tablespoons olive oil
- 8-ounce tempeh, crumbled

- 8 ounces white mushrooms, chopped
- 1/2 cup dried red lentils
- 28-ounce crushed tomatoes
- 28-ounce whole tomatoes, chopped
- 1 teaspoon dried oregano
- 1/2 teaspoon fennel seed
- 1/2 teaspoon ground black pepper
- 1/2 teaspoon salt
- 1 teaspoon dried basil
- 1/4 cup chopped parsley
- 1 bay leaf
- 6-ounce tomato paste
- 1 cup dry red wine

Directions:
1. Take a Dutch oven, place it over medium heat, add oil, and when hot, add the first six ingredients, stir and cook: for 5 minutes until sauté.
2. Then switch heat to medium-high level, add two ingredients after olive oil, stir and cook for 3 minutes.
3. Switch heat to medium-low level, stir in tomato paste, and continue cooking for 2 minutes.
4. Add remaining ingredients except for lentils, stir and bring the mixture to boil.
5. Switch heat to the low level, simmer sauce for 10 minutes, covering the pan partially, then add lentils and continue cooking for 20 minutes until tender.
6. Serve sauce with cooked pasta.

Nutrition: Calories: 208.8 Cal Fat: 12 g Carbs: 17.8 g Protein: 10.6 g Fiber: 3.8 g

227. Chipotle Bean Cheesy Dip

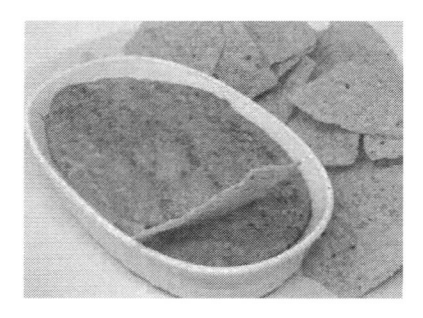

Cooking Time: 0 minutes
Servings: 3 cups
Ingredients:

- 2 cups pinto beans, cooked, mashed
- 1 tablespoon chipotle chiles in adobo, minced
- ¼ cup water
- ½ cup shredded vegan cheddar cheese
- ¾ cup tomato salsa
- 1 teaspoon chili powder
- Salt

Directions:
1. In a bowl combine the mashed beans, chipotle chile, salsa, chili powder and water in an instant pot.
2. Mix well and cover with lid.
3. Cook for about 5 minutes.
4. Add the cheddar cheese and salt and serve warm.
5. Drain the tomatoes and add to a blender.

Nutrition: Calories: 217, Fat: 19 g, Carbs: 3 g, Protein: 9 g Fiber: 1 g, Sugar 2 g, Sodium 636 mg.

228. Cilantro and Parsley Hot Sauce

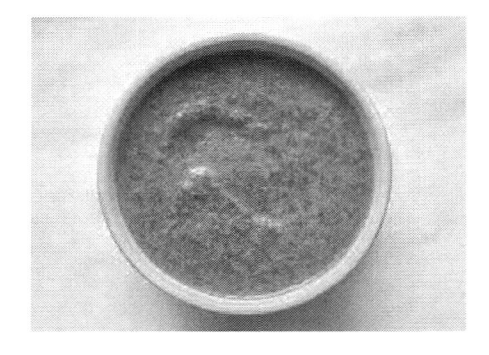

Cooking Time: 0 minutes
Servings: 4
Ingredients:

- 2 cups of parsley and cilantro leaves with stems
- 4 Thai bird chilies, destemmed, deseeded, torn
- 2 teaspoons minced garlic
- 1 teaspoon salt
- 1/4 teaspoon coriander seed, ground
- 1/4 teaspoon ground black pepper
- 1/2 teaspoon cumin seeds, ground
- 3 green cardamom pods, toasted, ground
- 1/2 cup olive oil

Directions:

1. Take a spice blender or a food processor, place all the ingredients in it, and process for 5 minutes until the smooth paste comes together.
2. Serve straight away.

Nutrition: Calories: 130 Cal Fat: 14 g Carbs: 2 g Protein: 1 g Fiber: 1 g

FISH AND SEAFOOD

229. Lemon-Caper Trout with Caramelized Shallots

Preparation Time: 10 minutes
Cooking Time: 20 minutes
Servings: 2
Ingredients:
- For the Shallots
- 2 shallots, thinly sliced
- 1 teaspoon ghee
- Dash salt
- For the Trout
- 1 tablespoon plus 1 teaspoon ghee, divided
- 2 (4-ounce) trout fillets
- ¼ cup freshly squeezed lemon juice
- 3 tablespoons capers
- ¼ teaspoon salt
- Dash freshly ground black pepper
- 1 lemon, thinly sliced

Directions:
1. To make the Shallot:
2. In a huge skillet on medium heat, cook the shallots, ghee, and salt for 20 minutes, stirring every 5 minutes, until the shallots have fully wilted and caramelized.
3. To make the Trout:
4. While the shallots cook, in another large skillet over medium heat, heat 1 teaspoon of ghee.
5. Add the trout fillets. Cook for at least 3 minutes on each side or until the center is flaky. Transfer to a plate and set aside.
6. In the skillet used for the trout, add lemon juice, capers, salt, and pepper. Bring it to a simmer. Whisk in the remaining 1 tablespoon of ghee. Spoon the sauce over the fish.
7. Garnish the fish with lemon slices and caramelized shallots before serving.

Nutrition: Calories: 399 | Total Fat: 22g | Saturated Fat: 10g | Cholesterol: 46mg | Carbohydrates: 17g | Fiber: 2g | Protein: 21g

230. Shrimp Scampi

Preparation Time: 10 minutes
Cooking Time: 15 minutes
Servings: 4
Ingredients:
- ¼ cup Extra Olive Oil
- 1 Onion, Finely Chopped
- 1 Red Bell Pepper, Chopped
- 1½ Pound Shrimp, Peeled and Tails Removed
- 6 Garlic Cloves, Minced
- 2 Lemon Juices
- 2 Lemon Zest
- ½ tsp. Sea Salt
- ⅛ tsp. Freshly Ground Black Pepper

Directions:
1. In a huge nonstick skillet on medium-high heat, warm the olive oil until it shimmers.
2. Add the onion and red bell pepper. Cook for about 6 minutes, occasionally stirring, until soft.
3. Add the shrimp and cook for about 5 minutes until pink.
4. Add the garlic. Cook for 30 seconds, stirring constantly.
5. Add the lemon juice and zest, salt, and pepper. Simmer for 3 minutes.

Nutrition: | Calories: 345 | Total Fat: 16 | Total Carbs: 10g | Sugar: 3g | Fiber: 1g | Protein: 40g | Sodium: 424mg

231. Shrimp with Spicy Spinach

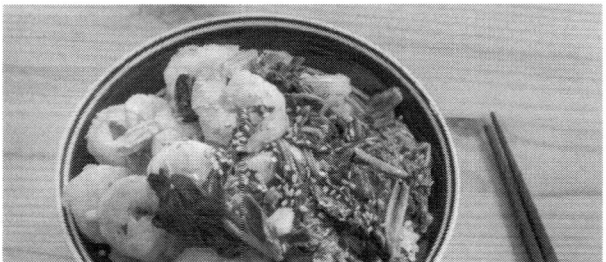

Preparation Time: 10 minutes
Cooking Time: 15 minutes

Servings: 4
Ingredients:
- ¼ cup Extra Olive Oil, divided
- 1½ Pound Peeled Shrimp
- 1 tsp. Sea Salt, divided
- 4 cups Baby Fresh Spinach
- 6 Garlic cloves, minced
- ½ cup Freshly Squeezed Orange Juice
- 1 tbsp. Sriracha Sauce
- ⅛ tsp. Freshly ground black pepper

Directions:
1. In a huge nonstick skillet on medium-high heat, heat 2 tablespoons of the olive oil until it shimmers.
2. Add the shrimp and ½ teaspoon salt. Cook for at least 4 minutes, occasionally stirring, until the shrimp are pink. Transfer the shrimp to a plate, tent with aluminum foil to keep warm, and set aside.
3. Put back the skillet to the heat and heat the remaining 2 tablespoons of olive oil until it shimmers.
4. Add the spinach. Cook for 3 minutes, stirring.
5. Add the garlic. Cook for 30 seconds, stirring constantly.
6. In a small bowl, put and mix together the orange juice, Sriracha, remaining ½ teaspoon of salt, and pepper. Add this to the spinach and cook for 3 minutes. Serve the shrimp with spinach on the side.

Nutrition: Calories: 317|**Total Fat:** 16|**Total Carbs:** 7g|**Sugar:** 3|**Fiber:** 1g|**Protein:** 38g|**Sodium:** 911mg

232. Shrimp with Cinnamon Sauce

Preparation Time: 10 minutes
Cooking Time: 10 minutes
Servings: 4
Ingredients:
- 2 tbsp. Extra Virgin Olive Oil
- 1½ Pound Peeled Shrimp
- 2 tbsp. Dijon Mustard
- 1 cup No Salt Added Chicken Broth
- 1 tsp. Ground Cinnamon
- 1 tsp. Onion Powder
- ½ tsp. Sea Salt
- ¼ tsp. Freshly Ground Black Pepper

Directions:
1. In a huge nonstick skillet at medium-high heat, heat the olive oil until it shimmers.
2. Add the shrimp. Cook for at least 4 minutes, occasionally stirring, until the shrimp is opaque.
3. Whisk the mustard, chicken broth, cinnamon, onion powder, salt, and pepper in a small bowl. Pour this into the skillet and continue to cook for 3 minutes, stirring occasionally.

Nutrition: Calories: 270|**Total Fat:** 11g|**Total Carbs:** 4g|**Sugar:** 1g|**Fiber:** 1g|**Protein:** 39g|**Sodium:** 664mg

233. Pan-Seared Scallops with Lemon-Ginger Vinaigrette

Preparation Time: 10 minutes
Cooking Time: 7 minutes
Servings: 4
Ingredients:
- 2 tbsp. Extra Virgin Olive Oil
- 1½ Pound Sea Scallop
- ½ tsp. Sea Salt
- ⅛ tsp. Freshly Ground Black Pepper
- ¼ cup Lemon Ginger Vinaigrette

Directions:
1. In a huge nonstick skillet at medium-high heat, heat the olive oil until it shimmers.
2. Season the scallops with pepper and salt and add them to the skillet. Cook for at least 3 minutes per side until just opaque.
3. Serve with the vinaigrette spooned over the top.

Nutrition: Calories: 280|**Total Fat:** 16|**Total Carbs:** 5g|**Sugar:** 1g|**Fiber:** 0g|**Protein:** 29g|**Sodium:** 508mg

234. Manhattan-Style Salmon Chowder

Preparation Time: 10 minutes
Cooking Time: 15 minutes
Servings: 4

Ingredients:
- ¼ cup Extra Virgin Olive Oil
- 1 Red Bell Pepper, Chopped
- 1 Pound Skinless Salmon. Pin Bones removed, chopped into ½ inch
- 2 (28 oz.) Cans Crushed Tomatoes, 1 Drained, 1 undrained
- 6 cups No salt added chicken broth
- 2 cups diced (1/2 inch) Sweet Potato
- 1 tsp. Onion Powder
- ½ tsp. Sea Salt
- ¼ tsp. Freshly Ground Black Pepper

Directions:
1. Add the red bell pepper and salmon. Cook for at least 5 minutes, occasionally stirring, until the fish is opaque and the bell pepper is soft.
2. Stir in the tomatoes, chicken broth, sweet potatoes, onion powder, salt, and pepper. Place to a simmer, then lower the heat to medium. Cook for at least 10 minutes, occasionally stirring, until the sweet potatoes are soft.

Nutrition: Calories: 570 | Total Fat: 42 | Total Carbs: 55g | Sugar: 24g | Fiber: 16g | Protein: 41g | Sodium: 1,249mg

235. Roasted Salmon and Asparagus

Preparation Time: 5 minutes
Cooking Time: 15 minutes
Servings: 4
Ingredients:
- 1-pound Asparagus Spears, trimmed
- 2 tbsp. Extra Virgin Olive Oil
- 1 tsp. Sea Salt, divide
- 1½ pound Salmon, cut into 4 fillets
- ⅛ tsp. freshly ground cracked black pepper
- 1 Lemon, zest, and slice

Directions:
1. Preheat the oven to 425°F.
2. Stir the asparagus with olive oil, then put ½ teaspoon of the salt. Place in a single layer in the bottom of a roasting pan.
3. Season the salmon with the pepper and the remaining ½ teaspoon of salt. Put skin-side down on top of the asparagus.
4. Sprinkle the salmon and asparagus with the lemon zest and place the lemon slices over the fish.
5. Roast at the oven for at least 12 to 15 minutes until the flesh is opaque.

Nutrition: Calories: 308 | Total Fat: 18g | Total Carbs: 5g | Sugar: 2g | Fiber: 2 | Protein: 36g | Sodium: 545mg

236. Citrus Salmon on a Bed of Greens

Preparation Time: 10 minutes
Cooking Time: 19 minutes
Servings: 4
Ingredients:
- ¼ cup Extra Virgin Olive Oil, divided
- 1½ pound Salmon
- 1 tsp. Sea Salt, divided
- ½ tsp. Freshly ground black pepper, divided
- 1 Lemon Zest
- 6 cups Swiss Chard, stemmed and chopped
- 3 Garlic cloves, chopped
- 2 Lemon Juice

Directions:
1. In a huge nonstick skillet at medium-high heat, heat 2 tablespoons of the olive oil until it shimmers.
2. Season the salmon with ½ teaspoon of salt, ¼ teaspoon of pepper, and lemon zest. Put the salmon in the skillet, skin-side up, and cook for about 7 minutes until the flesh is opaque. Flip the salmon and cook for at least 3 to 4 minutes to crisp the skin. Set aside on a plate, cover using aluminum foil.
3. Put back the skillet to the heat, add the remaining 2 tablespoons of olive oil, and heat it until it shimmers.
4. Add the Swiss chard. Cook for about 7 minutes, occasionally stirring, until soft.
5. Add the garlic. Cook for 30 seconds, stirring constantly.
6. Sprinkle in the lemon juice, the remaining ½ teaspoon of salt, and the remaining ¼ teaspoon of pepper. Cook for 2 minutes.

7. Serve the salmon on the Swiss chard.

Nutrition: Calories: 363 | Total Fat: 25 | Total Carbs: 3 | Sugar: 1 | Fiber: 1 | Protein: 34g | Sodium: 662mg

237. Orange and Maple-Glazed Salmon

Preparation Time: 15 minutes
Cooking Time: 15 minutes
Servings: 4
Ingredients:
- 2 Orange Juice
- 1 Orange Zest
- ¼ cup Pure maple syrup
- 2 tbsp. Low Sodium Soy Sauce
- 1 tsp. Garlic Powder
- 4 4-6 oz. Salmon Fillet, Pin bones removed

Directions:
1. Preheat the oven to 400°F.
2. Whisk the orange juice and zest, maple syrup, soy sauce, and garlic powder in a small, shallow dish.
3. Put the salmon pieces, flesh-side down, into the dish. Let it marinate for 10 minutes.
4. Transfer the salmon, skin-side up, to a rimmed baking sheet and bake for about 15 minutes until the flesh is opaque.

Nutrition: Calories: 297 | Total Fat: 11 | Total Carbs: 18g | Sugar: 15g Fiber: 1g | Protein: 34 | Sodium: 528mg

238. Salmon Ceviche

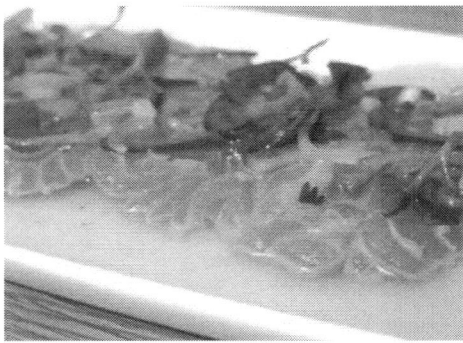

Preparation Time: 10 minutes +20 resting time
Cooking Time: 0 minutes

Ingredients:
- 1-pound Salmon, skinless & boneless, cut into bite-size pieces
- ½ cup Freshly squeezed lime juice
- 2 Tomatoes, diced
- ¼ cup Fresh Cilantro Leaves, chopped
- 1 Jalapeno Pepper, seeded and diced
- 2 tbsp. Extra Virgin Olive Oil
- ½ tsp. Sea Salt

Directions:
1. In a medium bowl, put and stir together the salmon and lime juice. Let it marinate for 20 minutes.
2. Stir in the tomatoes, cilantro, jalapeño, olive oil, and salt.

Nutrition: Calories: 222 | Total Fat: 14g | Total Carbs: 3g | Sugar: 2 | Fiber: 1 | Protein: 23 | Sodium: 288mg

239. Cod with Ginger

Preparation Time: 10 minutes
Cooking Time: 15 minutes
Servings: 4
Ingredients:
- 2 tbsp. Extra Virgin Olive Oil
- 4 (6 oz.) Cod Fillets
- 1 tbsp. Grated fresh ginger
- 1 tsp. Sea Salt, divided
- ¼ tsp. Freshly ground black pepper
- 5 Garlic cloves, minced
- ¼ cup Fresh Cilantro Leaves, chopped

Directions:
1. In a huge nonstick skillet at medium-high heat, heat the olive oil until it shimmers.
2. Season the cod with ginger, ½ teaspoon of salt, and pepper. Put it in the hot oil, then cook for at least 4 minutes per side until the fish is opaque. Take off the cod from the pan and set it aside on a platter tented with aluminum foil.
3. Put back the skillet to the heat and add the garlic. Cook for 30 seconds, stirring constantly.
4. Cook for 5 minutes, stirring occasionally.
5. Stir in the cilantro over the cod.

Nutrition: Calories: 41 | Total Fat: 2g | Total Carbs: 33 | Sugar: 1g | Fiber: 8 | Protein: 50g | Sodium: 605mg

240. Rosemary-Lemon Cod

Preparation Time: 5 minutes
Cooking Time: 10 minutes
Servings: 4
Ingredients:
- 2 tbsp. Extra Virgin Olive Oil
- 1½ pound Cod, Skin and Bone Removed, cut into 4 fillets
- 1 tbsp. Fresh Rosemary Leaves, chopped
- ½ tsp. Ground black pepper, or more to taste
- ½ tsp. Sea Salt
- 1 Lemon Juice

Directions:
1. In a huge nonstick skillet at medium-high heat, heat the olive oil until it shimmers.
2. Season the cod with rosemary, pepper, and salt. Put the fish in the skillet and cook for 3 to 5 minutes per side until opaque.
3. Pour the lemon juice over the cod fillets and cook for 1 minute.

Nutrition: Calories: 24|Total Fat: 9g|Total Carbs: 1g|Sugar: 1g|Fiber: 1g|Protein: 39g|Sodium: 370mg

241. Halibut Curry

Preparation Time: 10 minutes
Cooking Time: 10 minutes
Servings: 4
Ingredients:
- 2 tbsp. Extra Virgin Olive Oil
- 2 tsp. Ground Turmeric
- 2 tsp. Curry Powder
- 1½ pound Halibut, skin, and bones removed, cut into 1-inch pieces
- 4 cups No-salt added chicken broth
- 1 (14 oz.) can Lite coconut milk
- ½ tsp. Sea Salt
- ¼ tsp. Freshly ground black pepper

Directions:
1. In a huge nonstick skillet at medium-high, heat the olive oil until it shimmers.
2. Add the turmeric and curry powder. Cook for 2 minutes, constantly stirring, to bloom the spices.
3. Add the halibut, chicken broth, coconut milk, salt, and pepper. Place to a simmer, then lower the heat to medium. Simmer for 6 to 7 minutes, occasionally stirring, until the fish is opaque.

Nutrition: Calories: 429|Total Fat: 47g|Total Carbs: 5g|Sugar: 1g|Fiber: 1g|Protein: 27g|Sodium: 507mg

242. Lemony Mussels

Preparation Time: 5 minutes
Cooking Time: 5 minutes
Servings: 4
Ingredients:
- 1 tbsp. extra virgin extra virgin olive oil
- 2 minced garlic cloves
- 2 lbs. scrubbed mussels
- Juice of one lemon

Directions:
1. Put some water in a pot, add mussels, bring with a boil over medium heat, cook for 5 minutes, discard unopened mussels and transfer them with a bowl.
2. Mix the oil with garlic and freshly squeezed lemon juice in another bowl, whisk well, and add over the mussels, toss and serve.
3. Enjoy!

Nutrition: Calories: 140 | Fat: 4g|Carbs: 8g|Protein: 8g |Sugars: 4g|Sodium: 600 mg

243. Hot Tuna Steak

Preparation Time: 10 minutes
Cooking Time: 25 minutes
Servings: 6
Ingredients:
- 2 tbsps. Fresh lemon juice
- Pepper.
- Roasted orange garlic mayonnaise
- ¼ c. whole black peppercorns
- 6 sliced tuna steaks
- 2 tbsps. Extra-virgin olive oil
- Salt

Directions:
1. Bring the tuna in a bowl to fit. Put the oil, lemon juice, salt, and pepper. Turn the tuna to coat well in the marinade.

2. Rest for at least 15 to 20 minutes, turning once.
3. Put the peppercorns in a double thickness of plastic bags. Tap the peppercorns with a heavy saucepan or small mallet to crush them coarsely. Put on a large plate.
4. Once ready to cook the tuna, dip the edges into the crushed peppercorns. Heat a nonstick skillet over medium heat. Sear the tuna steaks, in batches if necessary, for 4 minutes per side for medium-rare fish, adding 2 to 3 tablespoons of the marinade to the skillet if necessary to prevent sticking.
5. Serve dolloped with roasted orange garlic mayonnaise

Nutrition: Calories: 124 | Fat: 0.4 g | Carbs: 0.6 g | Protein: 28 g | Sugars: 0 g | Sodium: 77 mg

244. Marinated Fish Steaks

Preparation Time: 10 minutes
Cooking Time: 15 minutes
Servings: 4
Ingredients:
- 4 lime wedges
- 2 tbsps. Lime juice
- 2 minced garlic cloves
- 2 tsp. Olive oil
- 1 tbsp. snipped fresh oregano
- 1 lb. fresh swordfish
- 1 tsp. lemon-pepper seasoning

Directions:
1. Rinse fish steaks; pat dry using paper towels. Cut into four serving-size pieces, if necessary.
2. Put and combine lime juice, oregano, oil, lemon-pepper seasoning, and garlic in a shallow dish. Add fish; turn to coat with marinade.
3. Cover and marinate in the refrigerator for 30 minutes to 1-1/2 hours, turning steaks occasionally. Drain fish, reserving marinade.
4. Put the fish on the greased, unheated rack of a broiler pan.
5. Broil 4 inches from the heat for at least 8 to 12 minutes or until fish starts to flake when tested with a fork, turning once and brushing with reserved marinade halfway through cooking.
6. Take off any remaining marinade.
7. Before serving, squeeze the lime juice on each steak.

Nutrition: Calories: 240 | Fat: 6 | Carbs: 19 g | Protein: 12 g | Sugars: 3.27 g | Sodium: 325 mg

245. Baked Tomato Hake

Preparation Time: 10 minutes
Cooking Time: 20-25 minutes
Servings: 4
Ingredients:
- ½ c. tomato sauce
- 1 tbsp. olive oil
- Parsley
- 2 sliced tomatoes
- ½ c. grated cheese
- 4 lbs. de-boned and sliced hake fish
- Salt.

Directions:
1. Preheat the oven to 400 0F.
2. Season the fish with salt.
3. In a skillet or saucepan, stir-fry the fish in the olive oil until half-done.
4. Take four foil papers to cover the fish.
5. Shape the foil to resemble containers; add the tomato sauce into each foil container.
6. Add the fish, tomato slices, and top with grated cheese.
7. Bake until you get a golden crust, for approximately 20-25 minutes.
8. Open the packs and top with parsley.

Nutrition: Calories: 265 | Fat: 15 g | Carbs: 18 g | Protein: 22 g | Sugars: 0.5 g | Sodium: 94.6 mg

246. Cheesy Tuna Pasta

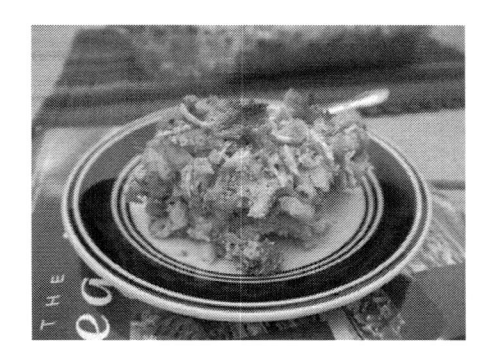

Preparation Time: 10 minutes
Cooking Time: 20 minutes
Servings: 2-4
Ingredients:
- 2 c. arugula
- ¼ c. chopped green onions
- 1 tbs. red vinegar
- 5 oz. drained canned tuna
- ¼ tsp. black pepper
- 2 oz. cooked whole-wheat pasta
- 1 tbsp. olive oil
- 1 tbsp. grated low-fat parmesan

Directions:
1. Cook the pasta in unsalted water until ready. Drain and set aside.
2. Thoroughly mix the tuna, green onions, vinegar, oil, arugula, pasta, and black pepper in a large-sized bowl.
3. Toss well and top with the cheese.
4. Serve and enjoy.

Nutrition: Calories: 566.3 | Fat: 42.4 g | Carbs: 18.6 | Protein: 29.8 g | Sugars: 0.4 g | Sodium: 688.6 mg

247. Salmon and Roasted Peppers

Preparation Time: 5 minutes
Cooking Time: 25 minutes
Servings: 4
Ingredients:
- 1 cup red peppers, cut into strips
- 4 salmon fillets, boneless
- ¼ cup chicken stock
- 2 tablespoons olive oil
- 1 yellow onion, chopped
- 1 tablespoon cilantro, chopped
- Pinch of sea salt
- Pinch black pepper

Directions:
1. Warm a pan with the oil on medium-high heat; add the onion and sauté for 5 minutes.
2. Put the fish and cook for at least 5 minutes on each side.
3. Add the rest of the ingredients, introduce the pan in the oven, and cook at 390 degrees F for 10 minutes.
4. Divide the mix between plates and serve.

Nutrition: Calories 265 | Fat 7 | Fiber | Carbs 1 | Protein 16

248. Shrimp and Beets

Preparation Time: 10 minutes
Cooking Time: 10 minutes
Servings: 4
Ingredients:
- 1-pound shrimp, peeled and deveined
- 2 tablespoons avocado oil
- 2 spring onions, chopped
- 2 garlic cloves, minced
- 1 beet, peeled and cubed
- 1 tablespoon lemon juice
- Pinch of sea salt
- Pinch of black pepper
- 1 teaspoon coconut aminos

Directions:
1. Warm a pan with the oil on medium-high heat, add the spring onions and the garlic and sauté for 2 minutes.
2. Add the shrimp and the other ingredients, toss, cook the mix for 8 minutes, divide into bowls and serve.

Nutrition: Calories 281 | Fat 6 | Fiber 7 | Carbs 11 | Protein 8

249. Shrimp and Corn

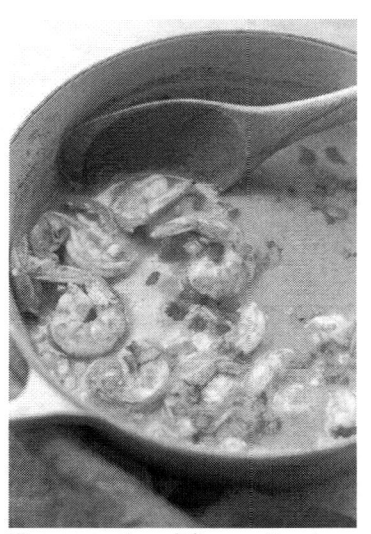

Preparation Time: 5 minutes

Servings: 4

Ingredients:
- 1-pound shrimp, peeled and deveined
- 2 garlic cloves, minced
- 1 cup corn
- ½ cup veggie stock
- 1 bunch parsley, chopped
- Juice of 1 lime
- 2 tablespoons olive oil
- Pinch of sea salt
- Pinch of black pepper

Directions:
1. Warm a pan with the oil on medium-high heat, then put the garlic and the corn and sauté for 2 minutes.
2. Add the shrimp and the other ingredients, toss, cook everything for 8 minutes more, divide between plates and serve.

Nutrition: Calories: 343 kcal | Protein: 29.12 g | Fat: 10.97 g | Carbohydrates: 34.25 g

250. Chili Shrimp and Pineapple

Preparation Time: 10 minutes
Cooking Time: 10 minutes
Servings: 4
Ingredients:
- 1-pound shrimp, peeled and deveined
- 2 tablespoons chili paste
- Pinch of sea salt
- Pinch of black pepper
- 1 tablespoon olive oil
- 1 cup pineapple, peeled and cubed
- ½ teaspoon ginger, grated
- 2 teaspoons almonds, chopped
- 2 tablespoons cilantro, chopped

Directions:
1. Warm a pan with the oil on medium-high heat, add the ginger and the chili paste, stir and cook for 2 minutes.
2. Add the shrimp and the other ingredients, toss, cook the mix for 8 minutes more, divide into bowls, and serve.

Nutrition: | Calories 261 Fat 4 | Fiber 7 | Carbs 15 | Protein 8

251. Balsamic Scallops

Preparation Time: 5 minutes
Cooking Time: 10 minutes
Servings: 4
Ingredients:
- 1-pound sea scallops
- 4 scallions, chopped
- 2 tablespoons olive oil
- 1 tablespoon balsamic vinegar
- 1 tablespoon cilantro, chopped
- A pinch of salt and black pepper

Directions:
1. Warm a pan with the oil on medium-high heat, add the scallops, the scallions, and the other ingredients, toss, cook for 10 minutes, divide into bowls and serve.

Nutrition: Calories 300 | Fat 4 | Fiber 4 | Carbs 14 | Protein 17

252. Whitefish Curry

Preparation Time: 10 minutes
Cooking Time: 15 minutes
Servings: 6
Ingredients:
- 1 chopped onion
- 1 lb. Firm white fish fillets
- ¼ c. chopped fresh cilantro
- 1 c. vegetable broth
- 2 minced garlic cloves
- 1 tbsp. Minced fresh ginger
- 1 tsp. Salt
- ¼ tsp. ground black pepper
- Lemon wedges
- 1 bruised lemongrass
- 2 c. cubed butternut squash
- 2 tsp. curry powder
- 2 tbsps. coconut oil
- 2 c. chopped broccoli
- oz. coconut milk
- 1 thinly sliced scallion

Directions:
1. In a pot, add coconut oil and melt.
2. Add onion, curry powder, ginger, garlic, and seasonings, then sauté for 5 minutes

3. Add broccoli, lemongrass and butternut squash and sauté for two more minutes
4. Stir in broth and coconut milk and bring to a boil. Lower the heat to simmer and add the fish.
5. Cover the pot, then simmer for 5 minutes, then discard the lemongrass.
6. Spoon the curry into a medium serving bowl.
7. Add scallion and cilantro to garnish before serving with lemon wedges.
8. Enjoy.

Nutrition: Calories: 218 kcal | Protein: 18.1 g | Fat: 8.57 g | Carbohydrates: 18.2 g

253. Swordfish with Pineapple and Cilantro

Preparation Time: 10 minutes
Cooking Time: 20 minutes
Servings: 4
Ingredients:
- 1 c. fresh pineapple chunks
- 1 tbsp. coconut oil
- 2 lbs. sliced swordfish
- 2 tbsps. Chopped fresh parsley
- ¼ tsp. Ground black pepper.
- 2 minced garlic cloves
- ¼ c. chopped fresh cilantro
- 1 tbsp. coconut aminos
- 1 tsp. Salt.

Directions:
1. Preheat the oven to 4000F.
2. Grease a baking tray with coconut oil
3. Add cilantro, swordfish, coconut aminos, pepper, salt, garlic, parsley, and pineapple to the dish, then mix well.
4. Put the dish in an already preheated oven and bake for 20 minutes.
5. Serve and enjoy.

Nutrition: Calories: 444 kcal | Protein: 47.53 g | Fat: 20.32 g | Carbohydrates: 16.44 g

254. Sesame-Tuna Skewers

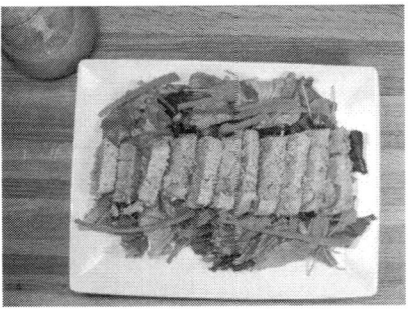

Preparation Time: 10 minutes
Servings: 6
Ingredients:
- 6 oz. cubed thick tuna steaks
- Cooking spray
- ¼ tsp. Ground black pepper.
- ¾ c. sesame seeds
- 1 tsp. Salt
- ½ tsp. Ground ginger.
- 2 tbsps. toasted sesame oil

Directions:
1. Preheat the oven to about 4000F.
2. Coat a rimmed baking tray with cooking spray.
3. Soak twelve wooden skewers in water
4. In a small mixing bowl, combine pepper, ground ginger, salt, and sesame seeds.
5. In another bowl, toss the tuna with sesame oil.
6. Press the oiled cubes into a sesame seed mixture and put the cubes on each skewer.
7. Put the skewers on a readily prepared baking tray and put the tray into the preheated oven.
8. Bake for 12 minutes and turn once.
9. Serve and enjoy.

Nutrition: Calories: 196 kcal | Protein: 14.47 g | Fat: 15.01 g | Carbohydrates: 2.48 g

255. Trout with Chard

Preparation Time: 10 minutes
Cooking Time: 15 minutes
Servings: 4
Ingredients:
- ½ c. vegetable broth
- 2 bunches of sliced chard

- 4 boneless trout fillets
- Salt
- 1 tbsp. extra-virgin olive oil
- 2 minced garlic cloves
- ¼ c. golden raisins
- Ground black pepper
- 1 chopped onion
- 1 tbsp. apple cider vinegar

Directions:
1. Preheat the oven to about 3750F.
2. Add seasonings to the trout
3. Add olive oil to a pan, then heat.
4. Add garlic and onion, then sauté for 3 minutes.
5. Add chard to sauté for 2 more minutes.
6. Add broth, raisins, and cedar vinegar to the pan.
7. Layer a topping of trout fillets
8. Cover the pan and put it in the preheated oven for 10 minutes.
9. Serve and enjoy.

Nutrition: Calories: 284 kcal | Protein: 2.07 g | Fat: 30.32 g | Carbohydrates: 3.49 g

256. Sole with Vegetables

Preparation Time: 10 minutes
Cooking Time: 15 minutes
Servings: 4
Ingredients:

- 4 tsp. divided extra-virgin olive oil
- 1 thinly sliced and divided carrot
- Salt
- Lemon wedges
- ½ c. divided vegetable broth
- 5 oz. sole fillets
- 2 sliced and thinly divided shallots
- Ground black pepper
- 2 tbsps. divided snipped fresh chives
- 1 thinly sliced and divided zucchini

Directions:
1. Preheat the oven to about 4250F.
2. Separate the aluminum foil into medium-sized pieces
3. Put a fillet on one half of the aluminum foil piece and add seasonings
4. Add shallots, zucchini, and ¼ each of the carrot on top of the fillet. Sprinkle with 1 ½ teaspoon of chives
5. Drizzle 2 tablespoons of broth and a tablespoon of olive oil over the fish and vegetables
6. Seal to make a packet and put the packet on a large baking tray.
7. Repeat for the rest of the ingredients and make more packets
8. Put the sheet in a preheated oven and bake the packets for 15 minutes
9. Peel back the foil and put the contents with the liquid onto a serving plate.
10. Garnish with lemon wedges before serving.
11. Enjoy.

Nutrition: Calories: 130 kcal | Protein: 9.94 g | Fat: 7.96 g Carbohydrates: 4.92 g

257. Poached Halibut and Mushrooms

Preparation Time: 5 minutes
Cooking Time: 30 minutes
Servings: 8
Ingredients:

- 1/8 teaspoon sesame oil
- 2 pounds' halibut, cut into bite-sized pieces
- 1 teaspoon fresh lemon juice
- ½ teaspoon soy sauce
- 4 cups mushrooms, sliced ¼ cup water
- Salt and pepper to taste ¾ cup green onions

Directions:
1. Place a heavy-bottomed pot on medium-high fire.
2. Add all ingredients and mix well.
3. Cover and bring to a boil. Once boiling, lower fire to a simmer. Cook for 25 minutes.
4. Adjust seasoning to taste.
5. Serve and enjoy.

Nutrition: Calories: 217 Ca | Fat 15.8 | Carbs: 1.1 g | Protein: 16.5 | Fiber: 0.4 g

258. Halibut Stir Fry

Preparation Time: 5 minutes
Cooking Time: 20 minutes
Servings: 6

Ingredients:
- 2 pounds' halibut fillets
- 2 tbsp. olive oil ½ cup fresh parsley
- 1 onion, sliced 2 stalks celery, chopped
- 2 tablespoons capers
- 4 cloves of garlic minced
- Salt and pepper to taste

Directions:
1. Place a heavy-bottomed pot on high fire and heat for 2 minutes. Add oil and heat for 2 more minutes.
2. Stir in garlic and onions. Sauté for 5 minutes. Add remaining ingredients except for the parsley and stir fry for 10 minutes or until fish is cooked.
3. Adjust seasoning to taste and serve with a sprinkle of parsley.

Nutrition: Calories 331 Cal |Fat 26 g| Carbs 2 g |Protein 22 g| Fiber 0.5 g

259. Steamed Garlic-Dill Halibut

Preparation Time: 5 minutes
Cooking Time: 25 minutes
Servings: 4
Ingredients:
- 1-pound halibut fillet
- 1 lemon, freshly squeezed
- Salt and pepper to taste
- 1 teaspoon garlic powder
- 1 tablespoon dill weed, chopped

Directions:
1. Place a large pot on medium fire and fill up to 1.5-inches of water. Place a trivet inside the pot.
2. In a baking dish that fits inside your large pot, add all ingredients and mix well. Cover dish with foil. Place the dish on top of the trivet inside the pot.
3. Cover pot and steam fish for 15 minutes.
4. Let fish rest for at least 10 minutes before removing from pot.
5. Serve and enjoy.

Nutrition: Calories: 270 Cal |Fat: 6.5 g |Carbs: 3.9 g |Protein: 47.8 g |Fiber: 2.1 g

260. Italian Halibut Chowder

Preparation Time: 5 minutes
Cooking Time: 20 minutes
Servings: 8
Ingredients:
- 2 tablespoons olive oil
- 1 onion, chopped
- 3 stalks of celery, chopped
- 3 cloves of garlic, minced
- 2 ½ pounds halibut steaks, cubed
- 1 red bell pepper, seeded and chopped
- 1 cup tomato juice
- ½ cup apple juice, organic and unsweetened
- ½ teaspoon dried basil
- 1/8 teaspoon dried thyme
- Salt and pepper to taste

Directions:
1. Place a heavy-bottomed pot on medium-high fire and heat pot for 2 minutes. Add oil and heat for a minute.
2. Sauté the onion, celery, and garlic until fragrant.
3. Stir in the halibut steaks and bell pepper. Sauté for 3 minutes.
4. Pour in the rest of the ingredients and mix well.
5. Cover and bring to a boil. Once boiling, lower the fire to a simmer and simmer for 10 minutes.
6. Adjust seasoning to taste.
7. Serve and enjoy.

Nutrition: Calories: 318 Cal |Fat: 23g |Carbs: 6g |Protein: 21g| Fiber: 1g

261. Dill Haddock

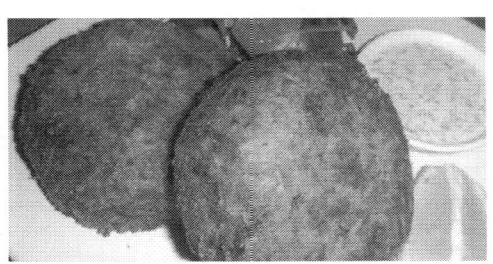

Preparation Time: 10 minutes

Servings: 4
Ingredients:

- 1-pound haddock fillets
- 3 teaspoons veggie stock
- 2 tablespoons lemon juice
- Salt and black pepper to the taste
- 2 tablespoons mayonnaise
- 2 teaspoons chopped dill
- A drizzle of olive oil

Directions:
1. Grease a baking dish with the oil, add the fish, and also add stock mixed with lemon juice, salt, pepper, mayo, and dill. Toss a bit and place in the oven at 350 degrees F to bake for 30 minutes. Divide between plates and serve.
2. Enjoy!

Nutrition: Calories: 214 cal | Fat: 12g | Fiber: 4g | Carbs: 7g | Protein: 17g

262. Chili Snapper

Preparation Time: 10 minutes
Cooking Time: 20 minutes
Servings: 2
Ingredients:

- 2 red snapper fillets, boneless and skinless
- 3 tablespoons chili paste
- A pinch of sea salt
- Black pepper
- 1 tablespoon coconut aminos
- 1 garlic clove, minced
- ½ teaspoon fresh grated ginger
- 2 teaspoons sesame seeds, toasted
- 2 tablespoons olive oil
- 1 green onion, chopped
- 2 tablespoons chicken stock

Directions:
1. Warm a pan with the oil on medium-high heat, add the ginger, onion, and garlic, stir and cook for 2 minutes. Add chili paste, aminos, salt, pepper, and the stock stir and cook for 3 minutes more. Add the fish fillets, toss gently, and cook for 5-6 minutes on each side.
2. Divide into plates, sprinkle sesame seeds on top, and serve.
3. Enjoy!

Nutrition: Calories 261 cal | Fat: 10 g | Fiber: 7 g | Carbs: 15 g | Protein: 16 g

263. Lemony Mackerel

Preparation Time: 10 minutes
Cooking Time: 15 minutes
Servings: 4
Ingredients:

- Juice of 1 lemon
- Zest of 1 lemon
- 4 mackerels
- 1 tablespoon minced chives
- Pinch of sea salt
- Pinch black pepper
- 2 tablespoons olive oil

Directions:
1. Warm a pan with the oil on medium-high heat, add the mackerel and cook for 6 minutes on each side. Add the lemon zest, lemon juice, chives, salt, and pepper, then cook for 2 more minutes on each side. Divide everything between plates and serve.
2. Enjoy!

Nutrition: Calories: 289 cal | Fat: 20 g | Fiber: 0 g | Carbs: 1 g | Protein: 21 g

264. Honey Crusted Salmon with Pecans

Preparation Time: 20 minutes
Cooking Time: 20 minutes
Servings: 6
Ingredients:

- 3 tablespoons olive oil
- 3 tablespoons mustard
- 5 teaspoons raw honey
- ½ cup chopped pecans
- 6 salmon fillets, boneless
- 3 teaspoons chopped parsley
- Salt and black pepper to the taste

Directions:
1. In a bowl, whisk the mustard with honey and oil. In another bowl, mix the pecans with parsley and stir. Season salmon fillets with salt and pepper, place them on a baking sheet, brush with mustard mixture, top with

the pecans mix, and place them in the oven at 400 degrees F to bake for 20 minutes. Divide into plates and serve with a side salad.
2. Enjoy!

Nutrition: Calories 200 kcal | Fat 10g | Fiber 5g | Carbs 12g | Protein 16g

POULTRY

265. Basic "Rotisserie" Chicken

Preparation Time: 15 minutes
Cooking Time: 6 to 8 hours
Servings: 6
Ingredients:
- 1 teaspoon garlic powder
- 1 teaspoon chili powder
- 1 teaspoon paprika
- 1 teaspoon dried thyme leaves
- 1 teaspoon sea salt
- Pinch cayenne pepper
- Freshly ground black pepper
- 1 (4-5 lb.) whole chicken, neck, and giblets removed
- ½ medium onion, sliced

Directions:
1. In a small bowl, stir together the garlic powder, chili powder, paprika, thyme, salt, and cayenne. Season with black pepper, and stir again to combine. Rub the spice mix all over the exterior of the chicken.
2. Place the chicken in the cooker with the sliced onion sprinkled around it.
3. Cover the cooker and set it to low. Cook for at least 6 to 8 hours, or until the internal temperature reaches 165°F on a meat thermometer and the juices run clear and serve.

Nutrition: Calories: 86| Total Fat: 59| Total Carbs: 7| Sugar: 6|Fiber: 0g|Protein: 86g|Sodium: 1,200mg

266. Hidden Valley Chicken Dummies

Preparation Time: 15 minutes
Cooking Time: 30 minutes
Servings: 4
Ingredients:
- 2 tbsps. Hot sauce
- ½ c. melted butter
- Celery sticks
- 2 packages Hidden Valley dressing dry mix
- 3 tbsps. Vinegar
- 12 chicken drumsticks
- Paprika

Directions:
1. Preheat the oven to 350 0F.
2. Rinse and pat dry the chicken.
3. In a bowl, blend the dry dressing, melted butter, vinegar, and hot sauce. Stir until combined.
4. Place the drumsticks in a large plastic baggie, pour the sauce over drumsticks. Massage the sauce until the drumsticks are coated.
5. Place the chicken in a single layer on a baking dish. Sprinkle with paprika.
6. Bake for 30 minutes, flipping halfway.
7. Serve with crudités or salad.

Nutrition: Calories: 155|Fat: 18 g|Carbs: 96 g|Protein:15 g|Sugars: 0.7 g|Sodium: 340 mg

267. Chicken Divan

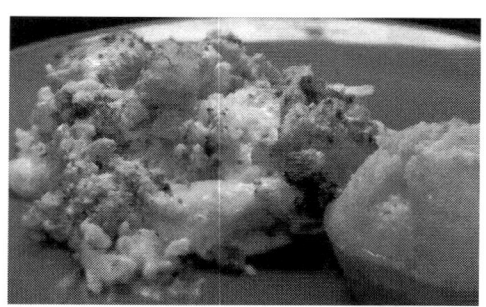

Preparation Time: 15 minutes
Cooking Time: 30 minutes

Ingredients:
- 1 c. croutons
- 1 c. cooked and diced broccoli pieces
- ½ c. water
- 1 c. grated extra sharp cheddar cheese
- ½ lb. de-boned and skinless cooked chicken pieces
- 1 can mushroom soup

Directions:
1. Preheat the oven to 350°F

2. In a large pot, heat the soup and water. Add the chicken, broccoli, and cheese. Combine thoroughly.
3. Pour into a greased baking dish.
4. Place the croutons over the mixture.
5. Bake for 30 minutes or until the casserole is bubbling and the croutons are golden brown.

Nutrition: Calories: 38|Fat: 22 g|Carbs: 10 g|Protein: 25 g|Sugars: 2 g|Sodium: 475 mg

268. Apricot Chicken Wings

Preparation Time: 15 minutes
Cooking Time: 45-60 minutes
Servings: 3-4
Ingredients:

- 1 medium jar apricot preserve
- 1 package Lipton onion dry soup mix
- 1 medium bottle Russian dressing
- 2 lbs. chicken wings

Directions:
1. Preheat the oven to 350°F.
2. Rinse and pat dry the chicken wings.
3. Bring the chicken wings on a baking pan, single layer.
4. Bake for 45 – 60 minutes, turning halfway.
5. In a medium bowl, combine the Lipton soup mix, apricot preserve, and Russian dressing.
6. Once the wings are cooked, toss with the sauce until the pieces are coated.
7. Serve immediately with a side dish.

Nutrition: Calories: 162|Fat: 17 g|Carbs: 76 | Protein: 13 g|Sugars: 24 g|Sodium: 700 mg

269. Champion Chicken Pockets

Preparation Time: 5 minutes
Cooking Time: 0 minutes
Servings: 4
Ingredients:

- ½ c. chopped broccoli
- 2 halved whole wheat pita bread rounds
- ¼ c. bottled reduced-fat ranch salad dressing
- ¼ c. chopped pecans or walnuts
- 1 ½ c. chopped cooked chicken
- ¼ c. plain low-fat yogurt
- ¼ c. shredded carrot

Directions:
1. In a bowl, put together yogurt and ranch salad dressing, then mix.
2. In a medium bowl, put then combine chicken, broccoli, carrot, and, if desired, nuts. Pour yogurt mixture over chicken; toss to coat.
3. Spoon chicken mixture into pita halves.

Nutrition: Calories: 384|Fat: 11.4 g| Carbs: 7.4 g | Protein: 59.3 g|Sugars: 1.3 |Sodium: 368.7 mg

270. Chicken-Bell Pepper Sauté

Preparation Time: 10 minutes
Cooking Time: 30 minutes
Servings: 6
Ingredients:

- 1 tbsp. olive oil
- 1 sliced large yellow bell pepper
- 1 sliced large red bell pepper
- 3 c. onion sliced crosswise
- 6 4-oz skinless, boneless chicken breast halves
- Cooking spray
- 20 Kalamata olives
- ¼ tsp. Freshly ground black pepper
- ½ tsp. salt
- 2 tbsps. finely chopped fresh flat-leaf parsley
- 2 1/3 c. coarsely chopped tomato
- 1 tsp. chopped fresh oregano

Directions:
1. Adjust your heat to medium-high and set non-stick frying in place. Heat the oil. Sauté the onions for 8 minutes once the oil is hot.
2. Add bell pepper and sauté for 10 more minutes.
3. Add tomato, salt, and black pepper to cook for about 7 minutes until the tomato juice has evaporated.
4. Add parsley, oregano, and olives to cooking for 2 minutes until heated. Set into a bowl and keep warm.
5. Using a paper towel, wipe the pam and grease with cooking spray. Set back to heat and add chicken breasts. Cook for 3 more minutes on each of the sides. You can opt to cook the chicken in batches

6. When cooking the last batch, add back the previous batch of chicken and onion-bell pepper mixture, then cook for a minute as you toss.
7. Serve warm and enjoy.

Nutrition: Calories: 223 kcal | Protein: 28.13 g | Fat: 7.82 g | Carbohydrates: 9.5 g

271. Avocado-Orange Grilled Chicken

Preparation Time: 10 minutes
Cooking Time: 12 minutes
Servings: 4
Ingredients:
- 1 c. low-fat yogurt
- Salt
- 4 pieces of 4-6oz boneless, skinless chicken breasts
- 2 tbsps. chopped cilantro
- 1 tbsp. honey
- 1 thinly sliced small red onion
- ¼ c. fresh lime juice
- 1 deseeded avocado, peeled and chopped
- 2 peeled and sectioned oranges
- Pepper
- ¼ c. minced red onion

Directions:
1. Set up a large mixing bowl and mix yogurt, minced red onion, cilantro, and honey
2. Add chicken into the mixture and marinate for half an hour
3. Grease grate and preheat the grill to medium-high heat.
4. Set the chicken aside and add seasonings
5. Grill for 6 minutes on each side
6. Set the avocado in a bowl.
7. Add lime juice and toss avocado to coat well.
8. Add oranges, thinly sliced onions, and cilantro into the bowl with avocado and combine well.
9. Serve avocado dressing alongside grilled chicken.
10. Enjoy.

Nutrition: Calories: 216 kcal | Protein: 8.83 g | Fat: 11.48 g | Carbohydrates: 21.86 g

272. Honey Chicken Tagine

Preparation Time: 60 minutes
Cooking Time: 25 minutes
Servings: 12
Ingredients:
- 1 tbsp. extra virgin olive oil
- 1 tsp. ground coriander
- 1 tbsp. Minced fresh ginger
- ½ tsp. ground pepper
- 2 thinly sliced onions
- 12-oz. seeded and roughly chopped kumquats
- 14-oz. vegetable broth
- 1/8 tsp. Ground cloves
- ½ tsp. salt
- 1 ½ tbsps. honey
- 1 tsp. ground cumin
- 2 lbs. boneless, skinless chicken thighs
- 4 slivered garlic cloves
- 15-oz rinsed chickpeas
- ¾ tsp. ground cinnamon

Directions:
1. Preheat the oven to about 375ºF.
2. Put a heatproof casserole on medium heat and heat the oil.
3. Add onions to sauté for 4 minutes
4. Add garlic and ginger to sauté for 1 minute
5. Add coriander, cumin, cloves, salt, pepper, and cloves seasonings. Sauté for a minute.
6. Add kumquats, broth, chickpeas, and honey, then bring to a boil before turning off the heat.
7. Set the casserole in the oven while covered. Bake for 15 minutes as you stir at a 15-minute interval.
8. Serve and enjoy

Nutrition: Calories: 586 kcal | Protein: 15.5 g | Fat: 40.82 g | Carbohydrates: 43.56 g

273. Roasted Chicken

Preparation Time: 60 minutes
Cooking Time: 60 minutes
Servings: 8
Ingredients:
- ½ tsp. thyme

- 3 lbs. whole chicken
- 1 bay leaf
- 3 garlic cloves
- 4 tbsps. Coarsely chopped orange peel
- ½ tsp. Black pepper
- ½ tbsp. salt

Directions:
1. Put the chicken under room temperature for about 1 hour.
2. Pat dries the inside and outside of the chicken using paper towels.
3. Preheat the oven to 4500F as soon as you start preparing the chicken seasoning.
4. Combine thyme, salt, and pepper in a small bowl.
5. Wipe inside using 1/3 of the seasoning. Inside the chicken, put the garlic, citrus peel, and bay leaf.
6. Tuck the tips of the wing and tie the legs together. Spread the rest of the seasoning all over the chicken and put it on a roasting pan.
7. Put in the oven to bake for 60 minutes at 1600F.
8. Set aside to rest for 15 minutes.
9. Cut up the roasted chicken and serve.
10. Enjoy.

Nutrition: Calories: 201 kcal | Protein: 35.48 g | Fat: 5.36 g | Carbohydrates: 0.5 g

274. Chicken in Pita Bread

Preparation Time: 10 minutes
Cooking Time: 10 minutes
Servings: 4
Ingredients:
- 1 tbsp. Greek seasoning blend
- Two lightly beaten large egg whites
- ½ c. chopped green onions
- ½ c. diced tomato
- 2 c. shredded lettuce
- 4 pieces of 6-inch halved pitas
- 2 tsp. Divided grated lemon rind
- ½ c. plain low-fat yogurt
- 1 tbsp. olive oil
- 1 ½ tbsp. chopped fresh oregano
- 1 lb. Ground chicken
- ½ tsp. coarsely ground black pepper

Directions:
1. Combine egg whites, Greek seasoning, a tablespoon of lemon rind, green onions, and black pepper. Separate into 8 parts and mold each into ¼ inch thick patty.
2. Adjust your heat to medium-high. Set a non-stick skillet in place and fry patties until browned.
3. Lower the heat to medium. Then, cover the skillet to cook for 4 more minutes.
4. Set up a small bowl and combine yogurt, oregano, and a tablespoon of lemon rind.
5. Spread the mixture on the pita and add ¼ cup lettuce and a tablespoon of tomato.

Nutrition: Calories: 421 kcal | Protein: 29.72 g | Fat: 23.37 g | Carbohydrates: 23.26 g

275. Skillet Chicken with Brussels Sprouts Mix

Preparation Time: 10 minutes
Cooking Time: 15 minutes
Servings: 4
Ingredients:
- 1½ pounds chicken thighs, skinless and boneless
- 1 tablespoon olive oil
- 2 teaspoons chopped thyme
- A pinch of salt and black pepper
- 12 ounces Brussel sprouts, shredded
- 1 apple, cored and sliced
- ½ red onion, sliced
- 1 garlic clove, minced
- 2 tablespoons balsamic vinegar
- ¼ cup walnuts, chopped

Directions:
1. Warm a pan with the oil over medium-high heat, then add the chicken thighs, season with salt, pepper, and thyme. Cook for 5 minutes on each side and transfer to a bowl. Heat the pan again over medium heat, add the onion, apple, sprouts, and garlic. Toss the mix and cook for 5 minutes. Add vinegar to the pan and return the chicken as well. Add the walnuts, toss, cook for 1-2 minutes more than divide between plates and serve.
2. Enjoy!

Nutrition: Calories: 211 | Fat: 4 | Fiber: 7 | Carbs:13 | Protein: 8

276. Spicy Chipotle Chicken

Preparation Time: 10 minutes
Cooking Time: 12 minutes
Servings: 4
Ingredients:

- 1-pound chicken breasts, skinless, boneless and cut into strips
- 1 teaspoon chili powder
- 1 teaspoon ground cumin
- A pinch of salt and black pepper
- 1 tablespoon olive oil
- 1 red bell pepper, sliced
- 1 cup halved mushrooms
- 1 yellow onion, chopped
- 3 garlic cloves, minced
- 1 tablespoon chopped chipotles in adobo
- 1½ tablespoons lime juice

Directions:

1. Warm a pan with the oil on medium-high heat and add the chicken. Mix and cook for 3-4 minutes. Add the chili powder, cumin, salt, pepper, bell pepper, mushrooms, onion, garlic, chipotles, and lime juice. Mix and cook for 7 minutes more, divide into bowls and serve.
2. Enjoy!

Nutrition: Calories: 241 | Fat: 4 | Fiber: 7 | Carbs: 14 | Protein: 7

277. Chicken with Fennel

Preparation Time: 10 minutes
Cooking Time: 8 minutes
Servings: 4
Ingredients:

- 1 ¼ pounds chicken cutlets
- 1 ½ teaspoon smoked paprika
- A pinch of salt and black pepper
- 3 tablespoons olive oil
- 1 fennel bulb, sliced
- ¾ cup fennel fronds
- 1/3 cup red onion, sliced
- 1 avocado, peeled, pitted, and sliced
- 2 tablespoons lemon juice

Directions:

1. Warm a pan with 1 tbsp Olive oil on medium-high heat temperature, then add the chicken, season with salt, pepper, and smoked paprika, and cook for 4 minutes on each side. In a bowl, mix the rest of the oil with the fennel, fennel fronds, onion, avocado, and lemon juice. Toss the salad and place it next to the chicken, then serve. Divide between plates.
2. Enjoy!

Nutrition: Calories: 288 | Fat: 4 | Fiber: 6 | Carbs: 12 | Protein: 7

278. Adobo Lime Chicken Mix

Preparation Time: 10 minutes
Cooking Time: 40 minutes
Servings: 6
Ingredients:

- 6 chicken thighs
- Salt and black pepper to the taste
- 1 tablespoon olive oil
- Zest of 1 lime
- 1½ teaspoons chipotle peppers in adobo sauce
- 1 cup sliced peach
- 1 tablespoon lime juice

Directions:

1. Warm a pan with the oil on medium-high heat and add the chicken thighs. Season with salt and pepper, then brown for 4 minutes on each side and bake in the oven at 375 degrees F for 20 minutes. In your food processor, mix the peaches with the chipotle, lime zest, and lime juice, then blend and pour over the chicken. Bake for 10 minutes more, divide everything between plates and serve.
2. Enjoy!

Nutrition: Calories: 309 | Fat: 6 | Fiber: 4 | Carbs: 16 | Protein: 15

279. Cajun Chicken & Prawn

Preparation Time: 5 minutes
Cooking Time: 35 minutes
Servings: 2

Ingredients:
- 2 Free-range Skinless Chicken breast, chopped
- 1 Onion, chopped
- 1 Red pepper, chopped
- 2 Garlic cloves, crushed
- 10 Fresh or frozen prawn
- 1 tsp. Cayenne powder
- 1 tsp. Chili powder
- 1 tsp. Paprika
- 1/4 tsp. Chili powder
- 1 tsp. Dried oregano
- 1 tsp. Dried thyme
- 1 cup Brown or wholegrain rice
- 1 tbsp. Extra Virgin olive oil
- 1 can Tomatoes, chopped
- 2 cups Homemade chicken stock

Directions:
1. Put all the spices and herbs in a bowl, then mix to form your Cajun spice mix.
2. Grab a large pan and add the olive oil, heating on medium heat.
3. Add the chicken and brown each side for around 4-5 minutes. Then place to one side.
4. Add the onion to the pan and fry until soft.
5. Add the garlic, prawns, Cajun seasoning, and red pepper to the pan and cook for around 5 minutes or until prawns become opaque.
6. Add the brown rice along with the chopped tomatoes, chicken, and chicken stock to the pan.
7. Cover the pan and allow to simmer for around 25 minutes or until the rice is soft.
8. Serve and enjoy!

Nutrition: Calories: 557 kcal | Protein: 18.96 g | Fat: 12.34 g | Carbohydrates: 93.28 g

280. <u>Healthy Turkey Gumbo</u>

Preparation Time: 5 minutes
Cooking Time: 2 hours
Servings: 1
Ingredients:
- 1 Whole Turkey
- 1 Onion, quartered
- Stalk of Celery, chopped
- 3 Cloves garlic, chopped
- 1/2 cup Okra
- 1 can chopped tomatoes
- 1 tbsp. Extra virgin olive oils
- 1-2 Bay leaves
- Black pepper to taste

Directions:
1. Take the first four ingredients and add 2 cups of water in a stockpot, heating on a high heat until boiling.
2. Lower the heat and simmer for 45-50 minutes or until turkey is cooked through.
3. Remove the turkey and strain the broth.
4. Grab a skillet, heat the oil on medium heat, and brown the rest of the vegetables for 5-10 minutes.
5. Stir until tender, and then add to the broth.
6. Add the tomatoes and turkey meat to the broth and stir.
7. Add the bay leaves and continue to cook for an hour or until the sauce has thickened.
8. Season with black pepper and enjoy.

Nutrition: Calories: 261 kcal | Protein: 11.72 g | Fat: 12.91 g | Carbohydrates: 28.33 g

281. <u>Chinese-Orange Spiced Duck Breasts</u>

Preparation Time: 4 minutes
Cooking Time: 20 minutes
Servings: 2
Ingredients:
- 1 tsp. EXTRA Virgin olive oil
- 2 Duck breasts, skin removed
- 1 White onion, sliced
- 3 Cloves garlic, minced
- 2 tsp. Ginger, grated
- 1 tsp. Cinnamon
- 1 tsp. Cloves
- 1 Orange-Zest and Juice (Reserved the wedges)
- 2 Bok or Pak Choy plants leaves separated

Directions:
1. Slice the duck breasts into strips and add to a dry, hot pan, cooking for 5-7 minutes on each side or until cooked through to your liking.
2. Remove to one side.

3. Add olive oil to a clean pan and sauté the onions with the ginger, garlic, and the rest of the spices for 1 minute.
4. Put the juice and zest of the orange and continue to sauté for 3-5 minutes.
5. Add the duck and bok choi and heat through until wilted and duck is piping hot.
6. Serve and garnish with the orange segments.

Nutrition: Calories: 267 kcal | Protein: 36.58 g | Fat: 11.1 g | Carbohydrates: 3.31 g

282. Super Sesame Chicken Noodles

Preparation Time: 10 minutes
Cooking Time: 10 minutes
Servings: 2
Ingredients:
- 2 Free-range skinless chicken breasts, chopped
- 1 cup Rice/Buckwheat noodles such as Japanese Udo
- 1 Carrot, chopped
- 1/2 orange juiced
- 1 tsp. Sesame Seed
- 2 tsp. Coconut Oil
- 1 Thumb size piece of ginger, minced
- 1/2 cup Sugar snap peas

Directions:
1. Warm 1 tsp oil on medium heat in a skillet.
2. Sauté the chopped chicken breast for about 10-15 minutes or until cooked through.
3. While cooking the chicken, place the noodles, carrots, and peas in a pot of boiling water for about 5 minutes. Drain.
4. In a bowl, mix the ginger, sesame seeds, 1 tsp oil, and orange juice to make your dressing.
5. Once the chicken is cooked and noodles are cooked and drained, add the chicken, noodles, carrots, and peas to the dressing and toss.
6. Serve warm or chilled.

Nutrition: Calories: 168 kcal | Protein: 5.31 g | Fat: 8.66 g | Carbohydrates: 19.34 g

283. Lebanese Chicken Kebabs and Hummus

Preparation Time: 10 minutes + 1 hour marinate
Cooking Time: 35 minutes
Servings: 4
Ingredients:
- For the Chicken:
- 1 cup Lemon Juice
- 8 Garlic cloves, minced
- 1 tbsp. Thyme, finely chopped
- 1 tbsp. Paprika
- 2 tsp. ground cumin
- 1 tsp. Cayenne pepper
- 4 Free-range skinless chicken breasts, cubed
- 4 Metal kebabs skewers
- Lemon wedges to garnish
- For the Hummus:
- 1 can Chickpeas/ 1 cup dried (soaked overnight)
- 2 tbsp. Tahini paste
- 1 Lemon juice
- 1 tsp. Turmeric
- 1 tsp. Black pepper
- 2 tbsp. Olive oil

Directions:
1. Whisk the lemon juice, garlic, thyme, paprika, cumin, and cayenne pepper in a bowl.
2. Skewer the chicken cubes using kebab sticks (metal).
3. Baste the chicken per side with the marinade, covering for as long as possible in the fridge (the lemon juice will tenderize the meat and means it will be more suitable for the anti-inflammatory diet).
4. When ready to cook, set the oven to 400°F/200 °C/Gas Mark 6 and bake for 20-25 minutes or until chicken is thoroughly cooked through.
5. Prepare the hummus by putting the ingredients into a blender and whizzing up until smooth. If it is a little thick and chunky, add a little water to loosen the mix.
6. Serve the chicken kebabs garnished with lemon wedges and the hummus on the side.

Nutrition: Calories: 576 kcal | Protein: 61.66 g | Fat: 18.55 g | Carbohydrates: 42.07 g

284. Nutty Pesto Chicken Supreme

Preparation Time: 10 minutes
Cooking Time: 30 minutes
Servings: 2
Ingredients:
- 2 Free ranges skinless chicken/ turkey breasts
- 1 bunch of fresh basil
- 1/2 cup raw spinach
- 1 cup Crashed macadamias/almonds/walnuts or a combination
- 2 tbsp. Extra virgin olive oil
- 1/2 cup low-fat hard cheese (optional)

Directions:
1. Set the oven to 350°F.
2. Get the chicken breasts and use a meat pounder to 'thin' each breast into a 1cm thick escalope.
3. Reserve a handful of the nuts before adding the rest of the ingredients and a little black pepper to a blender or pestle and mortar and blend until smooth (you can leave this a little chunky for a rustic feel if you wish).
4. Add a little water if the pesto needs loosening.
5. Coat the chicken in the pesto.
6. Bake for at least 30 minutes in the oven or until chicken is completely cooked through.
7. Top each chicken escalope with the remaining nuts and place under the broiler for 5 minutes for a crispy topping to complete.

Nutrition: Calories: 2539 kcal | Protein: 444.61 g | Fat: 71.66 g | Carbohydrates: 5.99 g

285. Delicious Roasted Duck

Preparation Time: 10 minutes
Cooking Time: 4 hours and 50 minutes
Servings: 4
Ingredients:
- 1 medium duck
- 1 celery stalk, chopped
- 2 yellow onions, chopped
- 2 teaspoons thyme, dried
- 8 garlic cloves, minced
- 2 bay leaves
- ¼ cup parsley, chopped
- A pinch of salt and black pepper
- One teaspoon herbs de Provence
- For the sauce:
- 1 tablespoon tomato paste
- 1 yellow onion, chopped
- ½ teaspoon sugar
- 3 cups water
- 1 cup chicken stock
- 1 and ½ cups black olives, pitted and chopped
- ¼ teaspoon herbs de Provence

Directions:
1. In a baking dish, arrange thyme, parsley, garlic, and 2 onions.
2. Add duck, season with salt, 1 teaspoon herbs de Provence and pepper.
3. Place in the oven at 475 degrees F and roast for 10 minutes.
4. Cover the dish, reduce heat to 275 degrees F, and roast duck for 3 hours and 30 minutes.
5. Meanwhile, heat a pan over medium heat, add 1 yellow onion, stir and cook for 10 minutes.
6. Add tomato paste, stock, sugar, ¼ teaspoon herbs de Provence, olives, and water, cover, reduce heat to low, and cook for 1 hour.
7. Transfer duck to a work surface, carve, discard bones, and divide between plates.
8. Drizzle the sauce all over and serve right away.

Nutrition: Calories: 254 | Fat: 3 | Fiber: 3 | Carbs: 8 | Protein: 13

286. Duck Breast with Apricot Sauce

Preparation Time: 10 minutes
Cooking Time: 20 minutes
Servings: 4
Ingredients:
- 4 duck breasts, boneless
- Salt and black pepper to taste
- ¼ teaspoon cinnamon, ground
- ¼ teaspoon coriander, ground

- 5 tablespoons apricot preserving
- 3 tablespoons chives, chopped
- 2 tablespoons parsley, chopped
- A drizzle of olive oil
- 3 tablespoons apple cider vinegar
- 2 tablespoons red onions, chopped
- 1 cup apricots, chopped
- ¾ cup blackberries

Directions:
1. Season duck breasts with salt, pepper, coriander, and cinnamon, place them on a preheated grill pan over medium-high heat, cook for 2 minutes, flip them and cook for 3 minutes more.
2. Flip duck breasts again, add 3 tablespoons apricot preserving, cook for 1 minute, transfer them to a cutting board, leave aside for 2-3 minutes, and slice.
3. Heat a pan over medium heat, add vinegar, onion, 2 tablespoons apricot preserving, apricots, blackberries, and chives, stir and cook for 3 minutes.
4. Divide sliced duck breasts between plates and serve with apricot sauce drizzled on top.

Nutrition: Calories: 275 | **Fat:** 4 | **Fiber:** 4 | **Carbs:** 7 | **Protein:** 12

287. Duck Breast Salad

Preparation Time: 10 minutes
Cooking Time: 20 minutes
Servings: 4
Ingredients:
- 2 tablespoons sugar
- 2 oranges, peeled and cut into segments
- 1 teaspoon orange zest, grated
- 1 tablespoon lemon juice
- 1 teaspoon lemon zest, grated
- 3 tablespoons shallot, minced
- tablespoons canola oil
- Salt and black pepper to taste
- 2 duck breasts, boneless but the skin on, cut into 4 pieces
- 1 head of fries, torn
- 2 small lettuce heads washed, torn into small pieces
- 2 tablespoons chives, chopped

Directions:
1. Warm a small saucepan on medium-high heat, add vinegar and sugar, stir and boil for 5 minutes and take off the heat.
2. Add orange zest, lemon zest and lemon juice, stir and leave aside for a few minutes.
3. Add shallot, salt, and pepper to taste and the oil, whisk well and leave aside.
4. Pat dry duck pieces' score skin, trim, and season with salt and pepper.
5. Warm a pan on medium-high heat for 1 minute, arrange duck breast pieces' skin side down, brown for 8 minutes, reduce heat to medium, and cook for 4 more minutes.
6. Flip pieces, cook for 3 minutes, transfer to a cutting board and cover them with foil.
7. Put fries and lettuce in a bowl, stir and divide between plates.
8. Slice duck, arrange on top, add orange segments, sprinkle chives, and drizzle the vinaigrette.

Nutrition: Calories: 320 | **Fat:** 4 | **Fiber:** 4 | **Carbs:** 6 | **Protein:** 14

288. Duck Breast and Blackberries Mix

Preparation Time: 10 minutes
Cooking Time: 25 minutes
Servings: 4
Ingredients:
- 4 duck breasts
- 2 tablespoons balsamic vinegar
- 3 tablespoons sugar
- Salt and black pepper to taste
- 1 ½ cups water
- 4 ounces' blackberries
- ¼ cup chicken stock
- 1 tablespoon butter
- 2 teaspoons cornflour

Directions:
1. Pat dry duck breasts with paper towels, score the skin, season with salt and pepper to taste, and set aside for 30 minutes.
2. Put breasts skin side down in a pan, heat over medium heat, and cook for 8 minutes.
3. Flip breasts and cook for 30 more seconds.

4. Transfer duck breasts to a baking dish skin side up, place in the oven at 425 degrees F and bake for 15 minutes.
5. Pull out the meat from the oven and leave it aside to cool down for 10 minutes before you cut them.
6. Meanwhile, put sugar in a pan, heat over medium heat, and melt it, stirring all the time.
7. Take the pan off the heat, add the water, stock, balsamic vinegar, and blackberries.
8. Heat this mix to medium temperature and cook until sauce is reduced to half.
9. Transfer sauce to another pan, add cornflour mixed with water, heat again, and cook for 4 minutes until it thickens.
10. Add salt and pepper, the butter, and whisk well. Slice the duck breasts, divide between plates and serve with the berries sauce on top.

Nutrition: Calories: 320 | Fat: 15 | Fiber: 15 | Carbs: 16 | Protein: 11

289. Chicken Piccata

Preparation Time: 15 minutes
Cooking Time: 30 minutes
Servings: 4
Ingredients:
- 4 boneless, skinless chicken breast
- 1 cup ground almond meal
- 1/4 cup grated Parmesan cheese
- 1/2 teaspoon Dijon mustard
- 1 yellow onion, chopped
- 1 teaspoon of sea salt
- 1/2 teaspoon ground black pepper
- 4 tablespoons olive oil
- 4 tablespoons organic unsalted butter
- 1/2 cup organic, gluten-free chicken broth
- 3 tablespoons lemon juice
- 2 tablespoons capers
- 3 tablespoons organic butter
- 1/4 cup fresh parsley, chopped

Directions:
1. Combine the almond meal, cheese, mustard, salt, and pepper spread the mixture on a shallow dish.
2. Wash the pounded chicken breasts in water and shake off the excess. Dredge the chicken in the flour mixture.
3. Add tablespoons of butter in a large saucepan over high heat; add the olive oil.
4. Cook chicken in butter and oil for approximately 3-4 minutes on each side until golden brown.
5. Place the cooked chicken on a serving dish and cover to keep warm.
6. Stir in the chicken broth, lemon juice, and capers, scraping up any brown bits in the pan.
7. Add the chicken broth, lemon juice, and capers to the skillet, stirring and scraping up any brown bits in the skillet. Simmer until the sauce is reduced and reaches a light syrup consistency. Reduce heat to low and stir in remaining butter.
8. Ladle the sauce over the chicken breasts and top with chopped parsley. Serve with lemon slices or wedges.

Nutrition: Calories: 357 kcal | Protein: 4.51 g | Fat: 35.73 g | Carbohydrates: 6.16 g

290. Honey-Mustard Lemon Marinated Chicken

Preparation Time: 10 minutes
Cooking Time: 20 minutes
Servings: 4
Ingredients:
- 1-pound lean chicken breast
- 1/4 cup Dijon mustard
- 1 tablespoon olive oil
- 1/4 cup rosemary leaves, chopped
- 1 lemon, zested and juiced
- 1 tablespoon cayenne pepper
- 1/2 teaspoon ground black pepper
- 1/2 teaspoon sea salt

Directions:
1. Place chicken breasts in a 7 x 11-inch baking dish.
2. Mix all ingredients except the chicken in a medium bowl.
3. Pour prepared marinade over chicken; turn sides to coat. Cover, place in the fridge, and marinate for an hour or overnight for the best flavor.

4. Bake at 350°F for 20 minutes.
5. Use the extra sauce over the top and serve.

Nutrition: Calories: 265 kcal | Protein: 26.12 g | Fat: 16.27 g | Carbohydrates: 3.08 g

291. Spicy Almond Chicken Strips with Garlic Lime Tartar Sauce

Preparation Time: 10 minutes
Cooking Time: 10 minutes
Servings: 4
Ingredients:
Chicken sticks:
- 1 ½ pounds chicken breast, cut into 1x5-inch pieces
- 2 organic free-range eggs, whisked
- 1/2 cup blanched almond flour
- 1/2 teaspoon ground cayenne pepper
- 1/4 cup dried basil
- 3 cloves garlic, finely chopped
- 1 teaspoon salt
- 1/4 teaspoon freshly ground black pepper
- 1/2 cup coconut oil

Garlic Lime Tartar Sauce:
- 1 cup mayonnaise
- 1 teaspoon garlic powder
- 2 tablespoons lime juice
- 1 1/2 tablespoon dill pickle relish
- 1 tablespoon dried onion flakes
- 1/2 teaspoon salt

Directions:
1. Whisk together all the ingredients for the tartar sauce until well-combined. Chill for at least 30 minutes until serving.
2. Whisk eggs in a medium bowl. Combine almond flour, cayenne pepper, basil, garlic, salt, and pepper in another bowl.
3. Dip chicken strips in egg, then flour mixture; coat well and place sticks on a plate.
4. Heat some coconut oil in a saucepan over medium-high heat. Add half of the chicken strips and cook for 2-3 minutes on each side until well-browned. Leave enough room around chicken strips so that they aren't overcrowded.
5. Drain sticks on paper towels on a plate. Heat another 1/4 cup coconut oil and cook the remaining half of the chicken strips. Serve with the prepared Garlic Lime Tartar Sauce.

Nutrition: Calories: 1092 kcal | Protein: 94.15 g | Fat: 75.01 g | Carbohydrates: 7.5 g

292. Chicken Scarpariello with Spicy Sausage

Preparation Time: 10 minutes
Cooking Time: 45 minutes
Servings: 6
Ingredients:
- 1-pound boneless chicken thighs
- Sea salt, for seasoning
- Freshly ground black pepper for seasoning
- 3 tablespoons good-quality olive oil, divided
- ½ pound Italian sausage (sweet or hot)
- 1 tablespoon minced garlic
- 1 pimiento, chopped
- 1 cup chicken stock
- 2 tablespoons chopped fresh parsley

Directions:
1. Preheat the oven. Set the oven temperature to 425°F.
2. Brown the chicken and sausage. Pat the chicken thighs to dry using paper towels and season them lightly with salt and pepper. In a large oven-safe skillet over medium-high heat, warm 2 tablespoons of olive oil. Add the chicken thighs and sausage to the skillet and brown them on all sides, turning them carefully, about 10 minutes.
3. Bake the chicken and sausage. Bring the skillet into the oven and bake for 25 minutes or until the chicken is cooked through. Take the skillet out of the oven, transfer the chicken and sausage to a plate, and put the skillet over medium heat on the stovetop.
4. Make the sauce. Warm the remaining 1 tablespoon of olive oil, add the garlic and pimiento, and sauté for 3 minutes. Deglaze the skillet by using a spoon to scrape up any browned bits from the bottom of the skillet. Pour in the chicken stock, bring it to a boil, then reduce the heat to low and simmer until

the sauce reduces by about half, about 6 minutes.
5. Finish and serve. Put back the chicken and sausage to the skillet, toss it to coat it with the sauce, and serve it topped with the parsley.

Nutrition: Calories: 370 | Total fat: 30g | Total carbs: 3g | Fiber: 0g | Net carbs: 3g | Sodium: 314mg | Protein: 19g

293. Almond Chicken Cutlets

Preparation Time: 10 minutes
Cooking Time: 15 minutes
Servings: 4
Ingredients:
- 2 eggs
- ½ teaspoon garlic powder
- 1 cup almond flour
- 1 tablespoon chopped fresh oregano
- 4 (4-ounce) boneless skinless chicken breasts, pounded to about ¼ inch thick
- ¼ cup good-quality olive oil
- 2 tablespoons grass-fed butter

Directions:
1. Bread the chicken. Whisk together the eggs, garlic powder in a medium bowl, and set it aside. Stir together the almond flour and oregano on a plate and set the plate next to the egg mixture. Pat the chicken breasts to dry using paper towels and dip them into the egg mixture. Remove excess egg, then roll the chicken in the almond flour until they are coated.
2. Fry the chicken. In a large skillet over medium-high heat, warm the olive oil and butter. Add the breaded chicken breasts and fry them, turning them once until they are cooked through, crispy, golden brown, and 14 to 16 minutes in total.
3. Serve. Place one cutlet on each of the four plates and serve them immediately.

Nutrition: Calories: 328 | Total fat: 23 | Total carbs: 0g | Fiber: 0g | Net carbs: 0g | Sodium: 75m | Protein: 28g

294. Cheesy Chicken Sun-Dried Tomato Packets

Preparation Time: 15 minutes
Cooking Time: 40 minutes
Servings: 4
Ingredients:
- 1 cup goat cheese
- ½ cup chopped oil-packed sun-dried tomatoes
- 1 teaspoon minced garlic
- ½ teaspoon dried basil
- ½ teaspoon dried oregano
- 4 (4-ounce) boneless chicken breasts
- Sea salt, for seasoning
- Freshly ground black pepper, for seasoning
- 3 tablespoons olive oil

Directions:
1. Preheat the oven. Set the oven temperature to 375°F.
2. Prepare the filling. Put the goat cheese, sun-dried tomatoes, garlic, basil, and oregano in a medium bowl, then mix until everything is well blended.
3. Stuff the chicken. Make a horizontal slice in the middle of each chicken breast to make a pocket, making sure not to cut through the sides or ends. Spoon one-quarter of the filling into each breast, folding the skin and chicken meat over the slit to form packets. Secure the packets with a toothpick. Lightly season the breasts with salt and pepper.
4. Brown the chicken. In a large oven-safe skillet over medium heat, warm the olive oil. Add the breasts and sear them, turning them once, until they are golden, about 8 minutes in total.
5. Bake the chicken. Bring the skillet into the oven and bake the chicken for 30 minutes or until it's cooked through.
6. Serve. Remove the toothpicks. Divide the chicken into 4 plates and serve them immediately.

Nutrition: Calories: 388 | Total fat: 29g | Total carbs: 4g | Fiber: 1g;
Net carbs: 3g | Sodium: 210mg | Protein: 28g

295. Tuscan Chicken Saute

Preparation Time: 10 minutes
Cooking Time: 35 minutes
Servings: 4
Ingredients:
- 1-pound boneless chicken breasts, each cut into three pieces
- Sea salt for seasoning
- Freshly ground black pepper for seasoning
- 3 tablespoons olive oil
- 1 tablespoon minced garlic
- ¾ cup chicken stock
- 1 teaspoon dried oregano
- ½ teaspoon dried basil
- ½ cup heavy (whipping) cream
- ½ cup shredded Asiago cheese
- 1 cup fresh spinach
- ¼ cup sliced Kalamata olives

Directions:
1. Prepare the chicken. Pat the chicken, breasts dry, and lightly season them with salt and pepper.
2. Sauté the chicken. In a large skillet over medium-high heat, warm the olive oil. Add the chicken and sauté until it is golden brown and just cooked through, about 15 minutes in total. Transfer the chicken to a plate and set it aside.
3. Make the sauce. Put the garlic to the skillet, then sauté until it's softened for about 2 minutes. Stir in the chicken stock, oregano, and basil, scraping up any browned bits in the skillet. Bring to a boil, then reduce the heat to low and simmer until the sauce is reduced by about one-quarter, about 10 minutes.
4. Finish the dish. Stir in the cream, Asiago, and simmer, stirring the sauce frequently, until it has thickened about 5 minutes. Put back the chicken to the skillet along with any accumulated juices. Stir in the spinach and olives and simmer until the spinach is wilted for about 2 minutes.
5. Serve. Divide the chicken and sauce between four plates and serve it immediately.

Nutrition: Calories: 483 | Total fat: 38g | Total carbs: 5g | Fiber: 1g; | Net carbs: 3g | Sodium: 332mg | Protein: 31g

296. Breaded Chicken Fillets

Preparation Time: 5 minutes
Cooking Time: 10-25 minutes
Servings: 4
Ingredients:
- 1-pound chicken fillets
- 3 bell peppers, quartered lengthwise
- 1/3 cup Romano cheese
- 2 teaspoons olive oil
- 1 garlic clove, minced
- Kosher salt, to taste
- Ground black pepper, to taste
- 1/3 cup crushed pork rinds

Directions:
1. Set oven to 410°F
2. Mix the crushed pork rinds, Romano cheese, olive oil, and minced garlic. Dredge the chicken into this mixture.
3. Bring the chicken into a lightly greased baking sheet. Sprinkle with salt and black pepper to taste.
4. Scatter the peppers around the chicken and bake in the preheated oven for 20 to 25 minutes or thoroughly cooked.

Nutrition: 367 Calories | 16.9g Fat | 6g Carbs | 43g Protein | 0.7g Fiber

297. Turkey Ham and Mozzarella Pate

Preparation Time: 10 minutes
Cooking Time: 0 minutes
Servings: 6
Ingredients:
- 4 ounces' turkey ham, chopped
- 2 tablespoons fresh parsley, roughly chopped
- 2 tablespoons flaxseed meal
- 4 ounces' mozzarella cheese, crumbled
- 2 tablespoons sunflower seeds

Directions:

1. Thoroughly combine the ingredients, except for the sunflower seeds, in your food processor.
2. Spoon the mixture into a serving bowl and scatter the sunflower seeds over the top.

Nutrition: 212 Calorie | 18.8g Fat | 2g Carbs | 10.6g Protein | 1.6g Fiber

298. Boozy Glazed Chicken

Preparation Time: 5 minutes
Cooking Time: 55 minutes
Servings: 4
Ingredients:
- 2 pounds' chicken drumettes
- 2 tablespoons ghee, at room temperature
- Sea salt, to taste
- Ground black pepper, to taste
- 1 teaspoon Mediterranean seasoning mix
- 2 vine-ripened tomatoes, pureed
- 3/4 cup rum
- 3 tablespoons coconut aminos
- A few drops of liquid Stevia
- 1 teaspoon chile peppers, minced
- 1 tablespoon minced fresh ginger
- 1 teaspoon ground cardamom
- 2 tablespoons fresh lemon juice, + wedges for serving

Directions:
1. Toss the chicken with the melted ghee, salt, black pepper, and Mediterranean seasoning mix until well coated on all sides.
2. In another bowl, thoroughly combine the pureed tomato puree, rum, coconut aminos, Stevia, chile peppers, ginger, cardamom, and lemon juice.
3. Pour the tomato mixture over the chicken drumettes; let it marinate for 2 hours. Bake in the preheated oven at 410 degrees F for about 45 minutes.
4. Add in the reserved marinade and place it under the preheated broiler for 10 minutes.

Nutrition: 307 Calories | 12.1g Fat | 2.7g Carbs | 33.6g Protein | 1.5g Fiber

299. Pan-Fried Chorizo Sausage

Preparation Time: 5 minutes
Cooking Time: 15 minutes
Servings: 4
Ingredients:
- 16 ounces smoked turkey chorizo
- 1 ½ cups Asiago cheese, grated
- 1 teaspoon oregano
- 1 teaspoon basil
- 1 cup tomato puree
- 4 scallion stalks, chopped
- 1 teaspoon garlic paste
- Sea salt, to taste
- Ground black pepper, to taste
- 1 tablespoon dry sherry
- 1 tablespoon extra-virgin olive oil
- 2 tablespoons fresh coriander, roughly chopped

Directions:
1. In a skillet, put oil and heat it over moderately high heat. Now, brown the turkey chorizo, crumbling with a fork for about 5 minutes.
2. Add in the other ingredients, except for cheese; continue to cook for 10 minutes more or until cooked through.

Nutrition: 330 Calories | 17.2g Fat | 4.5g Carbs | 34.4g Protein | 1.6g Fiber

300. Easy Chicken Tacos

Preparation Time: 5 minutes
Cooking Time: 27 minutes
Servings: 4
Ingredients:
- 1-pound ground chicken
- 1 ½ cups Mexican cheese blend
- 1 tablespoon Mexican seasoning blend
- 2 teaspoons butter, room temperature
- 2 small-sized shallots, peeled and finely chopped
- 1 clove garlic, minced
- 1 cup tomato puree
- 1/2 cup salsa
- 2 slices bacon, chopped

Directions:
1. In a saucepan, put butter, then melt in over a moderately high flame. Now, cook the shallots until tender and fragrant.

2. Then, sauté the garlic, chicken, and bacon for about 5 minutes, stirring continuously and crumbling with a fork. Add the in Mexican seasoning blend.
3. Fold in the tomato puree and salsa; continue to simmer for 5 to 7 minutes over medium-low heat; reserve.
4. Line a baking pan with wax paper. Place 4 piles of the shredded cheese on the baking pan and gently press them down with a wide spatula to make "taco shells."
5. Bake in the preheated oven at 365 degrees F for 6 to 7 minutes or until melted. Allow these taco shells to cool for about 10 minutes.

Nutrition: 535 Calories | 33.3g Fat | 4.8g Carbs | 47.9g Protein | 1.9g Fibe

301. Cheesy Bacon-Wrapped Chicken with Asparagus Spears

Preparation Time: 20 minutes
Cooking Time: 30 minutes
Servings: 4
Ingredients:

- 4 chicken breasts
- 8 bacon slices
- 1 pound (454 g) asparagus spears
- 2 tablespoons fresh lemon juice
- ½ cup Manchego cheese, grated
- From the cupboard
- 4 tablespoons olive oil, divided
- Salt, to taste
- Freshly ground black pepper, to taste

Directions:

1. Set the oven to 400°F. Line a baking sheet using parchment paper, then grease with 1 tablespoon olive oil.
2. Put the chicken breasts in a large bowl, and sprinkle with salt and black pepper. Toss to combine well.
3. Wrap every chicken breast with 2 slices of bacon. Place the chicken on the baking sheet, then bake in the preheated oven for 25 minutes or until the bacon is crispy.
4. Preheat the grill to high, then brush with the remaining olive oil.
5. Place the asparagus spears on the grill grate, and sprinkle with salt. Grill for 5 minutes or until fork-tender. Flip the asparagus frequently during the grilling.
6. Transfer the bacon-wrapped chicken breasts to four plates, drizzle with lemon juice, and scatter with Manchego cheese. Spread the hot asparagus spears on top to serve.

Nutrition: Calories: 455 | **Total fat: 38.1g** | **Net carbs: 2g** | **Protein: 26.1g**

302. Delightful Teriyaki Chicken Under Pressure

Preparation Time: 5 minutes
Cooking Time: 20 minutes
Servings: 8
Ingredients:

- 1 cup Chicken Broth
- ¾ cup Brown Sugar
- 2 tbsp. ground Ginger
- 1 tsp Pepper
- 3 pounds Boneless and Skinless Chicken Thighs
- ¼ cup Apple Cider Vinegar
- ¾ cup low-sodium Soy Sauce
- 20 ounces canned Pineapple, crushed
- 2 tbsp. Garlic Powder

Directions:

1. Mix all of the ingredients, excluding the chicken. Add the chicken meat and turn to coat. Seal the lid, press POULTRY, and cook for 20 minutes at High. Do a quick pressure release by turning the valve to an "open" position.

Nutrition: Calories 352 | Carbs 31g | Fat 11g | Protein 31g

303. Turkey and Potatoes with Buffalo Sauce

Preparation Time: 10 minutes
Cooking Time: 20 minutes
Servings: 2
Ingredients:

- 3 tbsps. Olive Oil

- 4 tbsp. Buffalo Sauce
- 1 pound Sweet Potatoes, cut into cubes
- 1 ½ pound Turkey Breast, cut into pieces
- ½ tsp Garlic Powder
- 1 Onion, diced
- ½ cup Water

Directions:
1. Heat 1 tbsp. Of olive oil on SAUTÉ mode at High. Stir-fry onion in hot oil for about 3 minutes. Stir in the remaining ingredients. Seal the lid, set it to PRESSURE COOK/MANUAL mode for 20 minutes at high pressure.
2. When cooking is over, do a quick pressure release by turning the valve to an "open" position.

Nutrition: Calories 377 | Carbs 32g | Fat 9g | Protein 14g

304. Exquisite Pear and Onion Goose

Preparation Time: 15 minutes
Cooking Time: 20 minutes
Servings: 8
Ingredients:
- 2 cups Chicken Broth
- 1 tbsp. Butter
- ½ cup slice Onions
- 1 ½ pounds Goose, chopped into large pieces
- 2 tbsp. Balsamic Vinegar
- 1 tsp Cayenne Pepper
- 3 Pears, peeled and sliced
- ¼ tsp Garlic Powder
- ½ tsp Pepper

Directions:
1. Melt the butter on SAUTÉ. Add the goose and cook until it becomes golden on all sides. Transfer to a plate. Add the onions and cook for 2 minutes. Return the goose to the cooker.
2. Add the rest of the ingredients, stir well to combine, and seal the lid. Select PRESSURE COOK/MANUAL mode, and set the timer to 18 minutes at High Pressure. Do a quick pressure release? Serve and enjoy!

Nutrition: Calories 313 | Carbs 14g | Fat 8g | Protein 38g

305. Turkey Breast with Fennel and Celery

Preparation Time: 10 minutes
Cooking Time: 15 minutes
Servings: 3
Ingredients:
- 2 pounds Boneless and Skinless Turkey Breast
- 1 cup Fennel Bulb, chopped
- 1 cup celery with leaves, chopped
- 2 ¼ cups Chicken Stock
- ¼ tsp Pepper
- ¼ tsp Garlic Powder

Directions:
1. Throw all ingredients in your pressure cooker. Give it a good stir and seal the lid. Press PRESSURE COOK/MANUAL, and cook for 15 minutes at High. Do a quick pressure release? Shred the turkey with two forks.

Nutrition: Calories 272 | Carbs 7g | Fat 4g | Protein 48g

306. Pancetta and Chicken Risotto

Preparation Time: 15 minutes
Cooking Time: 15 minutes
Servings: 2
Ingredients:
- 3/4-pound. Chicken meat, diced
- 2 to 3 slices pancetta; diced
- 3/4 cup risotto or Arborio rice
- 1 teaspoon fresh thyme
- 1 tablespoon lemon zest
- 1 tablespoon unsalted butter
- 1 tablespoon olive oil
- 2 tablespoon parmesan; grated
- 2 garlic cloves; chopped
- 1/2 onion; chopped
- 3 ½ cups chicken stock
- Salt and Pepper to taste

Directions:

1. Put oil and butter into Instant Pot and press the "Sauté" button (*Normal* preset). Wait till you see Hot on display.
2. Add onion, cook for 1 to 2 minutes. Add pancetta, chicken, and garlic. Cook for another 2 to 3 minutes.
3. Add rice and mix well. The rice should be covered with an oil-butter mixture. Scrape the sides of the pot. Cook for 2 to 3 minutes, stirring constantly. Press the *Cancel* button.
4. Add chicken stock, thyme, lemon zest, salt, and pepper. Seal the lid and turn the vent to *Sealed*. Press the *Pressure Cook* (Manual) button, use the *+* or *-* button to set the timer for 6 minutes. Use the *Pressure level* button to set Pressure to *HIGH*.
5. When the timer is up, press the *Cancel* button and allow the pressure to be released naturally; until the float valve drops down.
6. Open the lid; Add parmesan cheese to the pot and stir well until it melts. Serve topped with extra parmesan and lemon zest.

Nutrition: Calories: 586 g| Total Fat: 22.5 g|Total Carbohydrate: 23.6 g|Protein: 45

MEAT

307. Beef with Carrot & Broccoli

Preparation Time: 15 minutes
Cooking Time: 14 minutes
Servings: 4
Ingredients:
- 2 tbsp. coconut oil, divided
- 2 medium garlic cloves, minced
- 1 lb. beef sirloin steak, sliced into thin strips
- Salt, to taste
- ¼ cup chicken broth
- 2 tsp. fresh ginger, grated
- 1 tbsp. Ground flax seeds
- ½ tsp. Red pepper flakes, crushed
- ¼ tsp. freshly ground black pepper
- 1 large carrot, peeled and sliced thinly
- 2 cups broccoli florets
- 1 medium scallion, sliced thinly

Directions:
1. In a skillet, warm 1 tbsp. of oil on medium-high heat.
2. Put garlic and sauté for approximately 1 minute.
3. Add beef and salt and cook for at least 4-5 minutes or till browned.
4. Using a slotted spoon, transfer the beef in a bowl.
5. Take off the liquid from the skillet.
6. Put together broth, ginger, flax seeds, red pepper flakes, and black pepper, then mix in a bowl.
7. In the same skillet, warm the remaining oil on medium heat.
8. Put the carrot, broccoli, and ginger mixture, then cook for at least 3-4 minutes or till the desired doneness.
9. Mix in beef and scallion, then cook for around 3-4 minutes.

Nutrition: Calories: 41 | **Fat:** 13g | **Carbohydrates:** 28g | **Fiber:** 9g | **Protein:** 35g

308. Beef with Mushroom & Broccoli

Preparation Time: 15 minutes
Cooking Time: 12 minutes
Servings: 4
Ingredients:
- For Beef Marinade:
- 1 garlic clove, minced
- 1 (2-inch piece fresh ginger, minced
- Salt, to taste
- Freshly ground black pepper, to taste
- ¾ cup beef broth
- 1 lb. flank steak, trimmed and sliced into thin strips
- For Vegetables:
- 2 tbsp. coconut oil, divided
- 2 minced garlic cloves
- 3 cups broccoli rabe, chopped
- 4 oz. shiitake mushrooms halved
- 8 oz. cremini mushrooms, sliced

Directions:
1. For marinade in a bowl, put together all ingredients except beef, then mix.
2. Add beef and coat with marinade.
3. Bring in the fridge to marinate for at least 15 minutes.
4. In the skillet, warm oil on medium-high heat.
5. Take off beef from the bowl, reserving the marinade.
6. Put beef and garlic and cook for about 3-4 minutes or till browned.
7. Using a slotted spoon, transfer the beef in a bowl.
8. Put the reserved marinade, broccoli, and mushrooms in the same skillet and cook for at least 3-4 minutes.
9. Stir in beef and cook for at least 3-4 minutes.

Nutrition: Calories: 417 | **Fat:** 10g | **Carbohydrates:** 23g | **Fiber:** 11g | **Protein:** 33g

309. Citrus Beef with Bok Choy

Preparation Time: 15 minutes
Cooking Time: 11 minutes
Servings: 4
Ingredients:
- For Marinade:
- 2 minced garlic cloves
- 1 (1-inch piece fresh ginger, grated
- 1/3 cup fresh orange juice
- ½ cup coconut aminos
- 2 tsp. fish sauce
- 2 tsp. Sriracha
- 1¼ lb. sirloin steak, sliced thinly

For Veggies:
- 2 tbsp. coconut oil, divided
- 3-4 wide strips of fresh orange zest
- 1 jalapeño pepper, sliced thinly
- 1 tbsp. arrowroot powder
- ½ pound Bok choy, chopped
- 2 tsp. sesame seeds

Directions:
1. In a big bowl, put together garlic, ginger, orange juice, coconut aminos, fish sauce, and Sriracha for marinade, then mix.
2. Put the beef and coat with marinade.
3. Place in the fridge to marinate for around a couple of hours.
4. In a skillet, warm oil on medium-high heat.
5. Add orange zest and sauté for approximately 2 minutes.
6. Take off the beef from a bowl, reserving the marinade.
7. In the skillet, add beef and increase the heat to high.
8. Stir fry for at least 2-3 minutes or till browned.
9. With a slotted spoon, transfer the beef and orange strips right into a bowl.
10. With a paper towel, wipe out the skillet.
11. In a similar skillet, heat the remaining oil on medium-high heat.
12. Add jalapeño pepper and stir fry for about 3-4 minutes.
13. Meanwhile, add arrowroot powder in reserved marinade and stir to mix.
14. In the skillet, add marinade mixture, beef, and Bok choy and cook for about 1-2 minutes.
15. Serve hot with garnishing of sesame seeds.

Nutrition: Calories: 39| Fat: 11| Carbohydrates: 20|Fiber: 6g| Protein: 34g

310. Beef with Zucchini Noodles

Preparation Time: 15 minutes
Cooking Time: 9 minutes
Servings: 4
Ingredients:
- 1 teaspoon fresh ginger, grated
- 2 medium garlic cloves, minced
- ¼ cup coconut aminos
- 2 tablespoons fresh lime juice
- 1½ pound NY strip steak, trimmed and sliced thinly
- 2 medium zucchinis, spiralized with Blade C
- Salt, to taste
- 3 tablespoons essential olive oil
- 2 medium scallions, sliced
- 1 teaspoon red pepper flakes, crushed
- 2 tablespoons fresh cilantro, chopped

Directions:
1. In a big bowl, mix ginger, garlic, coconut aminos, and lime juice.
2. Add beef and coat with marinade generously.
3. Refrigerate to marinate for approximately 10 minutes.
4. Place zucchini noodles over a large paper towel and sprinkle with salt.
5. Keep aside for around 10 minutes.
6. In a big skillet, heat oil on medium-high heat.
7. Add scallion and red pepper flakes and sauté for about 1 minute.
8. Add beef with marinade and stir fry for around 3-4 minutes or till browned.
9. Add zucchini and cook for approximately 3-4 minutes.
10. Serve hot with all the topping of cilantro.

Nutrition: Calories: 434| Fat: 17g|Carbohydrates: 23g| Fiber: 12g|Protein: 29g

311. Beef with Asparagus & Bell Pepper

Preparation Time: 15 minutes
Cooking Time: 13 minutes
Servings: 4-5
Ingredients:
- 4 garlic cloves, minced
- 3 tablespoons coconut aminos
- 1/8 teaspoon red pepper flakes, crushed
- 1/8 teaspoon ground ginger
- Freshly ground black pepper, to taste
- 1 bunch asparagus, trimmed and halved
- 2 tablespoons olive oil, divided
- 1-pound flank steak, trimmed and sliced thinly
- 1 red bell pepper, seeded and sliced
- 3 tablespoons water
- 2 teaspoons arrowroot powder

Directions:
1. Mix garlic, coconut aminos, red pepper flakes, crushed, ground ginger, and black pepper in a bowl. Keep aside.
2. In a pan of boiling water, cook asparagus for about 2 minutes.
3. Drain and rinse under cold water.
4. In a substantial skillet, heat 1 tablespoon of oil on medium-high heat.
5. Add beef and stir fry for around 3-4 minutes.
6. With a slotted spoon, transfer the beef to a bowl.
7. In a similar skillet, heat the remaining oil on medium heat.
8. Add asparagus and bell pepper and stir fry for approximately 2-3 minutes.
9. Meanwhile, in the bowl, mix water and arrowroot powder.
10. Stir in beef, garlic, and arrowroot mixture, and cook for around 3-4 minutes or desired thickness.

Nutrition: Calories: 399 | Fat: 17g | Carbohydrates: 27g | Fiber: 8g | Protein: 35g

312. Spiced Ground Beef

Preparation Time: 10 minutes
Cooking Time: 22 minutes
Servings: 5
Ingredients:
- 2 tablespoons coconut oil
- 2 whole cloves
- 2 whole cardamoms
- 1 (2-inch piece cinnamon stick
- 2 bay leaves
- 1 teaspoon cumin seeds
- 2 onions, chopped
- Salt, to taste
- ½ tablespoon garlic paste
- ½ tablespoon fresh ginger paste
- 1-pound lean ground beef
- 1½ teaspoons fennel seeds powder
- 1 teaspoon ground cumin
- 1½ teaspoons red chili powder
- 1/8 teaspoon ground turmeric
- Freshly ground black pepper, to taste
- 1 cup coconut milk
- ¼ cup water
- ¼ cup fresh cilantro, chopped

Directions:
1. In a sizable pan, heat oil on medium heat.
2. Add cloves, cardamoms, cinnamon sticks, bay leaves, and cumin seeds and sauté for about 20-a a few seconds.
3. Add onion and 2 pinches of salt and sauté for about 3-4 minutes.
4. Add garlic-ginger paste and sauté for about 2 minutes.
5. Add beef and cook for about 4-5 minutes, entering pieces using the spoon.
6. Cover and cook for approximately 5 minutes.
7. Stir in spices and cook, stirring for approximately 2-2½ minutes.
8. Stir in coconut milk and water and cook for about 7-8 minutes.
9. Season with salt and take away from heat.
10. Serve hot using the garnishing of cilantro.

Nutrition: Calories: 444 | Fat: 15g | Carbohydrates: 29g | Fiber: 11g | Protein: 39g

313. Ground Beef with Cabbage

Preparation Time: 10 minutes
Cooking Time: 15 minutes
Servings: 6
Ingredients:

- 1 tbsp. olive oil
- 1 onion, sliced thinly
- 2 teaspoons fresh ginger, minced
- 4 garlic cloves, minced
- 1-pound lean ground beef
- 1½ tablespoons fish sauce
- 2 tablespoons fresh lime juice
- 1 small head of purple cabbage, shredded
- 2 tablespoons peanut butter
- ½ cup fresh cilantro, chopped

Directions:
1. In a huge skillet, warm oil on medium heat.
2. Add onion, ginger, and garlic and sauté for about 4-5 minutes.
3. Add beef and cook for approximately 7-8 minutes, getting into pieces using the spoon.
4. Drain off the extra liquid in the skillet.
5. Stir in fish sauce and lime juice and cook for approximately 1 minute.
6. Add cabbage and cook around 4-5 minutes or till the desired doneness.
7. Stir in peanut butter and cilantro and cook for about 1 minute.
8. Serve hot.

Nutrition: Calories: 402| Fat: 13g|Carbohydrates: 21g| Fiber: 10g| Protein: 33g

314. Ground Beef with Veggies

Preparation Time: 15 minutes
Cooking Time: 20 minutes
Servings: 2-4
Ingredients:
- 1-2 tablespoons coconut oil
- 1 red onion, sliced
- 2 red jalapeño peppers, seeded and sliced
- 2 minced garlic cloves
- 1-pound lean ground beef
- 1 small head broccoli, chopped
- ½ of head cauliflower, chopped
- 3 carrots, peeled and sliced
- 3 celery ribs, sliced
- Chopped fresh thyme to taste
- Dried sage to taste
- Ground turmeric, to taste
- Salt, to taste
- Freshly ground black pepper, to taste

Directions:
1. In a huge skillet, melt coconut oil on medium heat.
2. Add onion, jalapeño peppers, and garlic and sauté for about 5 minutes.
3. Add beef and cook for around 4-5 minutes, entering pieces using the spoon.
4. Add remaining ingredients and cook, occasionally stirring for about 8-10 min.
5. Serve hot.

Nutrition: Calories: 453| Fat: 17g| Carbohydrates: 26g|Fiber: 8g,|Protein: 35g

315. Ground Beef with Cashews & Veggies

Preparation Time: 15 minutes
Cooking Time: 15 minutes
Servings: 4
Ingredients:
- 1½ pound lean ground beef
- 1 tablespoon garlic, minced
- 2 tablespoons fresh ginger, minced
- ¼ cup coconut aminos
- Salt, to taste
- Freshly ground black pepper, to taste
- 1 medium onion, sliced
- 1 can water chestnuts, drained and sliced
- 1 large green bell pepper, sliced
- ½ cup raw cashews, toasted

Directions:
1. Heat a nonstick skillet on medium-high heat.
2. Add beef and cook for about 6-8 minutes, breaking into pieces with all the spoons.
3. Add garlic, ginger, coconut aminos, salt, and black pepper and cook for approximately 2 minutes.
4. Put the vegetables and cook approximately 5 minutes or till the desired doneness.
5. Stir in cashews and immediately remove from heat.
6. Serve hot.

Nutrition: Calories: 452|Fat: 20g|Carbohydrates: 26g|Fiber: 9g|Protein: 36g

316. Ground Beef with Greens & Tomatoes

Preparation Time: 15 minutes
Cooking Time: 15 minutes
Servings: 4
Ingredients:
- 1 tbsp. organic olive oil
- ½ of white onion, chopped
- 2 garlic cloves, chopped finely
- 1 jalapeño pepper, chopped finely
- 1-pound lean ground beef
- 1 teaspoon ground coriander
- 1 teaspoon ground cumin
- ½ teaspoon ground turmeric
- ½ teaspoon ground ginger
- ½ teaspoon ground cinnamon
- ½ teaspoon ground fennel seeds
- Salt, to taste
- Freshly ground black pepper, to taste
- 8 fresh cherry tomatoes, quartered
- 8 collard greens leave, stemmed, and chopped
- 1 teaspoon fresh lemon juice

Directions:
1. In a huge skillet, warm oil on medium heat.
2. Put onion and sauté for approximately 4 minutes.
3. Add garlic and jalapeño pepper and sauté for approximately 1 minute.
4. Add beef and spices and cook for approximately 6 minutes, breaking into pieces while using a spoon.
5. Stir in tomatoes and greens and cook, stirring gently for about 4 minutes.
6. Stir in lemon juice and take away from heat.

Nutrition: Calories: 432 | Fat: 16g | Carbohydrates: 27g | Fiber: 12g | Protein: 39g

317. Beef & Veggies Chili

Preparation Time: 15 minutes
Cooking Time: 1 hour
Servings: 6-8
Ingredients:
- 2 pounds lean ground beef
- ½ head cauliflower, chopped into large pieces
- 1 onion, chopped
- 6 garlic cloves, minced
- 2 cups pumpkin puree
- 1 teaspoon dried oregano, crushed
- 1 teaspoon dried thyme, crushed
- 1 teaspoon ground cumin
- 1 teaspoon ground turmeric
- 1-2 teaspoons chili powder
- 1 teaspoon paprika
- 1 teaspoon cayenne pepper
- ¼ teaspoon red pepper flakes, crushed
- Salt, to taste
- Freshly ground black pepper, to taste
- 1 (26 oz.) can tomatoes, drained
- ½ cup water
- 1 cup beef broth

Directions:
1. Heat a substantial pan on medium-high heat.
2. Add beef and stir fry for around 5 minutes.
3. Add cauliflower, onion, and garlic and stir fry for approximately 5 minutes.
4. Add spices and herbs and stir to mix well.
5. Stir in remaining ingredients and provide to a boil.
6. Reduce heat to low and simmer, covered approximately 30-45 minutes.
7. Serve hot.

Nutrition: Calories: 453 | Fat: 10g | Carbohydrates: 20g | Fiber: 8g | Protein: 33g

318. Ground Beef & Veggies Curry

Preparation Time: 15 minutes
Cooking Time: 36 minutes
Servings: 6-8
Ingredients:
- 2-3 tablespoons coconut oil
- 1 cup onion, chopped
- 1 garlic clove, minced
- 1-pound lean ground beef
- 1½ tablespoons curry powder
- 1/8 teaspoon ground ginger
- 1/8 teaspoon ground cinnamon

- 1/8 teaspoon ground turmeric
- Salt, to taste
- 2½-3 cups tomatoes, chopped finely
- 2½-3 cups fresh peas shelled
- 2 sweet potatoes, peeled and chopped

Directions:
1. In a sizable pan, melt coconut oil on medium heat.
2. Add onion and garlic and sauté for around 4-5 minutes.
3. Add beef and cook for about 4-5 minutes.
4. Add curry powder and spices and cook for about 1 minute.
5. Stir in tomatoes, peas, and sweet potato and bring to your gentle simmer.
6. Simmer covered approximately 25 minutes.

Nutrition: Calorie: 432 | Fat: 16g | Carbohydrates: 21g | Fiber: 11g | Protein: 36g

319. Spicy & Creamy Ground Beef Curry

Preparation Time: 15 minutes
Cooking Time: 32 minutes
Servings: 4
Ingredients:
- 1-2 tablespoons coconut oil
- 1 teaspoon black mustard seeds
- 2 sprigs curry leaves
- 1 Serrano pepper, minced
- 1 large red onion, chopped finely
- 1 (1-inch) fresh ginger, minced
- 4 garlic cloves, minced
- 1 teaspoon ground coriander
- 1 teaspoon ground cumin
- ½ teaspoon ground turmeric
- ¼ teaspoon red chili powder
- Salt, to taste
- 1-pound lean ground beef
- 1 potato, peeled and chopped
- 3 medium carrots, peeled and chopped
- ¼ cup water
- 1 (14 oz.) can coconut milk
- Salt, to taste
- Freshly ground black pepper, to taste
- Chopped fresh cilantro for garnishing

Directions:
1. In a big pan, melt coconut oil on medium heat.
2. Add mustard seeds and sauté for about thirty seconds.
3. Add curry leaves and Serrano pepper and sauté for approximately half a minute.
4. Add onion, ginger, and garlic and sauté for about 4-5 minutes.
5. Add spices and cook for about 1 minute.
6. Add beef and cook for about 4-5 minutes.
7. Stir in potato, carrot, and water and provide with a gentle simmer.
8. Simmer, covered for around 5 minutes.
9. Stir in coconut milk and simmer for around fifteen minutes.
10. Stir in salt and black pepper and remove from heat.
11. Serve hot while using garnishing of cilantro.

Nutrition: Calories: 432 | Fat: 14g | Carbohydrates: 22g | Fiber: 8 | Protein: 39g

320. Curried Beef Meatballs

Preparation Time: 20 minutes
Cooking Time: 22 minutes
Servings: 6
Ingredients:
- For Meatballs:
- 1-pound lean ground beef
- 2 organic eggs, beaten
- 3 tablespoons red onion, minced
- ¼ cup fresh basil leaves, chopped
- 1 (1-inch fresh ginger piece, chopped finely
- 4 garlic cloves, chopped finely
- 3 Thai bird's eye chilies, minced
- 1 teaspoon coconut sugar
- 1 tablespoon red curry paste
- Salt, to taste
- 1 tablespoon fish sauce
- 2 tablespoons coconut oil
- For Curry:
- 1 red onion, chopped
- Salt, to taste
- 4 garlic cloves, minced
- 1 (1-inch) fresh ginger piece, minced
- 2 Thai bird's eye chilies, minced

- 2 tablespoons red curry paste
- 1 (14 oz.) coconut milk
- Salt, to taste
- Freshly ground black pepper, to taste
- Lime wedges, for

Directions:
1. For meatballs in a huge bowl, put all together with the ingredients except oil and mix till well combined.
2. Make small balls from the mixture.
3. In a huge skillet, melt coconut oil on medium heat.
4. Add meatballs and cook for about 3-5 minutes or till golden brown all sides.
5. Transfer the meatballs right into a bowl.
6. In the same skillet, add onion and a pinch of salt and sauté for around 5 minutes.
7. Add garlic, ginger, and chilies, and sauté for about 1 minute.
8. Add curry paste and sauté for around 1 minute.
9. Add coconut milk and meatballs and convey to some gentle simmer.
10. Reduce the warmth to low and simmer, covered for around 10 minutes.
11. Serve using the topping of lime wedges.

Nutrition: Calories: 44 | Fat: 15g | Carbohydrates: 20g | Fiber: 2 | Protein: 37g

321. Beef Meatballs in Tomato Gravy

Preparation Time: 20 minutes
Cooking Time: 37 minutes
Servings: 4
Ingredients:
- For Meatballs:
- 1-pound lean ground beef
- 1 organic egg, beaten
- 1 tablespoon fresh ginger, minced
- 1 garlic oil, minced
- 2 tablespoons fresh cilantro, chopped finely
- 2 tablespoons tomato paste
- 1/3 cup almond meal
- 1 tablespoon ground cumin
- Pinch of ground cinnamon
- Salt, to taste
- Freshly ground black pepper, to taste
- ¼ cup coconut oil
- For Tomato Gravy:
- 2 tablespoons coconut oil
- ½ small onion, chopped
- 2 garlic cloves, chopped
- 1 teaspoon fresh lemon zest, grated finely
- 2 cups tomatoes, chopped finely
- Pinch of ground cinnamon
- 1 teaspoon red pepper flakes, crushed
- ¾ cup chicken broth
- Salt, to taste
- Freshly ground black pepper, to taste
- ¼ cup fresh parsley, chopped

Directions:
1. For meatballs in a sizable bowl, add all ingredients except oil and mix till well combined.
2. Make about 1-inch sized balls from the mixture.
3. In a substantial skillet, melt coconut oil on medium heat.
4. Add meatballs and cook for approximately 3-5 minutes or till golden brown on all sides.
5. Transfer the meatballs into a bowl.
6. For gravy in a big pan, melt coconut oil on medium heat.
7. Add onion and garlic and sauté for approximately 4 minutes.
8. Add lemon zest and sauté for approximately 1 minute.
9. Add tomatoes, cinnamon, red pepper flakes, and broth and simmer for approximately 7 minutes.
10. Stir in salt, black pepper, and meatballs and reduce the warmth to medium-low.
11. Simmer for approximately twenty minutes.
12. Serve hot with all the garnishing of parsley.

Nutrition: Calories: 40 | Fat: 11g | Carbohydrates: 27g | Fiber: 4g | Protein: 38g

322. Pork with Lemongrass

Preparation Time: 10 minutes
Cooking Time: 30 minutes
Servings: 4

Ingredients:
- 4 pork chops
- 2 tablespoons olive oil
- 2 spring onions, chopped
- A pinch of salt and black pepper
- ½ cup vegetable stock
- 1 stalk lemongrass, chopped
- 2 tablespoons coconut aminos
- 2 tablespoons cilantro, chopped

Directions:
1. Warm a pan with the oil on medium-high heat, add the spring onions and the meat, and brown for 5 minutes.
2. Add the rest of the ingredients, toss, and cook everything over medium heat for 25 minutes.
3. Divide the mix between plates and serve.

Nutrition: Calories 290 | Fat | Fiber 6 | Carbs 8 | Protein 14

323. Pork with Olives

Preparation Time: 10 minutes
Cooking Time: 40 minutes
Servings: 4
Ingredients:
- 1 yellow onion, chopped
- 4 pork chops
- 2 tablespoons olive oil
- 1 tablespoon sweet paprika
- 2 tablespoons balsamic vinegar
- ¼ cup kalamata olives, pitted and chopped
- 1 tablespoon cilantro, chopped
- Pinch of Sea Salt
- Pinch black pepper

Directions:
1. Warm a pan with the oil on medium heat; add the onion and sauté for 5 minutes.
2. Add the meat and brown for a further 5 minutes.
3. Put the rest of the ingredients, toss, cook over medium heat for 30 minutes, divide between plates and serve.

Nutrition: Calories 280 | Fat 11 | Fiber 6 | Carbs 10 | Protein 21

324. Pork Chops with Tomato Salsa

Preparation Time: 10 minutes
Cooking Time: 15 minutes
Servings: 4
Ingredients:
- 4 pork chops
- 1 tablespoon olive oil
- 4 scallions, chopped
- 1 teaspoon cumin, ground
- ½ tablespoon hot paprika
- 1 teaspoon garlic powder
- Pinch of sea salt
- Pinch of black pepper
- 1 small red onion, chopped
- 2 tomatoes, cubed
- 2 tablespoons lime juice
- 1 jalapeno, chopped
- ¼ cup cilantro, chopped
- 1 tablespoon lime juice

Directions:
1. Warm a pan with the oil on medium heat, add the scallions and sauté for 5 minutes.
2. Add the meat, cumin paprika, garlic powder, salt, and pepper, toss, cook for 5 minutes on each side, and divide between plates.
3. Combine the tomatoes with the remaining ingredients in a bowl, toss, divide next to the pork chops, and serve.

Nutrition: Calories 313 | Fat 23.7 | Fiber 1. | Carbs 5. | Protein 19.2

SALAD RECIPES

325. Loaded Kale Salad

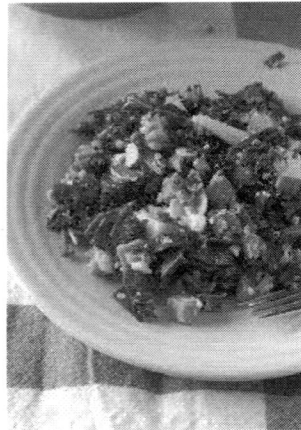

Preparation time: 10 minutes
Cooking Time: 0 minutes
Servings: 4
Ingredients:

- ¾ cups quinoa, cooked and drained

Vegetables:
- 4 large carrots, halved and chopped
- 1 whole beet, sliced
- 2 tablespoons water
- 1 pinch salt
- ½ teaspoon curry powder
- 8 cups kale, chopped
- ½ cups cherry tomatoes, chopped
- 1 ripe avocado, cubed
- ¼ cup hemp seeds
- ½ cup sprouts

Dressing:
- ⅓ cup tahini
- 3 tablespoons lemon juice
- 1-2 tablespoons maple syrup
- 1 pinch salt
- ¼ cup water

Directions:
1. Combine all the dressing ingredients in a small bowl.
2. In a salad bowl, toss in all the vegetables, quinoa, and dressing.
3. Mix them well then refrigerate to chill.
4. Serve.

Nutrition: Calories 72 Total Fat 15.4 g Saturated Fat 4.2 g Cholesterol 168 mg Sodium 203 mg Total Carbs 28.5 g Sugar 1.1 g Fiber 4 g Protein 7.9 g

326. Avocado Kale Salad

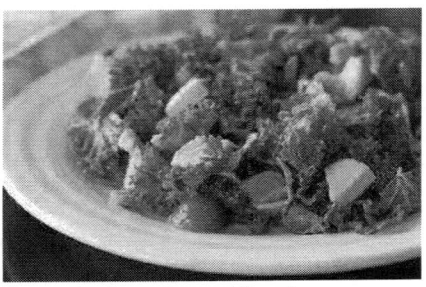

Preparation time: 10 minutes
Cooking Time: 0 minutes
Servings: 4
Ingredients:

- ⅓ cup tahini
- 2 teaspoons garlic, chopped
- 1 medium lemon juiced
- 1½ tablespoons maple syrup
- Water

Salad:
- 1 large bundle kale, chopped
- 1 tablespoon grapeseed oil
- 1 tablespoon lemon juice
- 1 medium beet

Directions:
1. Combine all the dressing ingredients in a small bowl.
2. In a salad bowl, toss in all the salad ingredients and dressing.
3. Mix them well then refrigerate to chill.
4. Serve.

Nutrition: Calories 201 Total Fat 8.9 g Saturated Fat 4.5 g Cholesterol 57 mg Sodium 340 mg Total Carbs 24.7 g Fiber 1.2 g Sugar 1.3 g Protein 15.3 g

327. Broccoli Sweet Potato Chickpea Salad

Preparation time: 35 minutes
Cooking Time: 0 minutes
Servings: 6

Ingredients:

Vegetables:
- 1 large, sweet potato, peeled and diced
- 1 head broccoli
- 2 tablespoons olive or grapeseed oil
- 1 pinch each salt and black pepper
- 1 teaspoon dried dill
- 1 medium red bell pepper

Chickpeas:
- 1 (15 ouncecan chickpeas, drained
- 1 tablespoon olive or grapeseed oil
- 1 tablespoon tandoori masala spice
- 1 pinch salt
- 1 teaspoon coconut sugar
- 1 pinch cayenne pepper

Garlic dill sauce:
- ⅓ cup hummus
- 3 large cloves garlic, minced
- 1 teaspoon dried dill
- 2 tablespoons lemon juice
- Water

Directions:
1. Preheat your oven to 400 degrees F.
2. In a greased baking sheet, toss sweet potato with salt and oil.
3. Bake the sweet potatoes for 15 minutes in the oven.
4. Toss all chickpea ingredients and spread in a tray.
5. Bake them for 7 minutes in the oven.
6. Combine all the sauce ingredients in a small bowl.
7. In a salad bowl, toss in all the vegetables, roasted potato, chickpeas, and sauce.
8. Mix them well then refrigerate to chill. Serve.

Nutrition: Calories 231 Total Fat 20.1 g Saturated Fat 2.4 g Cholesterol 110 mg Sodium 941 mg Total Carbs 20.1 g Fiber 0.9 g Sugar 1.4 g Protein 4.6 g

328. Broccoli, Kelp, And Feta Salad

Preparation Time: 15 minutes
Cooking Time: 0 minutes
Servings: 4

Ingredients:
- 2 tbsp olive oil
- 1 tbsp white wine vinegar
- 2 tbsp chia seeds
- Salt and freshly ground black pepper to taste
- 2 cups broccoli slaw
- 1 cup chopped kelp, thoroughly washed and steamed
- 1/3 cup chopped pecans
- 1/3 cup pumpkin seeds
- 1/3 cup blueberries
- 2/3 cup ricotta cheese

Directions:
1. In a small bowl, whisk olive oil, white wine vinegar, chia seeds, salt, and black pepper. Set aside.
2. In a large salad bowl, combine the broccoli slaw, kelp, pecans, pumpkin seeds, blueberries, and ricotta cheese.
3. Drizzle dressing on top, toss, and serve.

Nutrition: Calories 397, Total Fat 3.87g, Total Carbs 8.4g, Fiber 3.5g, Net Carbs 4.9g, Protein 8.93g

329. Cauliflower & Lentil Salad

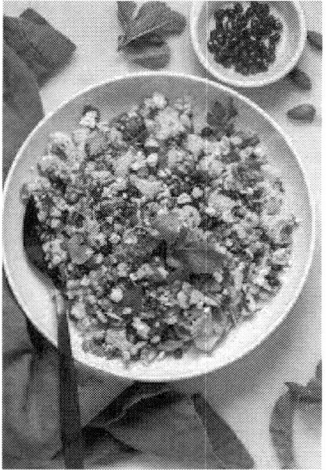

Preparation time: 35 minutes
Cooking Time: 0 minutes

Servings: 4
Ingredients:
Cauliflower:
- 1 head cauliflower, florets
- 1½ tablespoons melted coconut oil
- 1½ tablespoons curry powder
- ¼ teaspoon salt

Salad:
- 5 cups mixed greens
- 1 cup cooked lentils
- 1 cup red or green grapes, halved
- Fresh cilantro

Tahini Dressing:
- 4½ tablespoons green curry paste
- 2 tablespoons tahini
- 2 tablespoons lemon juice
- 1 tablespoon maple syrup
- 1 pinch salt
- 1 pinch black pepper
- Water to thin

Directions:
1. Preheat your oven to 400 degrees F.
2. On a greased baking sheet, toss cauliflower with salt, curry powder, and oil.
3. Bake the cauliflower for 25 minutes in the oven.
4. Combine all the dressing ingredients in a small bowl.
5. In a salad bowl, toss in all the vegetables, roasted cauliflower, and dressing.
6. Mix them well then refrigerate to chill.
7. Serve.

Nutrition: Calories 212 Total Fat 7 g Saturated Fat 1.3 g Cholesterol 25 mg Sodium 101 mg Total Carbs 32.5 g Sugar 5.7 g Fiber 6 g Protein 4 g

330. Cherry Tomato Salad with Soy Chorizo

Preparation Time: 10 minutes
Cooking Time: 0 minutes
Servings: 4
Ingredients:
- 2 ½ tbsp olive oil
- 4 soy chorizo, chopped
- 2 tsp red wine vinegar
- 1 small red onion, finely chopped
- 2 ½ cups cherry tomatoes, halved
- 2 tbsp chopped cilantro
- Salt and freshly ground black pepper to taste
- 3 tbsp sliced black olives to garnish

Directions:
1. Over medium fire, heat half tablespoon of olive oil in a skillet and fry soy chorizo until golden. Turn heat off.
2. In a salad bowl, whisk remaining olive oil and vinegar. Add onion, cilantro, tomatoes, and soy chorizo. Mix with dressing and season with salt and black pepper.
3. Garnish with olives and serve.

Nutrition: Calories 138, Total Fat 8.95g, Total Carbs 5.63g, Fiber 0.4g, Net Carbs 5.23g, Protein 7.12g

331. French Style Potato Salad

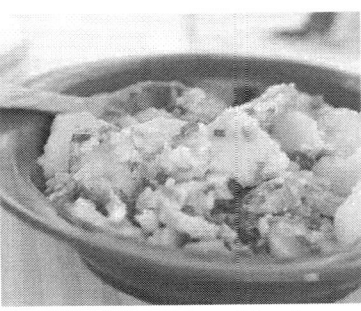

Preparation time: 10 minutes
Cooking Time: 0 minutes
Servings: 4
Ingredients:

- 2 pounds baby yellow potatoes, boiled, peeled, and diced
- 1 pinch salt and black pepper
- 1 tablespoon apple cider vinegar
- 1 cup green onion, diced
- ¼ cup fresh parsley, chopped

Dressing:
- 2½ tablespoons brown mustard
- 3 cloves garlic, minced
- ¼ teaspoon salt and black pepper
- 3 tablespoons red wine vinegar
- 1 tablespoon apple cider vinegar
- 3 tablespoons olive oil
- ¼ cup dill, chopped

Directions:

1. Combine all the dressing ingredients in a salad bowl.
2. In a salad bowl, toss in all the vegetables, seasonings, and dressing.
3. Mix them well then refrigerate to chill.
4. Serve.

Nutrition: Calories 197 Total Fat 4 g Saturated Fat 0.5 g Cholesterol 135 mg Sodium 790 mg Total Carbs 31 g Fiber 12.2 g Sugar 2.5 g Protein 11 g

332. Kale Salad with Tahini Dressing

Preparation time: 30 minutes
Cooking Time: 0 minutes
Servings: 4
Ingredients:
Roasted vegetables:
- 1 medium zucchini, chopped
- 1 medium sweet potato, chopped
- 1 cup red cabbage, chopped
- 1 tablespoon melted coconut oil
- 1 pinch salt
- ½ teaspoon curry powder

Dressing:
- ⅓ cup tahini
- ½ teaspoon garlic powder
- 1 tablespoon coconut aminos
- 1 pinch salt
- 1 large clove garlic, minced
- ¼ cup water

Salad:
- 6 cups mixed greens
- 4 small radishes, sliced
- 3 tablespoons hemp seeds
- 2 tablespoons lemon juice
- ½ ripe avocado, to garnish
- 2 tablespoons vegan feta cheese, crumbled
- Pomegranate seeds, to garnish
- Pecans, to garnish

Directions:
1. Preheat your oven at 375 degrees F.
2. On a greased baking sheet, toss zucchini, sweet potato, and red cabbage with salt, curry powder, and oil.
3. Bake the zucchini cabbage mixture for 20 minutes in the oven.
4. Combine all the dressing ingredients in a small bowl.
5. In a salad bowl, toss in all the vegetables, roasted vegetables, and dressing.
6. Mix them well then refrigerate to chill.
7. Garnish with feta cheese, pecans, pomegranate seeds and avocado.
8. Serve.

Nutrition: Calories 201 Total Fat 8.9 g Saturated Fat 4.5 g Cholesterol 57 mg Sodium 340 mg Total Carbs 24.7 g Fiber 1.2 g Sugar 1.3 g Protein 15.3 g

333. Almond-Goji Berry Cauliflower Salad

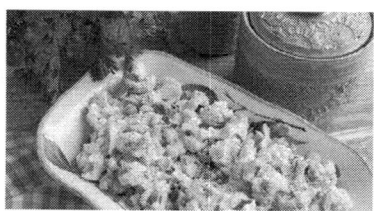

Preparation Time: 10 minutes
Cooking Time: 2 minutes
Serving: 4
Ingredients:

- 8 sun-dried tomatoes in olive oil, drained
- 12 pitted green olives, roughly chopped
- 1 lemon, zested and juiced
- 3 tbsp chopped green onions
- A handful chopped almonds
- ¼ cup goji berries
- 1 tbsp sesame oil
- ½ cup watercress
- 3 tbsp chopped parsley
- Salt and freshly ground black pepper to taste
- Lemon wedges to garnish

Directions:
1. Pour cauliflower into a large safe-microwave bowl, sprinkle with some water, and steam in microwave for 1 to 2 minutes or until softened.
2. In a large salad bowl, combine cauliflower, tomatoes, olives, lemon zest and juice, green onions, almonds, goji berries, sesame oil,

watercress, and parsley. Season with salt and black pepper, and mix well.
3. Serve with lemon wedges.

Nutrition: Calories 203, Total Fat 15.28g, Total Carbs 9.64g, Fiber 3.2g, Net Carbs 6.44g, Protein 6.67g, Protein 2.54g

334. Mango Salad with Peanut Dressing

Preparation time: 10 minutes
Cooking Time: 0 minutes
Servings: 4
Ingredients:
Salad:
- 1 head butter lettuce, washed and chopped
- 1½ cups carrot, shredded
- 1¼ cups red cabbage, shredded
- 1 large ripe mango, cubed
- ½ cup fresh cilantro, chopped

Dressing:
- ⅓ cup creamy peanut butter
- 2½ tablespoons lime juice
- 1½ tablespoons maple syrup
- 2 teaspoon chili garlic sauce
- 3 tablespoons coconut aminos

Directions:
1. Combine all the dressing ingredients in a small bowl.
2. In a salad bowl, toss in all the vegetables, seasonings, and dressing.
3. Mix them well then refrigerate to chill.
4. Serve.

Nutrition: Calories 305 Total Fat 11.8 g Saturated Fat 2.2 g Cholesterol 56 mg Sodium 321 mg Total Carbs 34.6 g Fibers 0.4 g Sugar 2 g Protein 7 g

335. Niçoise Salad

Preparation time: 25 minutes
Cooking Time: 0 minutes
Servings: 4
Ingredients:
Salad:
- 6 small red potatoes, peeled, boiled, and diced
- 1 cup green beans, chopped
- 1 head lettuce, chopped
- ½ cup pitted kalamata olives
- ½ cup tomato, sliced
- ½ medium red beet

Chickpeas:
- 1 (15 ounce can chickpeas
- 1 teaspoon Dijon mustard
- 1 teaspoon maple syrup
- 1 teaspoon dried dill
- 1 pinch salt
- 1 tablespoon roasted sunflower seeds

Dressing:
- 3 tablespoons minced shallot
- 1 heaping teaspoon Dijon mustard
- 1 teaspoon fresh thyme, chopped
- ⅓ cup red wine vinegar
- ¼ teaspoon salt and black pepper
- ¼ cup olive oil

Directions:
1. Preheat your oven to 400 degrees F.
2. In a greased baking sheet, toss chickpeas with salt and all the chickpea ingredients.
3. Bake the chickpeas for 15 minutes in the oven.
4. Combine all the dressing ingredients in a small bowl.
5. In a salad bowl, toss in all the vegetables, roasted chickpeas, and dressing.
6. Mix them well then refrigerate to chill. Serve.

Nutrition: Calories 205 Total Fat 22.7 g Saturated Fat 6.1 g Cholesterol 4 mg Sodium 227 mg Total Carbs 26.1 g Fiber 1.4 g Sugar 0.9 g Protein 5.2 g

336. Penne Pasta Salad

Preparation time: 30 minutes
Cooking Time: 0 minutes
Servings: 4
Ingredients:
Salad:
- 2 cups roasted tomatoes
- 12 ounces penne pasta

Pesto:
- 2 cups fresh basil
- 4 cloves garlic, minced
- ¼ cup toasted pine nuts

- 1 medium lemon, juice
- ¼ cup vegan cheese, shredded
- 1 pinch salt
- ¼ cup olive oil

Directions:
1. In a blender, add all the pesto ingredients.
2. Blend them well until it is lump free.
3. In a salad bowl toss in pasta, roasted tomatoes, and pesto.
4. Mix them well then refrigerate to chill.
5. Serve.

Nutrition: Calories 361 Total Fat 16.3 g Saturated Fat 4.9 g Cholesterol 114 mg Sodium 515 mg Total Carbs 29.3 g Fiber 0.1 g Sugar 18.2 g Protein 3.3 g

337. Maple Rice

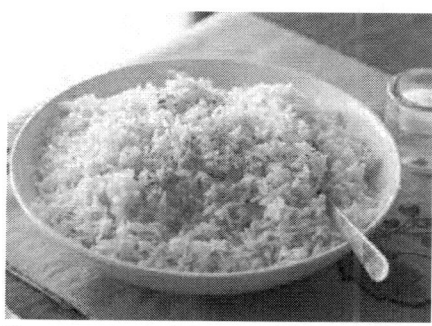

Preparation Time: 20 minutes, plus overnight soaking
Cooking Time: 5 minutes
Servings: 4

- Rice: 250g
- Maple syrup: 2 tsp
- Water: 500 ml

Directions:
1. Toast rice in the pan lightly and soak overnight in 250ml water
2. Add maple syrup, rice, and 250ml water to the blender and blend till smoothen
3. Strain and discard the puree
4. Shake before serving

Nutrition: Carbs: 7.5g Protein: 0.4g Fats: 0.1g Calories: 33Kcal

338. Rainbow Vegetable Bowl

Preparation Time: 25 minutes
Cooking Time: 0 minutes
Servings: 4

Ingredients
- Red bell Pepper: 1
- Yellow bell pepper: 1
- Smoked Paprika: ½ tsp
- Potatoes: 3 medium
- Mushrooms: 8 oz
- Yellow Onion: 1
- Zucchini: 1
- Cumin Powder: ½ tsp
- Garlic Powder: ½ tsp
- Salt and Pepper: as per your taste
- Cooking oil: 2 tbsp (optional)

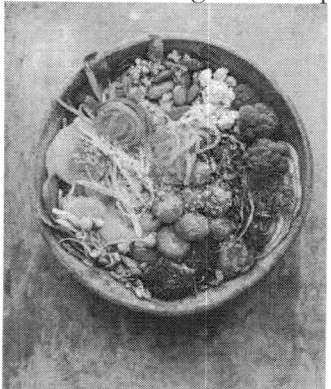

Directions:
1. Heat a large pan on medium flame, add oil and put the sliced potatoes
2. Cook the potatoes till they change color
4. Cook till veggies are soften

Nutrition: Carbs: 29.9g Protein: 5.9g Fats: 10g Calories: 227 Kcal

339. Red Bell Pepper Hummus

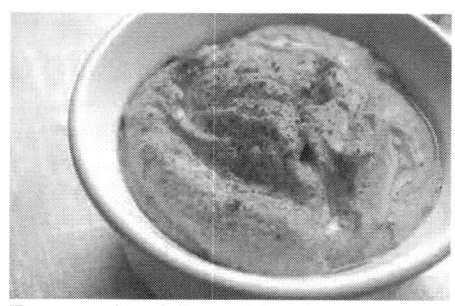

Preparation Time: 10 minutes
Cooking Time: 0 minutes
Servings: 4

- Chickpeas: 2 cups can rinsed and drained
- Red bell pepper: 1 cup diced
- Tahini: 3 tbsp
- Garlic: 1 clove
- Lemon: 2 tbsp
- Extra-virgin olive oil: 3 tbsp, plus extra to serve
- Salt: as per your need
- Cayenne pepper: 1 tsp

Directions:
1. Blend red bell pepper, chickpeas, tahini, olive oil, salt, and garlic together in a blender
2. Add in lemon juice and mix
3. Add to the serving bowl and top with extra olive oil and cayenne pepper

Nutrition: Carbs: 27.1g Protein: 9.8g Fats: 18.7g Calories: 302Kcal

340. Roasted Asparagus with Feta Cheese Salad

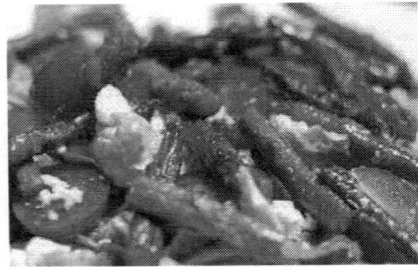

Preparation Time: 30 minutes
Cooking Time: 0 minutes
Servings: 4

- 1 lb asparagus, trimmed and halved
- 2 tbsp olive oil
- ½ tsp dried basil
- ½ tsp dried oregano
- Salt and freshly ground black pepper to taste
- ½ tsp hemp seeds
- 1 tbsp maple (sugar-free syrup
- ½ cup arugula
- 4 tbsp crumbled feta cheese
- 2 tbsp hazelnuts
- 1 lemon, cut into wedges

Directions:
1. Preheat oven to 350oF.
2. Pour asparagus on a baking tray, drizzle with olive oil, basil, oregano, salt, black pepper, and hemp seeds. Mix with your hands and roast in oven for 15 minutes.
3. Remove, drizzle with maple syrup, and continue cooking until slightly charred, 5 minutes.
4. Spread arugula in a salad bowl and top with asparagus. Scatter with feta cheese, hazelnuts, and serve with lemon wedges.

Nutrition: Calories 146, Total Fat 12.87g, Total Carbs 5.07g, Fiber 1.6g, Net Carbs 3.47g, Protein 4.44g

341. Roasted Bell Pepper Salad with Olives

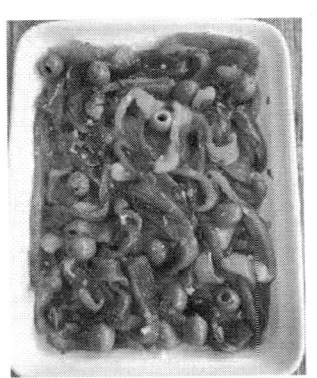

Preparation Time: 30 minutes
Cooking Time: 0 minutes
Servings: 4

- 8 large red bell peppers, deseeded and cut in wedges
- ½ tsp erythritol
- 2 ½ tbsp olive oil
- 1/3 cup arugula
- 1 tbsp mint leaves
- 1/3 cup pitted Kalamata olives
- 3 tbsp chopped almonds
- ½ tbsp balsamic vinegar
- Crumbled feta cheese for topping
- Toasted pine nuts for topping

Directions:
1. Preheat oven to 400° F.
2. Pour bell peppers on a roasting pan; season with erythritol and drizzle with half of olive oil. Roast in oven until slightly charred, 20 minutes. Remove from oven and set aside.

3. Arrange arugula in a salad bowl, scatter bell peppers on top, mint leaves, olives, almonds, and drizzle with balsamic vinegar and remaining olive oil. Season with salt and black pepper.
4. Toss: top with feta cheese and pine nuts and serve.

Nutrition: Calories 163, Total Fat 13.3g, Total Carbs 6.53g, Fiber 2.2g, Net Carbs 4.33g, Protein 3.37g

342. Roasted Broccoli with Peanuts and Kecap Manis

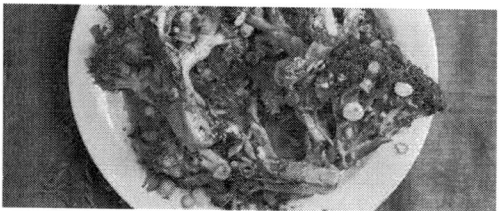

Preparation Time: 40 minutes
Cooking Time: 0 minutes
Servings: 4

- Broccoli: a large head diced
- Vegetable oil: 1 tbsp
- Kecap manis: 4 tbsp
- Spring onions: 2 sliced
- Grated garlic: 2 cloves
- Sesame oil: 2 tbsp
- Ginger: 1 tbsp grated
- Dried chili flakes: a pinch
- Salted peanuts: a handful roughly chopped
- Rice vinegar: 3 tbsp
- Coriander: ½ cup chopped
- Ready-made crispy onions: 3 tbsp
- Water: 50ml
- Cooked jasmine rice to serve

Directions:
1. Preheat the oven to 180C
2. Take a large pan and add oil and fry broccoli in batches and spread on baking sheet
3. In the same pan, fry garlic, ginger, and chili flakes for a minute and then add rice vinegar, manis, sesame oil, and water
4. Pour all this mixture over broccoli and cover with foil
5. Roast the broccoli for 20 minutes in the oven
6. Mix crispy onion and salted peanuts together and sprinkle over cooked broccoli
7. Top with coriander and serve with rice

Nutrition: Carbs: 22.5 g Protein: 9.4 g Fats: 12.8 g Calories:258 Kcal

343. Roasted Chili Potatoes

Preparation Time: 35 minutes
Cooking Time: 25 minutes
Servings: 2

Ingredients
- Olive oil: 1 tbsp
- Potatoes: 2 cups cut like fries
- Salt: as per your taste
- Pepper: as per your taste
- Red chili flakes: 1 tsp

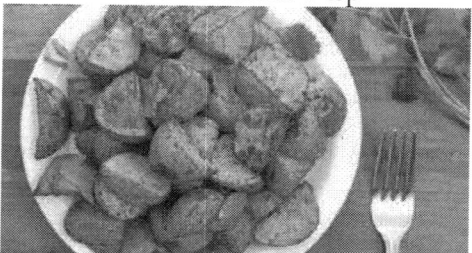

Directions:
1. Preheat the oven 200C
2. Add potatoes to the baking sheet and sprinkle seasoning and brush with olive oil
4. Remove from the oven and sprinkle red chili flakes
5. Serve as the side dish

Nutrition: Carbs: 26 g Protein: 3g Fats: 7.2g Calories: 178Kcal

VEGETABLE AND VEGAN RECIPES

344. Lentils with Tomatoes and Turmeric

Preparation Time: 10 minutes
Cooking Time: 10 minutes
Servings: 4
Ingredients:
- 2 tbsp. Extra Olive Virgin Oil, plus extra for garnish
- 1 Onion, finely chopped
- 1 tbsp. Ground turmeric
- 1 tsp. Garlic powder
- 1 (14 oz.) can Lentils, drained
- 1 (14 oz.) can Chopped tomatoes, drained
- ½ tsp. Sea salt
- ¼ tsp. Freshly ground black pepper

Directions:
1. In a huge pot on medium-high heat, warm the olive oil until it shimmers.
2. Add the onion and turmeric, and cook for about 5 minutes, occasionally stirring, until soft.
3. Add the garlic powder, lentils, tomatoes, salt, and pepper. Cook for 5 minutes, stirring occasionally. Serve garnished with additional olive oil, if desired

Nutrition: Calories: 24 | Total Fat: 8g | Total Carbs: 34g | Sugar: 5g | Fiber: 15g | Protein: 12g | sodium 243mg

345. Whole-Wheat Pasta with Tomato-Basil Sauce

Preparation Time: 15 minutes
Cooking Time: 10 minutes
Servings: 4
Ingredients:
- 2 tbsp. Extra Olive virgin oil
- 1 Onion, minced
- 6 Garlic cloves, minced
- 2 (28 oz.) can crushed tomatoes, undrained
- ½ tsp. Sea salt
- ¼ tsp. Ground black pepper
- ¼ cup Basil leaves, chopped
- 1 (8 oz.) Package whole-wheat pasta

Directions:
1. In a huge pot on medium-high heat, warm the olive oil until it shimmers.
2. Add the onion. Cook for about 5 minutes, occasionally stirring, until soft.
3. Add the garlic. Cook for 30 seconds, stirring constantly.
4. Stir in the tomatoes, salt, and pepper. Bring it to a simmer. Reduce the heat to medium and cook for 5 minutes, stirring occasionally.
5. Pull it out from the heat then stir in the basil. Toss with the pasta.

Nutrition: Calories: 330 | Total Fat: 8g | Total Carbs: 56g | Sugar: 24g

346. Fried Rice with Kale

Preparation Time: 10 minutes
Cooking Time: 12 minutes
Servings: 4
Ingredients:
- 2 tbsp. Extra olive virgin oil
- 8 oz. Tofu, chopped
- 6 Scallion, white and green parts, thinly sliced
- 2 cups Kale, stemmed and chopped
- 3 cups cooked brown rice
- ¼ cup Stir fry sauce

Directions:
1. In a huge skillet on medium-high heat, warm the olive oil until it shimmers.
2. Add the tofu, scallions, and kale. Cook for 5 to 7 minutes, frequently stirring, until the vegetables are soft.
3. Add the brown rice and stir-fry sauce. Cook for 3 to 5 minutes, occasionally stirring, until heated through.

Nutrition: Calories: 301 | Total Fat: 11g | Total Carbs: 36g | Sugar: 1g

347. Nutty and Fruity Garden Salad

Preparation Time: 10 minutes
Cooking Time: 0 minutes
Servings: 2
Ingredients:
- 6 cups baby spinach
- ½ cup chopped walnuts, toasted
- 1 ripe red pear, sliced
- 1 ripe persimmon, sliced
- 1 teaspoon garlic minced
- 1 shallot, minced
- 1 tablespoon extra-virgin olive oil
- 2 tablespoons fresh lemon juice
- 1 teaspoon wholegrain mustard

Directions:
1. Mix well garlic, shallot, oil, lemon juice, and mustard in a large salad bowl.
2. Add spinach, pear, and persimmon. Toss to coat well.
3. To serve, garnish with chopped pecans.

Nutrition: Calories 332 | Total Fat 21 | Saturated Fat 2g | Total Carbs 37g | Net Carbs 28g | Protein 7g

348. Stir-Fried Brussels Sprouts and Carrots

Preparation Time: 10 minutes
Cooking Time: 15 minutes
Servings: 6
Ingredients:
- 1 tbsp. cider vinegar
- 1/3 cup water
- 1 lb. Brussels sprouts halved lengthwise
- 1 lb. carrots cut diagonally into ½-inch thick lengths
- 3 tbsp. olive oil, divided
- 2 tbsp. chopped shallot
- ½ tsp pepper
- ¾ tsp salt

Directions:
1. On medium-high fire, place a nonstick medium fry pan and heat 2 tbsp. oil.
2. Ass shallots and cook until softened, around one to two minutes while occasionally stirring.
3. Add pepper salt, Brussels sprouts, and carrots. Stir fry until vegetables start to brown on the edges, around 3 to 4 minutes.
4. Add water, cook, and cover.
5. After 5 to 8 minutes, or when veggies are already soft, add the remaining butter.
6. If needed, season with more pepper and salt to taste.
7. Turn off fire, transfer to a platter, serve and enjoy.

Nutrition: Calories 9 | Total Fat 4 | Saturated Fat 2 | Total Carbs 14g | Net Carbs 9g | Protein 3g

349. Curried Veggies and Poached Eggs

Preparation Time: 10 minutes
Cooking Time: 50 minutes
Servings: 4
Ingredients:
- 4 large eggs
- ½ tsp white vinegar
- 1/8 tsp crushed red pepper – optional
- 1 cup water
- 14-oz can chickpeas, drained
- 2 medium zucchinis, diced
- ½ lb. sliced button mushrooms
- 1 tbsp. yellow curry powder
- 2 cloves garlic, minced
- 1 large onion, chopped
- 2 tsp extra virgin olive oil

Directions:
1. On medium-high fire, place a large saucepan and heat oil.
2. Sauté onions until tender, around four to five minutes.
3. Put the garlic and continue sautéing for another half minute.
4. Add curry powder, stir and cook until fragrant, around one to two minutes.
5. Add mushrooms, mix, cover, and cook for 5 to 8 minutes or until mushrooms are tender and have released their liquid.

6. Add red pepper if using water, chickpeas, and zucchini. Mix well to combine and bring to a boil.
7. Once boiling, reduce fire to a simmer, cover, and cook until zucchini is tender, around 15 to 20 minutes of simmering.
8. Meanwhile, in a small pot filled with 3-inches deep water, bring to a boil on a high fire.
9. When boiling, lower the heat temperature to a simmer and add vinegar.
10. Slowly add one egg, slipping it gently into the water. Allow simmering until egg is cooked, around 3 to 5 minutes.
11. Please take off the egg using a slotted spoon and transfer it to a plate: one plate, one egg.
12. Repeat the process with the remaining eggs.
13. Once the veggies are done cooking, divide evenly into 4 servings and place one serving per plate of the egg.
14. Serve and enjoy.

Nutrition: Calories 254| Total Fat 9g| Saturated Fat 2|Total Carbs 30g |Net Carbs 21g| Protein 16g

350. Braised Kale

Preparation Time: 10 minutes
Cooking Time: 15 minutes
Servings: 3
Ingredients:
- 2 to 3 tbsp. water
- 1 tbsp. coconut oil
- ½ sliced red pepper
- 2 stalk celery (sliced to ¼-inch thick)
- 5 cups of chopped kale

Directions:
1. Heat a pan over medium heat.
2. Add coconut oil and sauté the celery for at least five minutes.
3. Add the kale and red pepper.
4. Add a tablespoon of water.
5. Let the vegetables wilt for a few minutes. Add a tablespoon of water if the kale starts to stick to the pan.
6. Serve warm.

Nutrition: Calories 61|Total Fat 5g|Saturated Fat 1g|Total Carbs 3g | Net Carbs 2g|Protein 1g

351. Braised Leeks, Cauliflower and Artichoke Hearts

Preparation Time: 10 minutes
Cooking Time: 10 minutes
Servings: 4
Ingredients:
- 2 tbsp. coconut oil
- 2 garlic cloves, chopped
- 1 ½ cup artichoke hearts
- 1 ½ cups chopped leeks
- 1 ½ cups cauliflower flowerets

Directions:
1. In a skillet, warm oil at medium-high heat temperature.
2. Put the garlic and sauté for one minute. Add the vegetables and constantly stir until the vegetables are cooked.
3. Serve with roasted chicken, fish, or pork.

Nutrition: Calories 111|Total Fat 7g|Saturated Fat 1g|Total Carbs 12 |Net Carbs 8g

352. Celery Root Hash Browns

Preparation Time: 10 minutes
Cooking Time: 10 minutes
Servings: 4
Ingredients:
- 4 tbsp. coconut oil
- ½ tsp sea salt
- 2 to 3 medium celery roots

Directions:
1. Scrub the celery root clean and peel it using a vegetable peeler.
2. Grate the celery root in a manual grater.
3. In a skillet, add oil and heat it over medium heat.
4. Place the grated celery root on the skillet and sprinkle with salt.
5. Let it cook for 10 minutes on each side or until the grated celery turns brown.
6. Serve warm.

Nutrition: Calories 160|Total Fat 14g|Saturated Fat 3g |Total Carbs 10g|Net Carbs 7g Protein 1.5g

353. Braised Carrots 'n Kale

Preparation Time: 10 minutes
Cooking Time: 10 minutes
Servings: 2
Ingredients:
- 1 tablespoon coconut oil
- 1 onion, sliced thinly
- 5 cloves of garlic, minced
- 3 medium carrots, sliced thinly
- 10 ounces of kale, chopped
- ½ cup water
- Salt and pepper to taste
- A dash of red pepper flakes

Directions:
1. Warm oil in a skillet over medium flame and sauté the onion and garlic until fragrant.
2. Toss in the carrots and stir for 1 minute. Add the kale and water. Season with salt and pepper to taste.
3. Close the lid and allow to simmer for 5 minutes.
4. Sprinkle with red pepper flakes.
5. Serve and enjoy.

Nutrition: Calories 161 | Total Fat 8g | Saturated Fat 1g | Total Carbs 20g | Net Carbs 14g | Protein 8g

354. Stir-Fried Gingery Veggies

Preparation Time: 10 minutes
Cooking Time: 10 minutes
Servings: 4
Ingredients:
- 1 tablespoon oil
- 3 cloves of garlic, minced
- 1 onion, chopped
- 1 thumb-size ginger, sliced
- 1 tablespoon water
- 1 large carrot, peeled and julienned and seedless
- 1 large green bell pepper, julienned and seedless
- 1 large yellow bell pepper, julienned and seedless
- 1 large red bell pepper, julienned and seedless
- 1 zucchini, julienned
- Salt and pepper to taste

Directions:
1. Heat oil in a nonstick saucepan over a high flame and sauté the garlic, onion, and ginger until fragrant.
2. Stir in the rest of the ingredients.
3. Keep on stirring for at least 5 minutes until vegetables are tender.
4. Serve and enjoy.

Nutrition: Calories 70 | Total Fat 4g | Saturated Fat 1g | Total Carbs 9g | Net Carbs 7g | Protein 1g

355. Cauliflower Fritters

Preparation Time: 10 minutes
Cooking Time: 15 minutes
Servings: 6
Ingredients:
- 1 large cauliflower head, cut into florets
- 2 eggs, beaten
- ½ teaspoon turmeric
- ½ teaspoon salt
- ¼ teaspoon black pepper
- 1 tablespoon coconut oil

Directions:
1. Put the cauliflower florets in a pot with water and bring them to a boil. Cook until tender, around 5 minutes of boiling. Drain well.
2. Place the cauliflower, eggs, turmeric, salt, and pepper into the food processor.
3. Pulse until the mixture becomes coarse.
4. Transfer into a bowl. Using your hands, form six small flattened balls and place them in the fridge for at least 1 hour until the mixture hardens.
5. Warm the oil in a nonstick pan and fry the cauliflower patties for 3 minutes on each side.
6. Serve and enjoy.

Nutrition: Calories 53 | Total Fat 6g | Saturated Fat 2g | Total Carbs | Net Carbs 1g | Protein 3g

356. Stir-Fried Squash

Preparation Time: 10 minutes
Cooking Time: 10 minutes
Servings: 4

Ingredients:
- 1 tablespoon olive oil
- 3 cloves of garlic, minced
- 1 butternut squash, seeded and sliced
- 1 tablespoon coconut aminos
- 1 tablespoon lemon juice
- 1 tablespoon water
- Salt and pepper to taste

Directions:
1. Heat oil over medium flame and sauté the garlic until fragrant.
2. Stir in the squash for another 3 minutes before adding the rest of the ingredients.
3. Close the lid and allow to simmer for 5 more minutes or until the squash is soft.
4. Serve and enjoy.

Nutrition: Calories 83 | Total Fat 3g | Saturated Fat 0.5 | Total Carbs 14g | Net Carbs 12g | Protein 2g

357. Cauliflower Hash Brown

Preparation Time: 10 minutes
Cooking Time: 20 minutes
Servings: 6
Ingredients:
- 4 eggs, beaten
- ½ cup coconut milk
- ½ teaspoon dry mustard
- Salt and pepper to taste
- 1 large head cauliflower, shredded

Directions:
1. Place all together ingredients in a mixing bowl and mix until well combined.
2. Place a nonstick frypan and heat over medium flame.
3. Add a large dollop of cauliflower mixture in the skillet.
4. Fry one side for 3 minutes, flip and cook the other side for a minute, like a pancake. Repeat process to remaining ingredients.
5. Serve and enjoy.

Nutrition: Calories 102 | Total Fat 8g | Saturated Fat 1g | Total Carbs 4g | Net Carbs 3g

358. Sweet Potato Puree

Preparation Time: 10 minutes
Cooking Time: 15 minutes
Servings: 5
Ingredients:
- 2 pounds sweet potatoes, peeled
- 1 ½ cups water
- 5 Medjool dates, pitted and chopped

Directions:
1. Place water and potatoes in a pot.
2. Close the lid and boil for at least 15 minutes until the potatoes are soft.
3. Drain the potatoes and place them in a food processor together with the dates.
4. Pulse until smooth.
5. Serve and enjoy.

Nutrition: Calories 112 | Total Fat 8g | Saturated Fat 1g | Total Carbs 4g | Net Carbs 3g

359. Curried Okra

Preparation Time: 10 minutes
Cooking Time: 12 minutes
Servings: 4
Ingredients:
- 1 lb. small to medium okra pods, trimmed
- ¼ tsp curry powder
- ½ tsp kosher salt
- 1 tsp finely chopped serrano chile
- 1 tsp ground coriander
- 1 tbsp. canola oil
- ¾ tsp brown mustard seeds

Direction:
1. Place a large and heavy skillet on medium-high fire and cook mustard seeds until fragrant, around 30 seconds.
2. Add canola oil. Add okra, curry powder, salt, chile, and coriander. Sauté for a minute while stirring every once in a while.
3. Cover and cook low fire for at least 8 minutes. Stir occasionally.
4. Uncover, increase the fire to medium-high and cook until okra is lightly browned, around 2 minutes more.
5. Serve and enjoy.

Nutrition: Calories 102 | Total Fat 7g | Saturated Fat 1g | Total Carbs 4g | Net Carbs 3g

360. Vegetable Potpie

Preparation Time: 10 minutes
Cooking Time: 10 minutes
Servings: 8
Ingredients:
- 1 recipe pastry for double-crust pie
- 2 tbsp. cornstarch
- 1 tsp ground black pepper
- 1 tsp kosher salt
- 3 cups vegetable broth
- 2 cups cauliflower florets
- 2 stalks celery, sliced ¼ inch wide
- 2 potatoes, peeled and diced
- 2 large carrots, diced
- 1 clove garlic, minced
- 8 oz. mushroom
- 1 onion, chopped
- 2 tbsp. olive oil

Directions:
1. In a large saucepan, sauté garlic in oil until lightly browned, add onions and continue sautéing until soft and translucent.
2. Add celery, potatoes, and carrots, and sauté for 3 minutes.
3. Add vegetable broth and cauliflower and bring to a boil. Slow fire and simmer until vegetables are slightly tender. Season with pepper and salt.
4. Mix ¼ cup water and cornstarch in a small bowl. Stir until the mixture is smooth and has no lumps. Then pour into the vegetable pot while mixing constantly.
5. Continue mixing until soup thickens, around 3 minutes. Remove from fire.
6. Meanwhile, roll out pastry dough and place it on an oven-safe 11x7 baking dish. Pour the vegetable filling and then cover with another pastry dough. Seal and flute the edges of the dough and prick the top dough with a fork in several places.
7. Bake the dish in a preheated oven of 425oF for 30 minutes or until the crust has turned a golden brown.

Nutrition: Calories 202 | Total Fat 10g | Saturated Fat 2g | Total Carbs 26g | Net Carbs 23g | Protein 4g

361. Grilled Eggplant Roll-Ups

Preparation Time: 5 minutes
Cooking Time: 3 minutes
Servings: 8
Ingredients:
- 1 tomato
- 2 tbsps. chopped fresh basil
- 2 tbsps. olive oil
- 4 oz. mozzarella cheese
- 1 eggplant, sliced

Directions:
1. Thinly slice the tomato and mozzarella and reserve.
2. Rub the eggplant slices with olive oil and grill them in a skillet for 3 minutes per side.
3. Lay a slice of cheese and tomato on top of each zucchini.
4. Sprinkle basil and black pepper and grill for 3 minutes to soften the cheese.
5. Remove the slices and set them on a plate.
6. Roll each of the slices before serving.
7. Enjoy.

Nutrition: Calories: 50 kcal | Protein: 6.12 g | Fat: 0.92 g | Carbohydrates: 5.14 g

362. Eggplant Gratin

Preparation Time: 10 minutes
Cooking Time: 40 minutes
Servings: 6
Ingredients:
- ¾ c. Gruyere cheese
- ½ tsp. black pepper
- 1 c. heavy cream
- 2 sliced eggplant
- 3 tbsps. Olive oil
- ½ c. tomato sauce
- ½ tsp. salt
- 3 oz. crumbled feta cheese
- 1 tsp. Chopped thyme
- ¼ c. chopped fresh basil
- 1 tbsp. chopped chives

Directions:
1. Heat the oven to about 375oF.

2. Cover the slices of eggplant with salt, pepper, and olive oil and bake them for 20 minutes on a baking pan.
3. Meanwhile, put feta cheese and heavy cream in a pot and boil them.
4. Remove the pot from heat and add chives and thyme, then stir before setting aside.
5. Spread the tomato sauce on a medium-sized pan and lay the eggplant slices over it.
6. Cover eggplant slices with basil and Gruyere cheese.
7. Add another layer of the remaining eggplant and cover it with the heavy cream mixture.
8. Bake for about 20 minutes and serve.

Nutrition: Calories: 217 kcal | **Protein:** 8.37 g | **Fat: 15.47 g** | **Carbohydrates: 13.66 g**

363. Veggie Stuffed Peppers

Preparation Time: 5 minutes
Cooking Time: 0 minutes
Servings: 6
Ingredients:

- 1 c. quartered cherry tomatoes
- 1 tsp. black pepper
- 3 tbsps. Dijon mustard
- ¼ c. chopped fresh parsley
- 3 halved green bell peppers
- ½ peeled and sliced cucumber
- 1 bunch sliced scallions
- ½ tsp. Salt
- ½ c. Greek yogurt
- 4 diced celery stalks

Directions:

1. In a medium bowl, combine salt, pepper, yogurt, and mustard.
2. Add cucumbers, celery, tomatoes, and scallions and combine well.
3. Stuff the mix into the pepper halves.
4. Add the chopped parsley to garnish.
5. Serve immediately and enjoy

Nutrition: Calories: 41 kcal | **Protein:** 2.49 g | **Fat: 1.78 g** | **Carbohydrates: 4.3 g**

364. Cheesy Gratin Zucchini

Preparation Time: 15 minutes
Cooking Time: 45 minutes
Servings: 9
Ingredients:

- Spray oil
- ½ c. heavy cream
- 1 tsp. rosemary
- 1 tsp. turmeric
- 1 tsp. black pepper
- 2 tbsps. olive oil
- 1 peeled and sliced small white onion
- 4 c. sliced raw zucchini
- 1 tbsp. garlic powder
- 2 c. shredded pepper jack cheese
- ½ tsps. salt

Directions:

1. Heat the oven to about 375ºF.
2. Grease the baking tray with cooking oil
3. Add a third of the zucchini and onion slices on the pan and sprinkle seasonings and half of the pepper jack cheese.
4. Add one more layer of zucchini slices, and onion then season with pepper, salt, and the remaining pepper jack cheese.
5. Lay on the remaining zucchini slices and onions.
6. Microwave garlic powder, butter, and heavy cream for a minute to melt the butter and mix well.
7. Pour the mixture over the top layer of slices
8. Bake uncovered for 45 minutes
9. Serve and enjoy

Nutrition: Calories: 151 kcal | **Protein:** 8.49 g | **Fat: 12.08 g** | **Carbohydrates: 2.49 g**

365. Korean Barbecue Tofu

Preparation Time: 10 minutes
Cooking Time: 15 minutes
Servings: 3
Ingredients:

- 1 tbsps. olive oil
- 2 tsp onion powder
- 4 garlic cloves, minced
- 2 tsp dry mustard
- 3 tbsp. brown sugar
- ½ cup soy sauce
- 1 ½ lb. firm tofu, sliced to ¼-inch cubes

Directions:
1. In a re-sealable bag, mix all ingredients except for tofu and oil. Mix well until sugar is dissolved.
2. Add sliced tofu and slowly turn bag to mix. Seal bag and place flatly inside the ref for an hour.
3. After an hour, turn the bag to the other side and marinate for another hour.
4. To cook, in a nonstick fry pan, heat oil on medium-high fire. Add tofu and stir fry until sides are browned.
5. Serve and enjoy.

Nutrition: Calories 437 | Fat 25g | Carbs 23g | Protein 40g | Fiber 6g

366. Fruit Bowl with Yogurt Topping

Preparation Time: 15 minutes
Cooking Time: 0 minutes
Servings: 6
Ingredients:
- ¼ cup golden brown sugar
- 2/3 cup minced fresh ginger
- 1 16-oz Greek yogurt
- ¼ tsp ground cinnamon
- 2 tbsp. honey
- ½ cup dried cranberries
- 3 navel oranges
- 2 large tangerines
- 1 pink grapefruit, peeled

Directions:
1. Into sections, break tangerines and grapefruit.
2. Slice tangerine sections in half and grapefruit sections into thirds. Place all sliced fruits and their juices in a large bowl.
3. Peel oranges, remove the pith, slice into ¼-inch thick rounds, and then cut into quarters. Transfer to the bowl of fruit along with juices. In a bowl, add cinnamon, honey, and ¼ cup of cranberries. Place in the ref for an hour. In a medium bowl, mix ginger and yogurt. Place on top of the fruit bowl, drizzle with remaining cranberries and brown sugar.
4. Serve and enjoy.

Nutrition: Calories 171 Fat 1g | Carbs 35g | Protein 9g | Fiber 3g

367. Collard Green Wrap

Preparation Time: 10 minutes
Cooking Time: 0 minutes
Servings: 4
Ingredients:
- ½ block feta, cut into 4 (1-inch thick) strips (4-oz)
- ½ cup purple onion, diced
- ½ medium red bell pepper, julienned
- 1 medium cucumber, julienned
- 4 large cherry tomatoes, halved
- 4 large collard green leaves, washed
- 8 whole kalamata olives, halved

Sauce
Ingredients:
- 1 cup low-fat plain Greek yogurt
- 1 tablespoon white vinegar
- 1 teaspoon garlic powder
- 2 tablespoons minced fresh dill
- 2 tablespoons olive oil
- 2.5-ounces cucumber, seeded and grated (¼-whole)
- Salt and pepper to taste

Directions:
1. Make the sauce first: make sure to squeeze out all the excess liquid from the cucumber after grating. In a small bowl, put all together with the sauce ingredients and mix thoroughly, then refrigerate.
2. Prepare and slice all wrap ingredients.
3. On a flat surface, spread one collard green leaf. Spread 2 tablespoons of Tzatziki sauce in the middle of the leaf.
4. Layer ¼ of each of the tomatoes, feta, olives, onion, pepper, and cucumber. Place them on the center of the leaf, like piling them high instead of spreading them.
5. Fold the leaf-like you would like a burrito. Repeat process for remaining ingredients.
6. Serve and enjoy.

Nutrition: Calories 463 | Fat 31g | Carbs 31g | Protein 20g | Fiber 7g

368. Zucchini Garlic Fries

Preparation Time: 10 minutes
Cooking Time: 20 minutes
Servings: 6
Ingredients:
- ¼ teaspoon garlic powder
- ½ cup almond flour
- 2 large egg whites, beaten
- 3 medium zucchinis, sliced into fry sticks
- Salt and pepper to taste

Directions:
1. Set the oven to 400F.
2. Mix the ingredients in a bowl until the zucchini fries are well coated.
3. Place fries on the cookie sheet and spread evenly.
4. Put in the oven and cook for 20 minutes.
5. Halfway through cooking time, stir-fries.

Nutrition: Calories 11 | Fat 0.1g, | Carbs 1g | Protein1.5 g | Fiber 0.5g

369. Stir-Fried Eggplant

Preparation Time: 10 minutes
Cooking Time: 10 minutes
Servings: 2
Ingredients:
- 1 tablespoon coconut oil
- 2 eggplants, sliced into 3-inch in length
- 4 cloves of garlic, minced
- 1 onion, chopped
- 1 teaspoon ginger, grated
- 1 teaspoon lemon juice, freshly squeezed
- ½ tsp salt
- ½ tsp pepper

Directions:
1. Heat oil in a nonstick saucepan.
2. Pan-fry the eggplants for 2 minutes on all sides.
3. Add the garlic and onions until fragrant, around 3 minutes.
4. Stir in the ginger, salt, pepper, and lemon juice.
5. Add a ½ cup of water and bring to a simmer. Cook until eggplant is tender.

Nutrition: Calories 232 | Fat 8g | Carbs 41g | Protein 7g | Fiber 18g

370. Sautéed Garlic Mushrooms

Preparation Time: 10 minutes
Cooking Time: 10 minutes
Servings: 4
Ingredients:
- 1 tablespoon olive oil
- 3 cloves of garlic, minced
- 16 ounces' fresh brown mushrooms, sliced
- 7 ounces fresh shiitake mushrooms, sliced
- ½ tsp salt
- ½ tsp pepper or more to taste

Directions:
1. Place a nonstick saucepan on medium-high fire and heat pan for a minute.
2. Add oil and heat for 2 minutes.
3. Stir in garlic and sauté for a minute.
4. Add remaining ingredients and stir fry until soft and tender, around 5 minutes.
5. Turn off fire, let mushrooms rest while the pan is covered for 5 minutes.
6. Serve and enjoy.

Nutrition: Calories 95 | Fat 4g | Carbs 14g | Protein 3g, | Fiber 4g

371. Stir-Fried Asparagus and Bell Pepper

Preparation Time: 10 minutes
Cooking Time: 10 minutes
Servings: 6
Ingredients:
- 1 tablespoon olive oil
- 4 cloves of garlic, minced
- 1-pound fresh asparagus spears, trimmed
- 2 large red bell peppers, seeded and julienned
- ½ teaspoon thyme
- 5 tablespoons water
- ½ tsp salt
- ½ tsp pepper or more to taste

Directions:
1. Place a nonstick saucepan on high fire and heat pan for a minute.
2. Add oil and heat for 2 minutes.
3. Stir in garlic and sauté for a minute.

4. Add remaining ingredients and stir fry until soft and tender, around 6 minutes.
  5. Turn off fire, let veggies rest while the pan is covered for 5 minutes.

Nutrition: Calories 45 | Fat 2g | Carbs 5g, Net | Protein 2g | Fiber 2g

372. Wild Rice with Spicy Chickpeas

Preparation Time: 15 minutes
Cooking Time: 60 minutes
Servings: 6-7
Ingredients:
- 1 cup basmati rice
- 1 cup wild rice
- Salt & pepper to taste
- 4tbsp Olive oil
- 1tbsp Garlic powder
- 2tsp cumin powder
- ¼ Cup sunflower oil
- 3 cups chickpeas
- 1tsp Flour
- 1tsp Curry powder
- 3tsp Paprika powder
- 1tsp Dill
- 3tbsp parsley (chopped)
- 1 medium onion (thinly sliced)
- 2 Cups currants

Directions:
1. For cooking wild rice, fill the half pot with water and bring it to a boil. Put the rice and let it simmer for at least 40 minutes.
2. Take olive in the pot and heat it on medium flame. Now add cumin powder, salt, and water and bring it to a boil. Then add basmati rice and cook for 20 minutes.
3. Leave rice for cooking and prepare spicy chickpeas. Heat 2tbsp of olive oil in the pan and toss chickpeas, garlic powder, salt & pepper, cumin, and paprika powder in it.
4. In another pan, cook onion with sunflower oil until it is golden brown and add flour.
5. Mix flour and onion with your hands.
6. For serving, place both types of rice in a bowl with spicy chickpeas and fry the onion. Garnish it with parsley and herbs.

Nutrition: Calories: 647 kcal | Protein: 25.43 g | Fat: 25.72 g | Carbohydrates: 88.3 g

373. Cashew Pesto & Parsley with veggies

Preparation Time: 15 minutes
Cooking Time: 10 minutes
Servings: 3-4
Ingredients:
- 3 Zucchini (sliced)
- 8 Soaked bamboo skewers
- 2 red capsicums
- ¼Cup olive oil
- 750grams Eggplant
- 4 Lemon cheeks

For Serving
- Couscous salad

For Preparing Cashew Pesto
- ½Cup cashew (roasted)
- ½ Cup parsley
- 2 cup grated parmesan
- 2tbsp Lime juice
- ¼Cup olive oil

Directions:
1. Toss capsicum, eggplant, and zucchini with oil and salt and thread them onto skewers.
2. Cook bamboo sticks for 6-8 minutes on a barbecue grill pan on medium heat.
3. Also, grill lemon cheeks from both sides.
4. For preparing cashew pesto, combine all ingredients in the food processor and blend.
5. Place grill skewers in a plate with grill lemon slices and drizzle some cashew pesto over it for serving.

Nutrition: Calories: 666 kcal | Protein: 23.96 g | Fat: 48.04 g | Carbohydrates: 41.4 g

374. Spicy Chickpeas with Roasted Vegetables

Preparation Time: 10 minutes
Cooking Time: 25 minutes
Servings: 2-3
Ingredients:
- 1 large carrot (peeled)
- 2tbsp Sunflower oil

- 1 Cauliflower head
- 1tbsp ground cumin
- ½ Red onions (diced)
- 1 Red pepper (deseeded)
- 400g Can chickpeas

Directions:
1. Line a large baking tine in the preheated oven (at 240C).
2. Cut all the vegetables and toss with salt, pepper, and onion.
3. In a bowl, whisk olive oil, pepper, and cumin powder.
4. Add all veggies to the bowl and toss.
5. Transfer vegetables to baking tin and bake it almost for 15 minutes.
6. Now add chickpeas and stir.
7. Return to the oven and bake it for the next 10 minutes.
8. Serve it with toast bread.

Nutrition: Calories: 348 kcal | Protein: 14.29 g | Fat: 15.88 g | Carbohydrates: 40.65 g

375. Special Vegetable Kitchree

Preparation Time: 10 minutes
Cooking Time: 46 minutes
Servings: 5-6
Ingredients:
- ½Cup brown grain rice
- 1 Cup dry lentil or split peas
- 1tsp Sea salt, cumin powder, ground turmeric, ground fenugreek, and ground coriander
- 3tbsp Coconut oil
- 1tbsp Ginger
- 5 cups vegetable stock
- 1 cup baby spinach
- 1 Medium Zucchini (roughly chopped)
- 1 Small crown broccoli (chopped)
- Greek Yogurt (for serving)

Directions:
1. In a saucepan, warm the coconut oil on medium flame and add ginger, cumin, coriander, fennel seeds, fenugreek, and turmeric and cook it for 1 minute.
2. Now add lentils and brown rice in the spices and stir. Pour the vegetable stock in it and simmer for 40 minutes.
3. Add broccoli in the tender rice and lentils and cook for another 5 minutes. Now add other vegetables and stir for 10 minutes.
4. For serving, pour some Greek yogurt over vegetable kitcheree and serve hot.

Nutrition: Calories: 1728 kcal | Protein: 4.13 g | Fat: 190.35 g | Carbohydrates: 17.31 g

376. Mashed Sweet Potato Burritos

Preparation Time: 15 minutes
Cooking Time: 60 minutes
Servings: 4
Ingredients:
- 4 Tortillas
- 1 Avocado
- 1tsp Capsicum, paprika powder, and oregano
- Salt & pepper as needed
- ½Cup sour cream
- 1 Can diced tomato
- 2 Sweet Potatoes (mashed)
- 2 Garlic cloves (minced)
- 1tbsp Cumin powder
- Fresh cilantro or parsley

Directions:
1. Before mashing, roast sweet potatoes for 45 minutes in an already preheated (at 160°C) oven.
2. Cook onion in a frying pan with oil on medium heat. Add garlic cloves and cook for 1 minute.
3. Add 1 tin of tomatoes and leave it to simmer for 10 minutes. In halfway through, add salt & pepper, paprika, cumin powder,
4. After 5 minutes, add avocado in it.
5. Now make burritos, mix one scoop of mashed potatoes with avocado filling.
6. Wrap your tortilla and grill it in the oven at 200C for 30seconds.
7. Serve it with sour cream and hot sauce.

Nutrition: Calories: 442 kcal | Protein: 12.05 g | Fat: 15.43 g | Carbohydrates: 66.85 g

SOUPS AND STEWS

377. Spring Soup with Gourmet Grains

Preparation Time: 10 minutes
Cooking Time: 25 minutes
Servings: 2
Ingredients:
- 2-tbsp olive oil
- 1-pc small onion, diced
- 6-cups chicken broth, homemade (refer to the recipe of Avgolemono Soup)
- 1-bay leaf
- ½-cup of fresh dill, chopped (divided)
- 1/3-cup Italian or Arborio whole grain rice
- 1-cup asparagus, chopped
- 1-cup carrots, diced
- 1½-cups cooked chicken, de-boned and diced or shredded
- ½-lemon, juice
- 1-pc large egg
- 2-tbsp water
- Kosher salt and fresh pepper to taste
- Fresh chives, minced for garnish

Directions:
1. Heat the olive oil and sauté the onions for 5 minutes in a large stockpot placed over medium heat. Pour in the chicken broth.
2. Add the bay leaf and half of the dill. Bring to a boil.
3. Add rice and turn the heat to medium-low. Simmer for 10 minutes.
4. Add the asparagus and carrots. Cook for 15 minutes until the vegetables are tender and the rice cooks through.
5. Add the cooked shredded chicken. Continue simmer over low heat.
6. In the meantime, combine the lemon juice and egg with water in a mixing bowl.
7. Take ½-cup of the simmering stock and pour it on the lemon-egg mixture, whisking gradually to prevent eggs from curdling.
8. Pour the lemon-egg broth into the stockpot, still whisking gradually. Soon as the soup thickens, turn off heat
9. Remove the bay leaf, and discard. Add the remaining dill, salt, and pepper.
10. To serve, ladle the creamy soup into bowls and garnish with minced chives.

Nutrition: Calories: 252.8, Fats: 8g, Dietary Fiber: 0.3g, Carbohydrates: 19.8g, Protein: 25.6g

378. Spiced Soup with Lentils & Legumes

Preparation Time: 15 minutes
Cooking Time: 35 minutes
Servings: 2
Ingredients:
- 2-tbsp extra-virgin olive oil
- 2-cloves garlic, minced
- 4-pcs large celery stalks, diced
- 2-pcs large onions, diced
- 6-cups water
- 1-tsp cumin
- ¾-tsp turmeric
- ½-tsp cinnamon
- ½-tsp fresh ginger, grated
- 1-cup dried lentils, rinsed and sorted
- 1-16-oz. can chickpeas (garbanzo beans), drained and rinsed
- 3-pcs ripe tomatoes, cubed
- ½-lemon, juice
- ½ cup fresh cilantro or parsley, chopped
- Salt

Directions:
1. Heat the olive oil and sauté the garlic, celery, and onion for 5 minutes in a large stockpot placed over medium heat.
2. Pour in the water. Add the spices and lentils. Cover the stockpot and simmer for 40 minutes until the lentils are tender.
3. Add the chickpeas and tomatoes. (Pour more water and additional spices, if desired.) Simmer for 15 minutes over low heat.

4. Pour in the lemon juice and stir the soup. Add the cilantro or parsley and salt to taste.

Nutrition: Calories: 123, Fats: 3g, Dietary Fiber: 5g, Carbohydrates: 19g, Protein: 5g

379. Lemon and Egg Pasta Soup

Preparation Time: 15 minutes
Cooking Time: 0 minutes
Servings: 2
Ingredients
- 4 ounces ditalini pasta
- 4 cups fat-free and low-sodium chicken broth
- 2 large whole eggs
- ½ cup fresh lemon juice
- 4 tablespoons chopped fresh parsley
- lemon, thinly sliced for garnish
- Salt and freshly ground pepper to taste

Directions
1. Place medium saucepan on medium-high heat. Add chicken broth to it and bring it to a boil, stirring it a couple of times.
2. Bring down the heat to low and allow the broth to simmer for about 5 minutes. Take the saucepan off the heat.
3. Take a bowl and add the eggs into it. Beat them well, add the lemon juice, and beat the eggs again
4. Use a ladle to transfer a single serving of the chicken broth into the egg bowl. Mix them well and then transfer the entire contents of the bowl into the saucepan.
5. Heat the soup while ensuring that the heat is still at low. Keep an eye out on the eggs because they tend to curdle and you need to prevent that from happening by gently stirring the soup.
6. Add salt and pepper to taste, if preferred.
7. Serve hot and garnish with lemon slices and parsley.

Nutrition: Calories: 161 Protein: 10 g Fat: 2 g Carbohydrate: 65 g

380. Roasted Vegetable Soup

Preparation Time: 15 minutes
Cooking Time: 20 minutes
Servings: 2
Ingredients:
- tablespoon olive oil
- 5 garlic cloves, peeled
- 0.3 lb. Potatoes diced (1 cm thick)
- yellow bell peppers, diced
- ½ teaspoons fresh rosemary, finely chopped
- carrot, halved lengthwise and cut into 1 cm piece
- 1 red onion, in chunks
- 0.4 quarts carrot juice
- 0.3 lb. Italian tomatoes, diced
- 1 teaspoon fresh tarragon
- Salt and pepper, to taste

Directions:
1. Preheat oven to 400° F.
2. In a baking tray place potatoes, peppers, garlic, carrot, onion, and tomatoes. Drizzle with olive oil and roast for 10-15 minutes.
3. In a saucepan add carrot juice, tarragon; let boil a little.
4. Add all roasted vegetables and stir well. Let it simmer for a few minutes.
5. Season with salt, pepper, and rosemary. Mix well.
6. Serve and enjoy.

Nutrition: Calories – 318, Fat – 97 g, Carbs – 60 g, Protein – 1.7 g

381. Mediterranean Tomato Soup

Preparation Time: 5 minutes
Cooking Time: 30 minutes
Servings: 2
Ingredient:
- 2 red bell peppers, unseeded, chopped
- 2 medium onions, chopped
- 2-3 garlic cloves, minced
- 7-8 tomatoes, chopped
- 0.4 quarts chicken broth
- Salt and pepper, to taste
- 3 tablespoons olive oil
- 2 tablespoon vinegar

Directions:

1. Heat oil in a saucepan and cook onion, garlic, and bell peppers for 5-6 minutes or until bell peppers is roasted well.
2. Add tomatoes, salt, pepper, and vinegar; stir fry for 4-5 minutes.
3. Add chicken broth and cover with lid. Let it cook for about 20 minutes on low heat.
4. When tomatoes are cooked well, puree the soup with the help of an electric beater.
5. Simmer for 1-2 minutes.
6. Add to a serving dish and top with desired herbs.
7. Serve and enjoy.

Nutrition: Calories – 318, Fat – 97 g, Carbs – 60 g, Protein – 1.7 g

382. Tomato and Cabbage Puree Soup

Preparation Time: 5 minutes
Cooking Time: 30 minutes
Servings: 2
Ingredients:
- 0.6 lb. Tomatoes, chopped
- 3-4 garlic cloves, minced
- 0.2 lb. Cabbage, chopped
- 4 tablespoons olive oil
- red onion, chopped
- Salt and pepper, to taste
- Spice mix of choice
- 4 quarts of vegetable broth

Directions:
1. Heat oil in a saucepan and cook onion, garlic, and cabbage for about 4-5 minutes. Make sure that cabbage is nicely softened.
2. Add tomatoes and stir fry until liquid is reduced and tomatoes are dissolved.
3. Add salt, pepper, spice mix, and vegetable broth.
4. Cover the saucepan with a lid and let the mixture cook on low flame for about 30 minutes.
5. Puree the soup with the help of an electric beater.
6. Serve and enjoy.

Nutrition: Calories – 218, Fat – 15 g, Carbs – 220 g, Protein – 2 g

383. Athenian Avgolemono Sour Soup

Preparation Time: 20 minutes
Cooking Time: 50 minutes
Servings: 2
Ingredients:
- 8-cups water
- 1-pc whole chicken, cut in pieces
- Salt and pepper
- 1-cup whole grain rice
- 4-pcs eggs, separated
- 2-pcs lemons, juice
- ¼-cup fresh dill, minced
- Dill sprigs and lemon slices for garnish

Directions:
1. Pour the water in a large pot. Add the chicken pieces, and cover the pot. Simmer for an hour
2. Remove the cooked chicken pieces from the pot and take 2-cups of the chicken broth. Set aside and let it cool
3. Bring to a boil the remaining. Add salt and pepper to taste. Add the rice and cover the pot. Simmer for 20 minutes
4. Meanwhile, de-bone the cooked chicken and tear the flesh into small pieces. Set aside.
5. Work on the separated egg whites and yolks: whisk the egg whites until stiff; whisk the yolks with the lemon juice.
6. Pour the egg yolk mixture to the egg white mixture. Whisk well until fully combined.
7. Add gradually the reserved 2-cups of chicken broth to the mixture, whisking constantly to prevent the eggs from curdling.
8. After fully incorporating the egg mixture and chicken broth, pour this mixture into the simmering broth and rice. Add the dill, and stir well. Simmer further without bringing it to a boil.
9. Add the chicken pieces to the soup. Mix until fully combined.
10. To serve, ladle the soup in bowls and sprinkle with fresh ground pepper. Garnish with lemon slices and dill sprigs.

Nutrition: Calories: 122.4, Fats: 1.2g, Dietary Fiber: 0.2g, Carbohydrates: 7.5g, Protein: 13.7g

384. Italian Bean Soup

Preparation Time: 15 minutes
Cooking Time: 15 minutes
Servings: 2
Ingredients:
- tablespoon virgin olive oil
- onion (diced)
- garlic cloves (minced)
- cups tomato sauce (homemade or 1 can of low-sodium organic canned tomato sauce)
- cups cooked cannellini beans (or about 24 ounces of canned beans that have been drained and rinsed)
- 2tablespoon basil (dried)
- ½ teaspoon oregano
- ¼ teaspoon black pepper

Directions:
1. Take a large soup or stockpot and place it on your stove. Turn the heat all the way up to medium-high and pour in the virgin olive oil.
2. Allow the oil to heat slightly before adding your diced onions to the pot. Sautee for 3 minutes and then adds the garlic. Let the flavors come together for 2 minutes.
3. Add the cannellini beans, basil, oregano, and black pepper to the pot. Stir everything together then pour over the tomato sauce.
4. Allow the sauce to come to a steady simmer. Reduce the heat to medium-low. Cover your pot so the flavors can simmer together for 5 minutes.
5. Uncover the pot and allow the aroma to fill your kitchen. Then, take a ladle and fill your soup bowls! Grab a soup spoon and enjoy

Nutrition: Calories – 164, Carbs - 25.6 g, Protein - 8.1 g, Fat - 3.8 g

385. Red Soup, Seville Style

Preparation Time: 15 minutes
Cooking Time: 15 minutes
Servings: 2
Ingredients:
- 2 ounces stale bread, crusts removed
- 3 tablespoons further virgin olive oil
- 3 tablespoons fortified wine vinegar
- 2 garlic cloves, crushed
- 2 teaspoon salt
- Teaspoon cayenne pepper pinch of cumin
- Little red onion, chopped
- Pound ripe tomatoes, peeled, seeded, and chopped
- Cucumber, peeled, seeded, and chopped
- Red peppers, cored, seeded, and chopped
- Cups ice water
- For the garnish:
- 4 tablespoons red peppers, cored, seeded, and finely chopped
- 4 tablespoons finely cut cucumber
- 4 tablespoons finely cut purple onion
- 2 tablespoons finely cut contemporary mint leaves

Directions
1. First of all, you should Soak the bread into water and after that squeeze dry.
2. Place in a blender or kitchen appliance
3. With the vegetable oil, vinegar, garlic, salt, and spices and method to a sleek cream.
4. Add the onion, tomatoes, cucumber, and peppers and 1/2 the drinking water and still method the vegetables till sleek.
5. Pour into a soup serving dish and add the remaining water.
6. Chill totally before serving. Place the garnishes in little dishes and serve with the soup.

Nutrition: Calories: 123, Fats: 3g, Dietary Fiber: 5g, Carbohydrates: 19g, Protein: 5g

386. Garlic Soup

Preparation Time: 15 minutes
Cooking Time: 0 minutes
Servings: **2**
Ingredients:
- 5 cups water
- Head garlic, unpeeled
- Sprigs fresh thyme
- Tablespoons further virgin olive oil
- Salt
- Freshly ground black pepper
- 2 egg yolks
- Slices of bread, gently toasted

Directions

1. Bring the water to boil with the garlic and thyme and simmer for twenty minutes.
2. Take away the garlic and peel. Place the flesh in an exceedingly bowl and mash with a fork.
3. Step by step add the vegetable oil and blend well. Return to the soup.
4. Take away the thyme and after that you should Season it with salt & black pepper.
5. Beat the egg yolks in another bowl and step by step add a ladleful of the soup.
6. Combine well and stir into the soup. Simmer for some minutes, however don't let it boil or the soup can curdle.
7. Place the slices of toasts in individual bowls and pour over the soup. Serve at once.

Nutrition: Calories: 123, Fats: 3g, Dietary Fiber: 5g, Carbohydrates: 19g, Protein: 5g

387. Dalmatian Cabbage, Potato, And Pea Soup

Preparation Time: 15 minutes
Cooking Time: 15 minutes
Servings: 2
Ingredients:
- 4 tablespoons further virgin olive oil
- Medium onion, chopped
- Carrots, coarsely grated
- Medium potatoes, peeled and diced into little items inexperienced cabbage, shredded
- Cup contemporary shelled peas, or frozen petit pois
- Quart water
- Salt
- Freshly ground black pepper

Directions
1. Heat the vegetable oil in an exceedingly massive pot and cook the onion over a moderate heat for three minutes.
2. Add the carrots, potatoes, and cabbage and still cook for an additional five minutes.
3. Add the peas and water and produce to a boil.
4. Cowl and simmer for thirty-five to forty minutes or till the vegetables are tender and also the soup is fairly thick.
5. Finally, you must season it with salt & black pepper and serve hot.

Nutrition: Calories: 123, Fats: 3g, Dietary Fiber: 5g, Carbohydrates: 19g, Protein: 5g

DRINKS AND SMOOTHIES

388. Key Lime Pie Smoothie

Preparation Time: 5 Minutes
Cooking Time: 0 Minutes
Servings: 2
Ingredients:
- ½ cup Cottage Cheese
- 1 tbsp. Sweetener of your choice
- ½ cup Water
- ½ cup Spinach
- 1 tbsp. Lime Juice
- 1 cup Ice Cubes

Directions:
1. 1.Spoon in the ingredients to a high-speed blender and blend until silky smooth.
2. 2.Transfer to a serving glass and enjoy it.

Nutrition: Calories: 180cal Carbohydrates: 7g Proteins: 36g Fat: 1g Sodium: 35mg

389. Herb And Melon Kefir Smoothie

Preparation Time: 10 minutes
Cooking Time: 15 minutes
Servings: 2-3
Ingredients:
- 4 ounces nonfat plain kefir
- ¼ cup nonfat plain Greek yogurt
- ¾ cup chopped honeydew melon
- 4 fresh mint leaves
- 2 fresh basil leaves
- 1 teaspoon honey
- ¼ teaspoon vanilla extract

Directions:
1. 1.In a blender, combine the kefir, yogurt, melon, mint, basil, honey, and vanilla.
2. 2.Blend until smooth, or until your desired consistency is reached. Pour into a glass and enjoy.

Nutrition: Protein: 11g; Calories: 159; Fat: 2g; Carbohydrates: 26g; Fiber: 1g; Total sugar: 25g; Added sugar: 6g; Sodium: 94mg

390. Kefir And Yogurt Banana Flaxseed Shake

Preparation Time: 10 minutes
Cooking Time: 8 minutes to chill
Servings: 2-3
Ingredients:
- ⅓ cup nonfat plain kefir
- 6 ounces nonfat plain Greek yogurt
- ½ banana, fresh or frozen
- 1 tablespoon ground flaxseed
- 1 tablespoon sunflower seed butter
- 1 teaspoon sugar-free vanilla syrup or honey (optional)

Directions:
1. 1.In a blender, combine the kefir, yogurt, banana, flaxseed, sunflower seed butter, and syrup (if using).
2. 2.Blend until smooth. Pour into a glass and enjoy.
3. 3.Alternatively, refrigerate for 10 to 15 minutes to chill before sipping.

Nutrition: Protein: 26g; Calories: 329; Fat: 14g; Carbohydrates: 28g; Fiber: 5g; Total sugar: 17g; Added sugar: 0g; Sodium: 157mg

391. Cinnamon Roll Smoothie

Preparation Time: 5 Minutes
Cooking Time: 0 Minutes
Servings: 2
Ingredients:
- 1 tsp. Flax Meal or oats, if preferred
- 1 cup Almond Milk
- ½ tsp. Cinnamon
- 2 tbsp. Protein Powder
- 1 cup Ice
- ¼ tsp. Vanilla Extract
- 4 tsp. Sweetener of your choice

Directions:

1. 1.Pour the milk into the blender, followed by the protein powder, sweetener, flax meal, cinnamon, vanilla extract, and ice.
2. 2.Blend for 40 seconds or until smooth.
3. 3.Serve and enjoy.

Nutrition: Calories: 145cal Carbohydrates: 1.6g Proteins: 26.5g Fat: 3.25g Sodium: 30mg

392. Strawberry Cheesecake Smoothie

Preparation Time: 5 Minutes
Cooking Time: 0 Minutes
Servings: 2
Ingredients:
- ¼ cup Soy Milk, unsweetened
- ½ cup Cottage Cheese, low-fat
- ½ tsp. Vanilla Extract
- 2 oz. Cream Cheese
- 1 cup Ice Cubes
- ½ cup Strawberries
- 4 tbsp. Low-carb Sweetener of your choice

Directions:
1. Add all the ingredients for making the strawberry cheesecake smoothie to a high-speed blender until you get the desired smooth consistency.
2. Serve and enjoy.

Nutrition: Calories: 347cal Carbohydrates: 10.05g Proteins: 17.5g Fat: 24g Sodium: 45mg

393. Peanut Butter Banana Smoothie

Preparation Time: 5 Minutes
Cooking Time: 5 Minutes
Servings: 2
Ingredients:
- ¼ cup Greek Yoghurt, plain
- ½ tbsp. Chia Seeds
- ½ cup Ice Cubes
- ½ of 1 Banana
- ½ cup Water
- 1 tbsp. Peanut Butter

Directions:

1. Place all the ingredients needed to make the smoothie in a high-speed blender and blend to get a smooth and luscious mixture.
2. Transfer the smoothie to a serving glass and enjoy it.

Nutrition: Calories: 202cal Carbohydrates: 14g Proteins: 10g Fat: 9g Sodium: 30mg

394. Avocado Turmeric Smoothie

Preparation Time: 5 Minutes
Cooking Time: 5 Minutes
Servings: 2
Ingredients:
- ½ of 1 Avocado
- 1 cup Ice, crushed
- ¾ cup Coconut Milk, full-fat
- 1 tsp. Lemon Juice
- ¼ cup Almond Milk
- ½ tsp. Turmeric
- 1 tsp. Ginger, freshly grated

Directions:
1. Place all the ingredients excluding the crushed ice in a high-speed blender and blend for 2 to 3 minutes or until smooth.
2. Transfer to a serving glass and enjoy it.

Nutrition: Calories: 232cal Carbohydrates: 4.1g Proteins: 1.7g Fat: 22.4g Sodium: 25mg

395. Blueberry Smoothie

Preparation Time: 5 Minutes
Cooking Time: 5 Minutes
Servings: 2
Ingredients:
- 1 tbsp. Lemon Juice
- 1 ¾ cup Coconut Milk, full-fat
- ½ tsp. Vanilla Extract
- 3 oz. Blueberries, frozen

Directions:
1. Combine coconut milk, blueberries, lemon juice, and vanilla extract in a high-speed blender.
2. Blend for 2 minutes for a smooth and luscious smoothie.
3. Serve and enjoy.

Nutrition: Calories: 417cal Carbohydrates: 9g Proteins: 4g Fat: 43g Sodium: 35mg

396. Peanut Butter Cup Smoothies

Preparation Time: 10 minutes
Cooking Time: 0 minutes
Servings: 2-3
Ingredients:
- 1/2 cups skim milk
- 1/2 cup plain Greek yogurt
- tablespoons creamy natural peanut butter
- tablespoons sifted unsweetened cocoa powder
- 8 to 10 ice cubes

Directions:
1. 1.Place all ingredients in a blender container and pulse until thoroughly blended and smooth.
2. 2.Pour into 2 large glasses to serve. Enjoy!

Nutrition: Calories: 175; Total Fat: 9g; Saturated Fat: 2g; Protein: 11g; Carbs: 15g; Fiber: 3g; Sugar: 11g

397. Berry Cheesecake Smoothies

Preparation Time: 10 minutes
Cooking Time: 0 minutes
Servings: 2-3
Ingredients:
- 8 to 10 ice cubes
- cup mixed berries
- tablespoons cream cheese
- cups skim milk
- 1/4 teaspoon vanilla extract

Directions:
1. 1.Place all ingredients in a blender container and pulse until thoroughly blended and smooth.
2. 2.Pour into 2 large glasses to serve. Enjoy!

Nutrition: Calories: 182; Total Fat: 5g; Saturated Fat: 3g; Protein: 10g; Carbs: 21g; Fiber: 3g; Sugar17g

398. Guava Smoothie

Preparation Time: 5-7 minutes
Cooking Time: 2 minutes
Servings: 2-3
Ingredients:
- 1 cup guava, seeds removed, chopped
- 1 cup baby spinach, finely chopped
- 1 banana, peeled and sliced
- 1 tsp. fresh ginger, grated
- ½ medium-sized mango, peeled and chopped
- 2 cups water

Directions:
1. 1.Peel the guava and cut in half. Scoop out the seeds and wash it. Cut into small pieces and set aside.
2. 2.Rinse the baby spinach thoroughly under cold running water. Drain well and torn into small pieces. Set aside.
3. 3.Peel the banana and chop into small chunks. Set aside.
4. 4.Peel the mango and cut into small pieces. Set aside.
5. 5.Now, combine guava, baby spinach, banana, ginger, and mango in a juicer and process until well combined. Gradually add water and blend until all combined and creamy.
6. 6.Transfer to a serving glass and refrigerate for 20 minutes before serving.

Nutrition: Net carbs 39.1 g Fiber 7.8 g Fats 1.4 g Sugar 2 g Calories 166

399. Watermelon, Cantaloupe and Mango Smoothie

Preparation Time: 5 minutes;
Cooking Time: 0 minutes;
Servings: 4-5
Ingredients:
- ½ of a large mango, peeled
- ½ of burro banana, peeled
- ½ cup cantaloupe, peeled
- ½ cup amaranth greens
- ½ cup watermelon chunks
- Extra:
- 1 cup soft jelly coconut water

Directions:
1. 1.Plug in a high-speed food processor or blender and add all the Ingredients: in its jar.

2. 2.Cover the blender jar with its lid and then pulse for 40 to 60 seconds until smooth.
3. 3.Divide the drink between two glasses and then serve.

Nutrition: 132 Calories; 1 g Fats; 3.5 g Protein; 30.1 g Carbohydrates; 3.2 g Fiber;

400. BlackBerry & Banana Smoothie

Preparation Time: 5 minutes;
Cooking Time: 0 minutes;
Servings: 2-3
Ingredients:
- 1 burro banana, peeled
- ½ cup blackberries
- 2 dates, pitted
- 1 cup mango chunks
- ¼ cup walnut milk, unsweetened
- Extra:
- ¾ cup of coconut water

Directions:
1. 1.Plug in a high-speed food processor or blender and add all the Ingredients: in its jar.
2. 2.Cover the blender jar with its lid and then pulse for 40 to 60 seconds until smooth.
3. 3.Divide the drink between two glasses and then serve.

Nutrition: 147.7 Calories; 0.7 g Fats; 5 g Protein; 34 g Carbohydrates; 4.1 g Fiber;

401. Green Smoothie with Raspberries

Preparation Time: 5 minutes;
Cooking Time: 5 minutes;
Servings: 2-3
Ingredients:
- 1 cup raspberries
- 1 cup kale leaves
- 1 tablespoon sea moss
- 2 tablespoons key lime juice
- 1 cup soft-jelly coconut milk

Directions:
1. 1.Plug in a high-speed food processor or blender and add all the Ingredients: in its jar.

2. 2.Cover the blender jar with its lid and then pulse for 40 to 60 seconds until smooth.
3. 3.Divide the drink between two glasses and then serve.

Nutrition: 151 Calories; 1.2 g Fats; 3 g Protein; 37 g Carbohydrates; 8 g Fiber;

402. Veggie-Ful Smoothie

Preparation Time: 5 minutes;
Cooking Time: 0 minutes;
Servings: 2-3
Ingredients:
- 1 pear, cored, deseeded
- ½ cup watercress
- ¼ of avocado, peeled
- ½ cup Romaine lettuce
- ½ of cucumber, peeled, deseeded
- Extra:
- 1 tablespoon date
- ½ cup spring water

Directions:
1. 1.Plug in a high-speed food processor or blender and add all the Ingredients: in its jar.
2. 2.Cover the blender jar with its lid and then pulse for 40 to 60 seconds until smooth.
3. 3.Divide the drink between two glasses and then serve.

Nutrition: 145 Calories; 6 g Fats; 1 g Protein; 25 g Carbohydrates; 6 g Fiber;

403. Apple Pie Smoothie

Preparation Time: 5 minutes;
Cooking Time: 0 minutes;
Servings: 2-3
Ingredients:
- ½ of a large apple, deseeded
- ¼ cup walnuts
- 2 figs
- 1 teaspoon Bromide Plus Powder
- Extra:
- 1 tablespoon date

Directions:
1. 1.Plug in a high-speed food processor or blender and add all the Ingredients: in its jar.
2. 2.Cover the blender jar with its lid and then pulse for 40 to 60 seconds until smooth.

3. 3.Divide the drink between two glasses and then serve.

Nutrition: 170 Calories; 8 g Fats; 2 g Protein; 26 g Carbohydrates; 8 g Fiber

404. Banana Almond Smoothie

Preparation Time: 5 minutes
Cooking Time: 2 minutes
Servings: 2-3
Ingredients:
- 15 almonds
- 1 cup unsweetened almond milk
- 1 apple, peeled
- 1 banana, frozen

Directions:
1. 1.Add all ingredients into the blender and blend until smooth and creamy.
2. 2.Serve and enjoy.

Nutrition: Calories 190 Fat 5 g Carbohydrates 61 g Sugar 41 g Protein 14 g Cholesterol 18 mg

405. Protein Spinach Shake

Preparation Time: 10 minutes
Cooking Time: 2 minutes
Servings: 2-3
Ingredients:
- 2/3 cup water
- ½ cup ice
- 5 drops liquid stevia
- ¼ cup vanilla protein powder
- ½ cup fat-free plain yogurt
- ½ tsp. vanilla extract
- 2 cups fresh spinach

Directions:
1. 1.Add all ingredients into the blender and blend until smooth.
2. 2.Serve and enjoy.

Nutrition: Calories 54 Fat 0.9 g Carbohydrates 5.5 g Sugar 4.6 g Protein 4.4 g Cholesterol 4 mg

406. Fresh Lemon Cream Shake

Preparation Time: 5 minutes
Cooking Time: 2 minutes
Servings: 2-3
Ingredients:
- ½ cup ice cubes
- 2 tsp. lemon zest, grated
- ½ cup fat-free plain yogurt
- 1 scoop vanilla protein powder
- 5 oz. water
- 5 drops liquid stevia

Directions:
1. 1.Add all ingredients into the blender and blend until smooth and creamy.
2. 2.Serve and enjoy.

Nutrition: Calories 175 Fat 0.1 g Carbohydrates 9.8 g Sugar 9 g Protein 33.1 g Cholesterol 4 mg

407. Avocado Banana Smoothie

Preparation Time: 10 minutes
Cooking Time: 2 minutes
Servings: 2-3
Ingredients:
- ½ tsp. vanilla
- 1 tbsp. honey
- 2 cups unsweetened coconut milk
- 1 cup ice cubes
- 1 cup baby spinach
- ½ avocado
- 3 bananas

Directions:
1. 1.Add all ingredients into the blender and blend until smooth and creamy.
2. 2.Serve and enjoy.

Nutrition: Calories 425 Fat 33 g Carbohydrates 33 g Sugar 19 g Protein 4 g Cholesterol 0 mg

408. Banana Cherry Smoothie

Preparation Time: 5 minutes
Cooking Time: 2 minutes
Servings: 2-3
Ingredients:
- ½ tsp. vanilla
- 2 tbsp. unsweetened cocoa powder
- 2 ½ tbsp. chia seeds
- 1 cup unsweetened almond milk
- 1 cup ice cubes
- 1 cup fresh spinach
- 1 banana

Directions:
1. 1.Add all ingredients into the blender and blend until smooth and creamy.
2. 2.Serve and enjoy.

Nutrition: Calories 135 Fat 5 g Carbohydrates 20 g Sugar 7 g Protein 4.6 g Cholesterol 0 mg

409. Banana and Kale Smoothie

Preparation Time: 5 minutes
Cooking Time: 0 minutes
Servings: 2-3

Ingredients:
- 2 cups unsweetened almond milk
- 2 cups kale, stemmed, leaves chopped
- 2 bananas, peeled
- 1 to 2 packets stevia, or to taste
- 1 teaspoon ground cinnamon
- 1 cup crushed ice

Directions:
1. 1.In a blender, combine the almond milk, kale, bananas, stevia, cinnamon, and ice. Blend until smooth.
2. 2.Serve immediately.

Nutrition: calories: 181 | total carbs: 37.0g | protein: 4.0g | total fat: 4.0g | sugar: 15.0g | fiber: 6.0g | sodium: 210mg

410. Blueberry and Spinach Smoothie

Preparation Time: 5 minutes
Cooking Time: 2 minutes
Servings: 2-3

Ingredients:
- 2 cups blueberries
- 3 cups chopped fresh spinach
- ½ cup chopped fresh coriander
- Juice of 1 lemon
- 1-inch fresh ginger, grated
- 2 cups water

Directions:
1. 1.Put all the ingredients in the blender, mix for 2 minutes or until smooth.
2. 2.Serve immediately.

Nutrition: calories: 121 | total carbs: 30.0g | protein: 1.6g | total fat: 0.6g | sugar: 26.6g | fiber: 2.6g | sodium: 25mg

411. Matcha Mango Smoothie

Preparation Time: 5 minutes
Cooking Time: 0 minutes
Servings: 2-3

Ingredients:
- 2 cups cubed mango
- 2 tablespoons matcha powder
- 2 teaspoons turmeric powder
- 2 cups almond milk
- 2 tablespoons honey
- 1 cup crushed ice

Directions:
1. 1.In a blender, combine the mango, matcha, turmeric, almond milk, honey, and ice. Blend until smooth.
2. 2.Serve immediately.

Nutrition: calories: 285 | total carbs: 68.0g | protein: 4.0g | total fat: 3.0g | sugar: 63.0g | fiber: 6.0g | sodium: 94mg

412. Avocado Milk Whip

Preparation Time: 10 minutes
Cooking Time: 0 minutes
Servings: 2-3

Ingredients:
- 1 avocado, peeled, pitted, diced
- 1 cup skimmed milk
- ½ cup non-fat cottage cheese
- ¼ cup fresh cilantro leaves, stems removed
- ½ teaspoon lime juice
- ¼ teaspoon garlic powder
- Chili powder, for garnish

Directions:
1. 1.Put all ingredients in a blender and blend until smooth.
2. 2.Divide the whip between two bowls and sprinkle with a dash of chili powder to serve.

Nutrition: calories: 317 | total carbs: 26.6g | protein: 11.5g | total fat: 20.0g | sugar: 17.7g | fiber: 6.8g | sodium: 241mg

DESSERTS

413. Carrot Cake

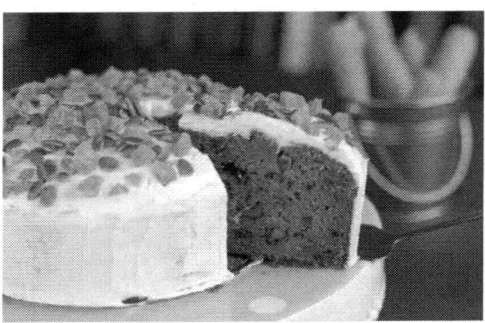

Preparation Time: 5 minutes + overnight
Cooking Time: 0 minutes
Servings: 1
Ingredients:

- 1 cup Coconut or almond milk
- 1 tbsp. Chia seeds
- 1 tsp. Cinnamon, ground
- ½ cup Raisins
- 2 tbsp. Cream cheese, low fat, at room temperature
- 1 Large Carrot, peel, and shred
- 2 tbsp. Honey

Directions:
1. Mix all of the listed ingredients and store them in a safe refrigerator container overnight. Eat cold in the morning if you choose to warm this; just microwave for one minute and stir well before eating.

Nutrition: Calories 340 |32 grams' sugar| 8 grams' protein |4 grams' fat| 9 grams' fiber| 70 grams' carbs

414. Lemon Vegan Cake

Preparation Time: 10 minutes
Cooking Time: 10 minutes
Servings: 3
Ingredients:

- 1 cup of pitted dates
- 2-1/2 cups pecans
- 1-1/2 cup agave
- 3 avocados, halved & pitted
- 3 cups of cauliflower rice, prepared
- 1 lemon juice and zest
- ½ lemon extract
- 1-1/2 cups pineapple, crushed
- 1-1/2 teaspoon vanilla extract
- Pinch of cinnamon
- 1-1/2 cups of dairy-free yogurt

Directions:
1. Line your baking sheet with parchment paper.
2. Pulse the pecans in your food processor.
3. Add the agave and dates. Pulse for a minute.
4. Transfer this mix to the baking sheet. Wipe the bowl of your processor.
5. Bring together the pineapple, agave, avocados, cauliflower, lemon juice, and zest in your food processor. Get a smooth mixture.
6. Now add the lemon extract, cinnamon, and vanilla extract. Pulse.
7. Pour this mix into your pan on the crust.
8. Refrigerate for 5 hours minimum.
9. Take out the cake and keep it at room temperature for 20 minutes.
10. Take out the cake's outer ring.
11. Whisk together the vanilla extract, agave, and yogurt in a bowl.
12. Pour on your cake.

Nutrition: Calories 688 |Carbohydrates 100g |Fat 28g |Protein 9g |Sugar 40g

415. Dark Chocolate Granola Bars

Preparation Time: 10 minutes
Cooking Time: 25 minutes
Servings: 12
Ingredients:

- 1 cup tart cherries, dried
- 2 cups buckwheat
- ¼ cup of flaxseed
- 1 cup of walnuts

- 2 eggs
- 1 teaspoon of salt
- ¼ cup dark cocoa powder
- 2/3 cup honey
- ½ cup dark chocolate chips
- 1 teaspoon of vanilla

Directions:
1. Preheat your oven to 350 degrees F.
2. Apply cooking spray lightly on your baking pan.
3. Pulse together the walnuts, wheat, tart cherries, salt, and flaxseed in your food processor. Everything should be chopped fine.
4. Whisk together the honey, eggs, vanilla, and cocoa powder in a bowl.
5. Add the wheat mix to your bowl. Stir to combine well.
6. Include the chocolate chips. Stir again.
7. Now pour this mixture into your baking dish.
8. Sprinkle some chocolate chips and tart cherries.
9. Bake for 25 minutes. Set aside for cooling before serving.

Nutrition: Calories 634 | Carbohydrates 100g | Fat 28g | Protein 9g | Sugar 40g

416. Blueberry Crisp

Preparation Time: 5 minutes
Cooking Time: 30 minutes
Servings: 4

Ingredients:
- ¼ cups pecans, chopped
- 1 cup buckwheat
- ½ teaspoon ginger
- 1 teaspoon of cinnamon
- 2 tablespoons olive oil
- ¼ teaspoon nutmeg
- 1 lb. blueberries
- 1 teaspoon of honey

Directions:
1. Preheat your oven to 350 degrees F.
2. Grease your baking dish.
3. Whisk together the pecans, wheat, oil, spices, and honey in a bowl.
4. Add the berries to your pan. Layer the topping on your berries.
5. Bake for 30 minutes at 350 F.

Nutrition: Calories 348 | Carbohydrates 40g | Fat 28g | Protein 9g | Sugar 40g

417. Chocolate Chip Quinoa Granola Bars

Preparation Time: 5 minutes
Cooking Time: 10 minutes
Servings: 16

Ingredients:
- ½ cup of chia seeds
- ½ cup walnuts, chopped
- 1 cup buckwheat
- 1 cup uncooked quinoa
- 2/3 cup dairy-free margarine
- ½ cup flax seed
- 1 teaspoon of cinnamon
- ½ cup of honey
- ½ cup of chocolate chips
- 1 teaspoon of vanilla
- ¼ teaspoon salt

Directions:
1. Preheat your oven to 350 degrees F.
2. Spread the walnuts, quinoa, wheat, flax, and chia on your baking sheet.
3. Bake for 10 minutes.
4. Line your baking dish with plastic wrap. Apply cooking spray. Keep aside.
5. Melt the margarine and honey in a saucepot.
6. Whisk together the vanilla, salt, and cinnamon into the margarine mix.
7. Keep the wheat mix and quinoa in a bowl. Pour the margarine sauce into it.
8. Stir the mixture. Coat well. Allow it to cool. Stir in the chocolate chips.
9. Spread your mixture into the baking dish. Press firmly into the pan.
10. Plastic wrap. Refrigerator overnight.
11. Slice into bars and serve.

Nutrition: Calories 408 | Carbohydrates 32g | Fat 18g | Protein 9g | Sugar 30g

418. Strawberry Granita

Preparation Time: 10 minutes

Cooking Time: 10 minutes
Servings: 8
Ingredients:
- 2 lb. strawberries, halved & hulled
- 1 cup of water
- Agave to taste
- ¼ teaspoon balsamic vinegar
- ½ teaspoon lemon juice
- Just a small pinch of salt

Directions:
1. Rinse the strawberries in water.
2. Keep in a blender. Add water, agave, balsamic vinegar, salt, and lemon juice.
3. Pulse many times so that the mixture moves. Blend to make it smooth.
4. Pour into a baking dish. The puree should be 3/8 inch deep only.
5. Refrigerate the dish uncovered till the edges start to freeze. The center should be slushy.
6. Stir crystals from the edges lightly into the center. Mix thoroughly.
7. Chill till the granite is almost completely frozen.
8. Scrape loose the crystals like before and mix.
9. Refrigerate again. Use a fork to stir 3-4 times till the granite has become light.

Nutrition: Calories 238 | Carbohydrates 10g | Fat 28g | Protein 5g | Sugar 34g

419. Apple Fritters

Preparation Time: 15 minutes
Cooking Time: 10 minutes
Servings: 4
Ingredients:
- 1 apple, cored, peeled, and chopped
- 1 cup all-purpose flour
- 1 egg
- ½ cup cashew milk
- 1-1/2 teaspoons of baking powder
- 2 tablespoons of stevia sugar

Directions:
1. Preheat your air fryer to 175 degrees C or 350 degrees F.
2. Keep parchment paper at the bottom of your fryer.
3. Apply cooking spray.
4. Mix together ¼ cup sugar, flour, baking powder, egg, milk, and salt in a bowl.
5. Combine well by stirring.
6. Sprinkle 2 tablespoons of sugar on the apples. Coat well.
7. Combine the apples into your flour mixture.
8. Use a cookie scoop and drop the fritters with it to the air fryer basket's bottom.
9. Now air fry for 5 minutes.
10. Flip the fritters once and fry for another 3 minutes. They should be golden.

Nutrition: Calories 348 | Carbohydrates 14g | Fat 18g | Protein 9g | Sugar 40g

420. Roasted Bananas

Preparation Time: 2 minutes
Cooking Time: 7 minutes
Servings: 1
Ingredients:
- 1 banana, sliced into diagonal pieces
- Avocado oil cooking spray

Directions:
1. Take parchment paper and line the air fryer basket with it.
2. Preheat your air fryer to 190 degrees C or 375 degrees F.
3. Keep your slices of banana in the basket. They should not touch.
4. Apply avocado oil to mist the slices of banana.
5. Cook for 5 minutes.
6. Take out the basket. Flip the slices carefully.
7. Cook for 2 more minutes. The slices of banana should be caramelized and brown. Take them out from the basket.

Nutrition: Calories 234 | Carbohydrates 16g | Fat 28g | Protein 9g | Sugar 20g

421. Berry-Banana Yogurt

Preparation Time: 10 minutes
Cooking Time: 0 minute
Servings: 1
Ingredients:
- ½ banana, frozen fresh
- 1 container 5.3ounes Greek yogurt, non-fat
- ¼ cup quick-cooking oats
- ½ cup blueberries, fresh and frozen

- 1 cup almond milk
- ¼ cup collard greens, chopped
- 5-6 ice cubes

Directions:
1. Take a microwave-safe cup and add 1 cup almond milk and ¼ cup oats
2. Place the cups into your microwave on high for 2.5 minutes
3. When oats are cooked and 2 ice cubes to cool
4. Mix them well
5. Add all ingredients in your blender
6. Blend it until it gets a smooth and creamy mixture
7. Serve chilled and enjoy!

Nutrition: Calories: 379| Fat: 10g |Carbohydrates: 63g| Protein: 13g

422. Avocado Chocolate Mousse

Preparation Time: 10 minutes
Cooking Time: 0 minute
Servings: 9
Ingredients:
- 3 ripe avocados, pitted and flesh scooped out
- 6 ounces plain Greek yogurt
- 1/8 cup almond milk, unsweetened
- ¼ cup of cocoa powder
- ½ teaspoon salt
- 2 tablespoons raw honey
- 1 bar dark chocolate
- 1 teaspoon vanilla extract

Directions:
1. Place all ingredients in your food processor
2. Pulse until smooth
3. Serve chilled and enjoy!

Nutrition: Calories: 208| Fat: 4g |Carbohydrates: 17g| Protein: 5g

423. Anti-Inflammatory Apricot Squares

Preparation Time: 20 minutes
Cooking Time: 0 minute
Servings: 8
Ingredients:
- 1 cup shredded coconut, dried
- 1 teaspoon vanilla extract
- 1 cup apricot, dried
- 1 cup macadamia nuts, chopped
- 1 cup apricot, chopped
- 1/3 cup turmeric powder

Directions:
1. Place all ingredients in your food processor
2. Pulse until smooth
3. Place the mixture into a square pan and press evenly
4. Serve chilled and enjoy!

Nutrition: Calories: 201| Fat: 15g| Carbohydrates: 17g| Protein: 3g

424. Raw Black Forest Brownies

Preparation Time: 2 hours and 10 minutes
Cooking Time: 0 minute
Servings: 6
Ingredients:
- 1 and ½ cups cherries, pitted, dried, and chopped
- 1 cup raw cacao powder
- ½ cup dates pitted
- 2 cups walnuts, chopped
- ½ cup almonds, chopped
- ¼ teaspoon salt

Directions:
1. Place all ingredients in your food processor
2. Pulse until small crumbs are formed
3. Press the brownie batter in a pan
4. Freeze for two hours
5. Slice before serving and enjoy!

Nutrition: Calories: 294 |Fat: 18g| Carbohydrates: 33g| Protein: 7g

425. Berry Parfait

Preparation Time: 10 min
Cooking Time: 10 min
Servings: 5
Ingredients:
- 7oz / 200g almond butter
- 3.5oz / 100g Greek yogurt
- 14oz / 400g mixed berries
- 2 tsp honey

Directions:

1. Mix the Greek yogurt, butter, and honey until it's smooth.
2. Add a layer of berries and a layer of the mixture in a glass until it's full.
3. Serve immediately

Nutrition: Calories: 394 |Fat: 18g| Carbohydrates: 35g| Protein: 8g

426. Sherbet Pineapple

Preparation Time: 20 Minutes
Cooking Time: 0 Minute
Servings: 4
Ingredients:
- 1 can of 8-ounce pineapple chunks
- 1/3 cup of orange marmalade
- ¼ teaspoon of ground ginger
- ¼ teaspoon of vanilla extract
- 1 can of 11-ounce orange sections
- 2 cups of pineapple, lemon or lime sherbet

Directions:
1. Drain the pineapple, ensure you reserve the juice.
2. Take a medium-sized bowl and add pineapple juice, ginger, vanilla, and marmalade to the bowl
3. Add pineapple chunks, drained mandarin oranges as well
4. Toss well and coat everything
5. Free them for 15 minutes and allow them to chill
6. Spoon the sherbet into 4 chilled stemmed sherbet dishes
7. Top each of them with a fruit mixture
8. Enjoy!

Nutrition: Calories: 204 |Fat: 17g| Carbohydrates: 32g| Protein: 6g

427. Easy Peach Cobbler

Preparation Time: 5 minutes
Cooking Time: 20 minutes
Servings: 6
Ingredients:
- 5 organic peaches, pitted and chopped
- ¼ cup coconut palm sugar, divided
- ½ teaspoon cinnamon
- ¾ cup chopped pecans
- ½ cup gluten-free oats
- ¼ cup ground flaxseeds
- ¼ brown rice flour
- ¼ cup extra virgin olive oil

Directions:
1. Preheat the oven to 3500F.
2. Grease the bottom of 6 ramekins.
3. In a bowl, mix the peaches, ½ of the coconut sugar, cinnamon, and pecans.
4. Distribute the peach mixture into the ramekins.
5. In the same bowl, mix the oats, flaxseed, rice flour, and oil. Add in the remaining coconut sugar. Mix until a crumbly texture is formed.
6. Top the mixture over the peaches.
7. Place for 20 minutes.

Nutrition: Calories: 194 |Fat: 15g| Carbohydrates: 32g| Protein: 7g

428. Thar She' Salts Peanut Butter Cookies

Preparation Time: 15 Minutes
Cooking Time: 0 0 Minute
Servings: 9
Ingredients:
- 1 cup of raw almonds
- ½ a cup of peanut butter (creamy and unsalted)
- 1 cup of pitted Medjool dates
- 1 and a ¼ teaspoon of vanilla extract
- Sea salt as needed

Directions:
1. Take a food processor and add almonds, peanut butter, vanilla, dates and blend the whole mixture until a dough-like texture comes (should take a few minutes)
2. If you want, add some more peanut butter to make the dough sticker.
3. Form balls using the dough and press down using a fork to create a crisscross pattern
4. Sprinkle salt generously
5. Serve immediately.

Nutrition: Calories: 214 |Fat: 16g| Carbohydrates: 32g| Protein: 6g

429. Almond Butter Balls Vegan

Preparation Time: 10 Minutes
Cooking Time: 0 0 Minute
Servings: 4
Ingredients:
- 12 dates, pitted and diced
- 1/3 cup of unsweetened shredded coconut
- 2 and a ½ tablespoon of almond butter

Directions:
1. Take a bowl and add dates, almond butter, and coconut
2. Mix well
3. Use the mixture to form small balls
4. Store them in your fridge and chill them
5. Enjoy!

Nutrition: Calories: 62Cal | Fats: 3g | Carbohydrates: 8 g | Protein: 1 g

430. Coffee Cream

Preparation Time: 10 minutes
Cooking Time: 15 minutes
Servings: 4
Ingredients:
- ¼ cup brewed coffee
- 2 tablespoons swerve
- 2 cups heavy cream
- 1 teaspoon vanilla extract
- 2 tablespoons ghee, melted
- 2 eggs

Directions:
1. In a bowl, combine the coffee with the cream and the other ingredients, whisk well and divide it into 4 ramekins and whisk well.
2. Introduce the ramekins in the oven at 350 degrees F and bake for 15 minutes.
3. Serve warm.

Nutrition: Calories 300 | Fat: 11g | Carbohydrates: 3g | Protein: 4g | Sugar: 12g

431. Almond Cookies

Preparation Time: 15 min
Cooking Time: 15 min
Servings: 12

Ingredients:
- 14oz / 400g non-wheat flour
- 1tsp baking soda
- 1tsp baking powder
- 3.5oz / 100g tahini
- 1.7oz / 50g coconut butter
- ½ tsp vanilla
- ½ tsp honey
- Salt

Directions:
1. Mix the flour, soda, salt, baking powder together.
2. Mix tahini and coconut butter and add 2 tbsp. Water in the same bowl.
3. Add honey, vanilla to the tahini mixture and blend it well with a mixer.
4. Preheat your oven (180C/356F) and put a baking sheet on it.
5. Add 24 tablespoons of the mixture onto the baking sheet and let it bake in the oven for 11-15 minutes.
6. Let it get cold a little bit and serve.

Nutrition: Calories: 114 | Fat: 16g | Carbohydrates: 22g | Protein: 6g

432. Chocolate Mousse

Preparation Time: 10 Minutes
Cooking Time: 0 Minute
Servings: 4
Ingredients:
- Coconut cream scraped from the upper side of 2 pieces of 13.5-ounce chilled cans of full-fat coconut milk
- 4 tablespoons of cocoa
- 3 tablespoons of Agave Nectar
- 1 teaspoon of vanilla extract

Directions:
1. Take a large bowl and scoop out the thick coconut cream from the can to the bowl
2. Add nectar, vanilla extract, and cocoa to the bowl
3. Beat it well using an electric mixer, starting from low and going to medium until a foamy texture appears
4. Divide the mix evenly amongst ramekins and chill to your desired level of cold
5. Enjoy!

Nutrition: Calories: 114 |Fat: 12g| Carbohydrates: 22g| Protein: 6g

433. Raspberry Diluted Frozen Sorbet

Preparation Time: 10 min
Cooking Time: 20 min
Servings: 4
Ingredients:

- 14oz / 400g frozen raspberry
- 4 fly oz. / 50g almond milk
- 1 tsp honey
- Mint

Directions:

1. Put the almond milk and raspberry in a mixer till it's smooth, and leave the consistency in the freezer for 20 minutes.
2. When serving, put them in ice cream bowls and serve with mint on top.

Nutrition: Calories: 224 |Fat: 16g| Carbohydrates: 22g| Protein: 4g

434. Chocolate Covered Strawberries

Preparation Time: 15 Minutes
Cooking Time: 0 Minute
Servings: 24
Ingredients:

- 16 ounces milk chocolate chips
- 2 tablespoons shortening
- 1-pound fresh strawberries with leaves

Directions:

1. In a bain-marie, melt chocolate and shorter, occasionally stirring until smooth. Hold them by the toothpicks and immerse the strawberries in the chocolate mixture.
2. Put toothpicks on the top of the strawberries.
3. Turn the strawberries and put the toothpick in the Styrofoam so that the chocolate cools.

Nutrition: Calories: 205 |Fat: 16g| Carbohydrates: 32g| Protein: 6g

435. Coconut Muffins

Preparation Time: 5 Minutes
Cooking Time: 25 Minutes
Servings: 8
Ingredients:

- ½ cup ghee, melted
- 3 tablespoons swerve
- ¼ teaspoon vanilla extract
- 1 cup coconut, unsweetened and shredded
- ¼ cup of cocoa powder
- eggs whisked
- 1 teaspoon baking powder

Directions:

1. In a bowl, combine the ghee with the swerve, coconut, and the other ingredients, stir well and divide it into a lined muffin pan. Bake at 370 degrees F for 25 minutes, cool down, and serve.

Nutrition: Calories: 324 Fat: 31g Carbohydrates: 8.3g Protein: 4g Sugar: 11g

436. Chocolate Cherry Chia Pudding

Preparation Time: 4 hours and 5 minutes
Cooking Time: 0 minutes
Servings: 4
Ingredients:

- 1 ½ cup Any non-dairy milk like coconut or almond milk
- 3 tbsp. Raw cacao powder
- ½ cup Sliced pitted cherries
- ¼ cup Chia seeds, you can also use chia seed powder.
- 3 tbsp. Maple syrup or honey
- Additional toppings:
- Raw cacao nibs
- Extra cherries
- Dark chocolate shavings (Preferably 70% dark chocolate or more)

Directions:

1. Use a mason jar or a bowl. If you're using a bowl, just pour in the milk, maple syrup, chia seeds or powder, and raw cacao. Stir thoroughly and place in the refrigerator for 4 hours or more.
2. If you decide to use a mason jar, just pour in the same ingredients, screw the lid on and shake vigorously!

3. Serve in separate dishes and top with any or all of the toppings I listed above.
4. Enjoy!

Nutrition: Calories: 404 | Fat: 16g | Carbohydrates: 12g | Protein: 6g

437. Strawberry Orange Sorbet

Preparation Time: 5 minutes
Cooking Time: 0 minutes
Servings: 3
Ingredients:
- 1 cup Orange juice or coconut water
- 1 pound Frozen strawberries

Direction:
1. Pour strawberries in a blender and pulse until all you have left are flakes. 2 minutes tops.
2. Now add the coconut water or orange juice and pulse until you get a nice and smooth puree. Have a spatula handy because you might need to scrape some of the purees off the walls of the blender sometimes.
3. Serve as soon as you're done or put in the freezer for 45 minutes for a sorbet feel.
4. Also, you can pour the smoothie into popsicle molds and freeze for hours or even overnight.
5. Enjoy!

Nutrition: Calories: 118 kcal | Protein: 2.88 g | Fat: 2.19 g | Carbohydrates: 23.25 g

438. Pineapple Cake

Preparation Time: 15 minutes
Cooking Time: 50 minutes
Servings: 8
Ingredients:
- 2 Whole medium eggs
- 5 tbsp. Raw honey
- 1 tbsp. Almond flour
- 1 tsp. Vanilla extract
- 15 pcs. Frozen sweet cherries
- 3 tbsp. Melted coconut oil
- 2 slices Fresh pineapples
- ½ tsp. Baking powder

Directions:
1. Prep oven by preheating to 350°F.
2. Remove the skin and core of the pineapples. Set aside.
3. Drizzle 1½ tablespoons of raw honey in a round cake tin.
4. Layer the pineapple rings and sweet cherries on the honey in a decorative fashion.
5. Bring the cake tin to the oven, then bake for 15 minutes.
6. While all that is going on, mix in the almond and baking powder.
7. In a separate bowl, combine the eggs and leftover honey. Drizzle in coconut oil and stir.
8. Now add the almond mix to the egg mix and stir thoroughly.
9. Take out the cake tin and drizzle batter over the top of the partially baked pineapple rings. Use a spatula to spread it evenly.
10. Put the cake tin back in the oven and bake for an additional 35 minutes.
11. When it's all set, take it out of the oven and leave it to sit for 10 minutes before placing it in a plate.
12. Serve with extra cherries if you like.

Nutrition: Calories: 120 kcal | Protein: 2.3 g | Fat: 6.99 g | Carbohydrates: 12.98 g

439. Mediterranean Rolled Baklava with Walnuts

Preparation Time: 20 minutes
Cooking Time: 40 minutes
Servings: 12
Ingredients:
- 2 cups Walnuts
- 1 Lemon zest
- 1 cup Cream of wheat or plain breadcrumbs
- 8 sheets Thawed phyllo dough
- 3 tbsp. Sugar
- 1/3 cup Milk
- 3 sticks Melted Unsalted butter
- Syrup:
- 1 medium Lemon
- 3 cups Granulated sugar
- 3 cups Water

Directions:
1. Mix 3 cups of sugar, 3 cups of water, and lemon slices in a pan and leave to boil

2. Lower the heat, then let it simmer until the sugar completely dissolves. It should take 15 minutes. You should have a nice smooth syrup now. Now leave it to cool for a bit.
3. Chop the walnuts in a blender into bits using short pulses.
4. Pour the walnuts in a bowl along with the cream of wheat, lemon zest, and 4 tablespoons of sugar.
5. Stir in milk and set aside.
6. Now, preheat your oven to 375°F.
7. Spread out the phyllo dough and fit it into a baking pan. Trim off the edges that don't fit with scissors. Cover the remaining phyllo sheets while you work so they don't dry out.
8. Place a sheet on a clean flat surface and glaze with melted butter. Do this for all the sheets until it's finished.
9. Arrange the walnut mixture on one side of the sheets and roll them up like you're trying to make a sausage. Do this for all the sheets and walnuts.
10. Arrange the walnut rolls on an ungreased baking pan and glaze with the leftover butter.
11. Bake for about 45 minutes. It's ready when it looks golden.
12. Turn off the oven, then pull out the baking pan. Drizzle syrup over the baklava, making sure the syrup gets everywhere.
13. Bring back the baking pan into the oven, then leave to sit for 5 minutes.
14. Take off from the oven and leave it to cool for a few hours. Slice the rolls into tiny bits and serve.

Nutrition: Calories: 488 kcal| Protein: 4.49 g| Fat: 36.89 g| Carbohydrates: 38.21 g

440. Mint Chocolate Chip Ice-cream

Preparation Time: 5 minutes
Cooking Time: 0 minutes
Servings: 2
Ingredients:
- 2 Frozen overripe bananas
- Pinch Spirulina or any natural food coloring, optional.
- 3 tbsp. Chocolate chips or sugar-free chocolate chips
- 1/8 tsp. Pure peppermint extracts
- ½ cup raw cashews or coconut cream, optional.
- Pinch Salt

Directions:
1. Mint or imitation peppermint won't be a substitute for this. Use pure peppermint extract and pour it all at once because a drop is more potent than you realize, so add slowly.
2. Peel and cut the bananas first. Place the slices in a Ziplock bag, then freeze.
3. For the ice cream, put all the ingredients in a blender and pulse. You can skip the chocolate chips and just add them after blending. It'll turn out delicious either way.
4. Serve as soon as it's ready or freeze until it's firm enough, then serve!

Nutrition: Calories: 250 kcal| Protein: 6.13 g| Fat: 24.37 g | Carbohydrates: 7.72 g

441. Flourless Sweet Potato Brownies

Preparation Time: 10 minutes
Cooking Time: 30 minutes
Servings: 9
Ingredients:
- ½ cup Cooked sweet potato
- 2 tsp. Vanilla extract
- ½ cup Almond butter
- 6 tbsp. Honey
- ½ tsp. Baking soda
- 1 large Whole egg
- ¼ cup Unsweetened Cocoa powder
- 3 tbsp. Dairy-free chocolate chips, optional.

Directions:
1. Prep your oven by preheating to 350°F.
2. Line a baking pan with parchment paper, leaving a few extra inches on the sides to make it easier to discard or remove
3. Blend all the ingredients, excluding the chocolate chips, until you get a very smooth and soft batter.
4. Transfer the creamy batter to your prepared baking pan and use a spatula to spread it around so it looks almost even.

5. Slide it in the oven, then bake for 30 minutes or until a knife inserted into the pan comes out clean.
6. Take off from the oven and leave to cool in the pan for 15 minutes before putting it up on a wire rack.
7. If you decide to use the chocolate chip topping, put the chips in a microwave-safe dish and heat until it completely melts. Take off from the microwave and drizzle over the brownies.
8. Serve or store!

Nutrition: Calories: 171 kcal| Protein: 5.17 g| Fat: 9.28 g| Carbohydrates: 20.01 g

442. Paleo Raspberry Cream Pie

Preparation Time: 20 minutes
Cooking Time: 0 minutes
Servings: 12
Ingredients:
- For the crust:
- 1 ½ tbsp. Maple syrup
- Pinch Salt
- ½ cup Unsweetened shredded coconut
- 1 tsp. Vanilla extract
- 1 cup Roasted or salted cashews
- Raspberry filling:
- ¾ cup Unrefined coconut oil
- 1 ½ cup Roasted or salted cashews
- ½ cup & 1 tbsp. Maple syrup
- ¼ cup & 2 tsp. Fresh lemon juice
- ¼ cup Coconut cream from the top solid part of a can of coconut milk that has been refrigerated overnight
- 2 tsp. Vanilla extract
- 3 cups Fresh raspberries
- Pinch Salt

Directions:
1. Prepare 12 muffin pans, line them with muffin liners, and set them aside.
2. Make the crust. Set a pan over medium heat and the coconut and stir until it's completely toasted. Stay by the pan because coconuts tend to burn very easily.
3. Transfer the toasted coconuts to a bowl and leave to cool for 5 minutes or so. Honestly, this toasting step isn't essential, but it adds incredible flavor to the crust.
4. To make the crust, put all the ingredients in a blender and pulse at the lowest speed until the mix gets all clumpy. Also, don't pulse for too long, or you might end up with a paste. To know if it's ready, put a bit of the mixture on your fingers and pinch. If it gets clumpy, you're on track. If not, add a little water and pulse at the lowest speed for further minutes.
5. Scoop the mix into the lined tins using your fingers to pack the mix tightly inside the pan.
6. Put the pans to refrigerate while you get to make the filling.
7. In a tiny pot set over low heat, stir in all the ingredients until the oil and coconut cream melts completely. Clean the blender using a paper towel and pour in the filling.
8. Pulse at high speed for like 60 seconds or until it's completely smooth. The only clumps we can forgive are the raspberry seeds.
9. Drizzle a quarter of the filling over the top of each crust. There should be extra filling; you can store and use that in another dish.
10. Place the coated muffins in the fridge to cool. This will take a few hours, like 6 hours, so put it in the freezer if you don't have time for that.
11. To serve, leave them to defrost for 80 minutes or until obviously creamy.

Nutrition: Calories: 565 kcal| Protein: 7.74 g| Fat: 43.72 g | Carbohydrates: 42.72 g

443. Caramelized Pears

Preparation Time: 20 minutes
Cooking Time: 5 minutes
Servings: 5
Ingredients:
- 1 Teaspoon Cinnamon
- 2 Tablespoon Honey, Raw
- 1 Tablespoon Coconut Oil
- 4 Pears, Peeled, Cored & Quartered
- 2 Cups Yogurt, Plain
- ¼ Cup Toasted Pecans, Chopped
- 1/8 Teaspoon Sea Salt

Directions:
1. Get out a large skillet, and then heat the oil over medium-high heat.
2. Add in your honey, cinnamon, pears, and salt. Cover, and allow it to cook for four to five minutes. Stir occasionally, and your fruit should be tender.
3. Uncover it, and allow the sauce to simmer until it thickens. This will take several minutes.
4. Soon your yogurt into four dessert bowls. Top with pears and pecans before serving.

Nutrition: Calories: 290 | Protein: 12 Grams | Fat: 11 Grams | Carbs: 41 Grams

444. Berry Ice Pops

Preparation Time: 3 Hours 5 Minutes
Cooking Time: 0 minutes
Servings: 4
Ingredients:
- 1 Cup Strawberries, Fresh or Frozen
- 2 Cups Whole Milk Yogurt, Plain
- 1 Cup Blueberries, Fresh or Frozen
- ¼ Cup Water
- 1 Teaspoon Lemon Juice, Fresh
- 2 Tablespoons Honey, Raw

Directions:
1. Place the ingredients in a blender, and blend until smooth.
2. Pour into your molds, and freeze for at least three hours before serving.

Nutrition: Calories: 140 | Protein: 5 Grams | Fat: 4 Grams | Carbs: 23 Grams

445. Fruit Cobbler

Preparation Time: 10 minutes
Cooking Time: 20 minutes
Servings: 8
Ingredients:
- 1 Teaspoon Coconut Oil
- ¼ Cup Coconut Oil, Melted
- 2 Cups Peaches, Fresh & Sliced
- 2 Cups Nectarines, Fresh & Sliced
- 2 Tablespoons Lemon Juice, Fresh
- ¾ Cup Rolled Oats
- ¾ Cup Almond Flour
- ¼ Cup Coconut Sugar
- ½ Teaspoon Vanilla Extract, Pure
- 1 Teaspoon Ground Cinnamon
- Dash Salt
- Filter Water for Mixing

Directions:
1. Start by heating your oven to 425.
2. Get out a cast-iron skillet, coating it with a teaspoon of coconut oil.
3. Mix your lemon juice, peaches, and nectarines together in the skillet.
4. Get out a food processor, mixing your almond flour, oats, coconut sugar, and remaining coconut oil. Add in your cinnamon, vanilla, and salt, pulsing until the oat mixture resembles a dry dough.
5. If you need more moisture, add filtered water a tablespoon at a time, and then break the dough into chunks, spreading it across the fruit.
6. Bake for twenty minutes before serving warm.

Nutrition: Protein: 4 Grams | Fat: 12 Grams | Carbs: 15 Grams

446. Watermelon and Avocado Cream

Preparation Time: 2 hours
Cooking Time: 0 minutes
Servings: 4
Ingredients:
- 2 cups coconut cream
- 1 watermelon, peeled and chopped
- 2 avocados, peeled, pitted, and chopped
- 1 tablespoon honey
- 2 teaspoons lemon juice

Directions:
1. In a blender, put the ingredients. Divide it into bowls, and keep it in the fridge for 2 hours before serving.

Nutrition: Calories 121| Fat 2| Fiber: 2| Carbs: 6| Protein: 5

447. Coconut and Chocolate Cream

Preparation Time: 2 hours

Cooking Time: 0 minutes
Servings: 4

Ingredients:
- 2 cups coconut milk
- 2 tablespoons ginger, grated
- 2 tablespoons honey
- 1 cup dark chocolate, chopped and melted
- ½ teaspoon cinnamon powder
- 1 teaspoon vanilla extract

Directions:
1. In a blender, put the ingredients and blend. Divide into bowls and place in the fridge for 2 hours before serving.

Nutrition: Calories: 200 | Fat: 3 | Fiber: 5 | Carbs: 12 | Protein: 7

448. Chocolate Bananas

Preparation Time: 5 Minutes
Cooking Time: 15 Minutes
Servings: 4
Ingredients:
- 3 Bananas, large & cut into thirds
- 12 oz. Dark Chocolate
- 1 tbsp. Coconut Oil

Directions:
1. Melt the chocolate and coconut oil in a double boiler for 3 to 4 minutes till you get a smooth and glossy mixture.
2. Next, keep the popsicles to the end of each of the bananas by inserting them.
3. After that, immerse the chocolate into the warm chocolate mixture.
4. Shake off the excess chocolate and place them on parchment paper.
5. Sprinkle with the topping of your choice.
6. Finally, place them in the freezer for a few hours or until set.
7. Tip: You can use topping like chopped pistachios or unsweetened chocolate sprinkles etc.

Nutrition: Calories: 427Kcal | Proteins: 5.9g | Carbohydrates: 80g | Fat: 15.6g

449. Watermelon Sorbet

Preparation Time: 5 Minutes
Cooking Time: 15 Minutes
Servings: 4
Ingredients:
- 1 Seedless Watermelon, cubed

Directions:
1. To start with, place the watermelon cubes in a baking sheet in an even layer.
2. After that, keep the sheet in the freezer for 2 hours or until the watermelon is solid.
3. Next, transfer the frozen watermelon cubes in the high-speed blender and puree them until you get a smooth puree.
4. Then, pour the puree among the two loaf pans.

Nutrition: Calories: 427Kcal | Proteins: 5.9g | Carbohydrates: 80g | Fat: 15.6g

450. Cinnamon Apple Chips

Preparation Time: 10 Minutes
Cooking Time: 2 Hours
Servings: 3
Ingredients:
- ¾ tsp. Cinnamon, grounded
- 3 Honey crisp Apple, large & sweet

Directions:
1. For making this dessert fare, preheat the oven to 200 ° F.
2. After that, keep a parchment paper-lined baking sheet in the middle and lower rack.
3. With the help of an apple corer, core the apples and then slice the apples into 1/8-inch-thick rounds.
4. Then, arrange the apples in the preheated baking sheet in a single layer.
5. Next, sprinkle the cinnamon over the apples.
6. Once sprinkled, bake them for 1 hour.
7. Remove the baking sheet and then switch its position.
8. Bake them for another 1 to 1 ½ hours or until the chips are crispy.
9. Finally, once they are crisp according to your liking, remove the apple chips from the oven.
10. Allow the chips to cool for one hour before serving.

11. Tip: You can top the apple crisps on top of ice creams or yogurt etc.

Nutrition: Calories: 96Kcal | Proteins: 0g | Carbohydrates: 25.5g | Fat: 0g

451. Avocado Brownies

Preparation Time: 10 Minutes
Cooking Time: 25 Minutes
Servings: 16
Ingredients:
- 1 tsp. Baking Soda
- 1 Avocado, large
- ¼ tsp. Sea Salt
- ½ cup Applesauce, unsweetened
- ½ cup Cocoa Powder, Dutch-processed & unsweetened
- ½ cup Maple Syrup
- ½ cup Coconut Flour
- 3 Eggs, large
- 1 tap. Vanilla Extract

Directions:
1. First, preheat the oven to 350 °F.
2. After that, place avocado, vanilla, applesauce, and maple syrup in a high-speed blender and blend for 2 minutes or until smooth.
3. Next, transfer the smooth mixture to a large mixing bowl.
4. To this, stir in the eggs and combine until whisked well.
5. Then, spoon in the coconut flour, sea salt, and cocoa powder to the mixture.
6. Give a good stir until everything comes together.
7. Now, pour the mixture into a greased baking dish and bake for 23 to 25 minutes or until cooked.
8. Lastly, take off from the oven and allow it to cool for 15 to 20 minutes before serving.

Nutrition: Calories: 91Kcal | Proteins: 1.9g | Carbohydrates: 12.1g | Fat: 4.3g

452. Fruit Salad

Preparation Time: 10 Minutes
Cooking Time: 20 Minutes
Servings: 2-3
Ingredients:
- ½ of 1 Watermelon, chopped into small pieces
- 1 Pineapple, cut into small pieces
- Dash of Turmeric
- 4 Strawberries, chopped
- 1 Red Papaya, cut into small pieces
- 1 tsp. Ginger, freshly grated
- 1 Pomegranate, small

Directions:
1. To start with, place all the fruits in a large-sized bowl.
2. After that, spoon in the turmeric and ginger over the fruits.
3. Toss well and serve.
4. Tip: Instead of ginger, you can use cinnamon or clove.

Nutrition: Calories: 118Kcal | Proteins: 1.6g | Carbohydrates: 36.6g | Fat: 0.5g

453. Chocolate Chip Cookies

Preparation Time: 10 Minutes
Cooking Time: 20 Minutes
Servings: 16
Ingredients:
- ½ cup Maple Syrup
- 2 cups Almond Flour, finely sifted
- ½ cup Almond Butter
- ½ cup Dark Chocolate Chips, sugar-free

Directions:
1. Preheat the oven to 350 °F.
2. Next, combine the almond flour, almond butter, and maple syrup in a medium-sized mixing bowl until mixed well.
3. To this, stir in the chocolate chips and mix again.
4. With the help of an ice cream scooper, scoop out the mixture to a greased baking sheet. Flatten the top slightly with your hand.
5. Finally, bake them for 10 to 12 minutes or until they are going to get browned.

Nutrition: Calories: 176Kcal | Proteins: 5g | Carbohydrates: 16g | Fat: 11g

SLOW COOKER RECIPES

454. Quinoa and Cauliflower Congee

Preparation Time: 10 minutes
Cooking Time: 1 hour
Servings: 8
Ingredients:
- 1 cauliflower head, minced
- 2 tablespoons red quinoa
- 2 leeks, minced
- 1 tablespoon fresh ginger, grated
- 2 garlic cloves, grated
- 6 cups of water
- 2 tablespoons brown rice
- 1 tablespoon olive oil
- 1 tablespoon fish sauce
- 2 onions, minced
- Pinch of white pepper
- For Garnish
- 4 eggs, soft-boiled
- 2 red chilies, minced
- 1 lime, sliced into wedges
- ¼ cup packed basil leaves, torn
- ¼ cup loosely packed cilantro leaves, torn
- ¼ cup loosely packed spearmint leaves, torn

Directions:
1. Put olive oil into a huge skillet on medium heat. Sauté shallots, garlic, and ginger until limp and aromatic; pour into a slow cooker set at medium heat.
2. Except for garnishes, pour remaining ingredients into slow cooker; stir. Put the lid on. Cook for 6 hours. Turn off heat. Taste; adjust seasoning if needed.
3. Ladle congee into individual bowls. Garnish with basil leaves, cilantro leaves, red chili, and spearmint leaves. Add 1 piece of soft-boiled egg on top of each; serve with a wedge of lime on the side. Slice egg just before eating so yolk runs into congee. Squeeze lime juice into congee just before eating.

Nutrition: Calories: 138 kcal | Protein: 7.23 g | Fat: 7.65 g | Carbohydrates: 10.76 g

455. Zucchini and Carrot Combo

Preparation Time: 10 minutes
Cooking Time: 8 hours
Serving: 3
Ingredients
- ½ cup steel cut oats
- 1 cup of coconut milk
- 1 carrot, grated
- ¼ zucchini, grated
- Pinch of nutmeg
- ½ teaspoon cinnamon powder
- 2 tablespoons brown sugar
- ¼ cup pecans, chopped

Directions:
1. Grease the Slow Cooker well.
2. Add oats, zucchini, milk, carrot, nutmeg, cloves, sugar, cinnamon, and stir well.
3. Place lid and cook on LOW for 8 hours.
4. Divide amongst serving bowls and enjoy!

Nutrition: Calories: 200 Fat: 4g Carbohydrates: 11g Protein: 5g

456. Salmon in Dill Sauce

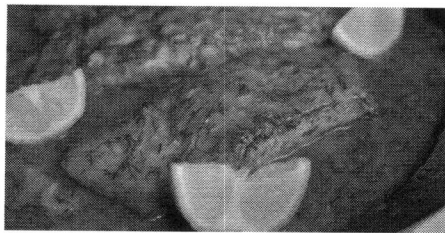

Preparation Time: 10 minutes
Cooking Time: 2 hours
Servings: 6
Ingredients:
- 2 cups water
- 1-cup homemade chicken broth
- 2 tablespoons fresh lemon juice
- ¼ cup fresh dill, chopped
- 6 salmon fillets
- 1 teaspoon cayenne pepper
- Salt and ground black pepper

Directions:
1. In the pot of Ninja Foody, mix the water, broth, lemon juice, lemon juice, and dill.
2. Organize the salmon fillets on top, skin side down, and sprinkle with cayenne pepper, salt black pepper.
3. Close the Ninja Foody with a crisping lid and select Slow Cooker.
4. Set on Low for 1-2 hours.
5. Press Start/Stop to begin cooking.
6. Serve hot.

Nutrition: Calories: 16 | Fats: 7.4 | Carbohydrates 1.6 g | Proteins: 23.3g

457. Parsley Tilapia

Preparation Time: 15 minutes
Cooking Time: 1 hour and 30 minutes
Servings: 6
Ingredients:
- 6 tilapia fillets
- Salt and ground black pepper
- ½ cup yellow onion, chopped
- 3 teaspoons fresh lemon rind, grated finely
- ¼ cup fresh parsley, chopped
- 2 tablespoons unsalted butter, melted

Directions:
1. Grease the pot of Ninja Foody.
2. Spice the tilapia fillets with salt and black pepper generously.
3. In the prepared pot of Ninja Foody, place the tilapia fillets.
4. Arrange the onion, lemon rind, and parsley over fillets evenly and drizzle with melted butter.
5. Close the Ninja Foody with a crisping lid and select Slow Cooker.
6. Set on Low for 1½ hours.
7. Press Start/Stop to begin cooking.
8. Serve hot.

Nutrition: Calories: 133 | Fats: 4.9g | Carbohydrates: 1.3g | Proteins: 21.3g

458. Cod with Bell Pepper

Preparation Time: 15 minutes
Cooking Time: 1 hour and 30 minutes
Servings: 4

Ingredients:
- 1 bell pepper, seeded and sliced
- ½ small onion, sliced
- 3 garlic cloves, minced
- 1 can sugar-free diced tomatoes
- 1 tablespoon fresh rosemary, chopped
- ¼ cup homemade fish broth
- ¼ teaspoon red pepper flakes
- Salt and ground black pepper
- 1-pound cod fillets

Directions:
1. In the pot of Ninja Foody, add all the ingredients except cod and stir to combine.
2. Season cod fillets with salt and black pepper evenly.
3. Arrange the cod fillets over broth mixture.
4. Close the Ninja Foody with a crisping lid and select Slow Cooker.
5. Set on High for 1½ hours.
6. Press Start/Stop to begin cooking.
7. Serve hot.

Nutrition: Calories: 12 | Fats: 1.6 | Carbohydrates 7.7 g | Proteins: 22.1

459. Tangy Barbecue Chicken

Preparation Time: 15 minutes
Cooking Time: 3-4 hours
Servings: 4
Ingredients:
- 4- 5 (2 lb.) boneless, skinless chicken breasts
- 2 cups Tangy Barbecue Sauce with Apple Cider Vinegar

Directions:
1. In your slow cooker, combine the chicken and barbecue sauce. Stir until the chicken breasts are well coated in the sauce.
2. Cover the cooker and set it to high. Cook for 3 to 4 hours, or until the internal temperature of the chicken reaches 165°F on a meat thermometer and the juices run clear.
3. Shred the chicken with a fork, mix it into the sauce, and serve.

Nutrition: Calories: 41 | Total Fat: 13g | Total Carbs: 22 | Sugar: 19 | Fiber: 0 | Protein: 51 | Sodium: 766mg

460. Salsa Verde Chicken

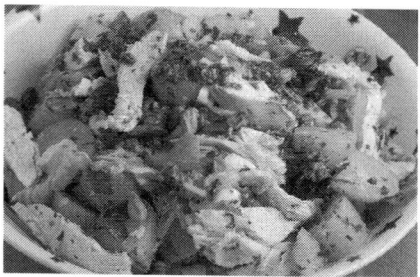

Preparation Time: 15 minutes
Cooking Time: 6 to 8 hours
Servings: 4
Ingredients:

- 4 to 5 boneless, skinless chicken breasts (about 2 pounds)
- 2 cups green salsa
- 1 cup chicken broth
- 2 tablespoons freshly squeezed lime juice
- 1 teaspoon sea salt
- 1 teaspoon chili powder

Directions:

1. In your slow cooker, combine the chicken, salsa, broth, lime juice, salt, and chili powder. Stir to combine.
3. Shred the chicken with a fork, mix it into the sauce, and serve.

Nutrition: Calories: 318 | Total Fat: 8g | Total Carbs: 6g | Sugar: 2g | Fiber: 1g | Protein: 52g | Sodium: 1,510mg

461. Lemon & Garlic Chicken Thighs

Preparation Time: 15 minutes
Cooking Time: 7 to 8 hours
Servings: 4
Ingredients:

- 2 cups chicken broth
- 1½ teaspoons garlic powder
- 1 teaspoon sea salt
- Juice and zest of 1 large lemon
- 2 pounds' boneless skinless chicken thighs

Directions:

1. Pour the broth into the slow cooker.
2. In a small bowl, put the garlic powder, salt, lemon juice, and lemon zest, then stir. Baste each chicken thigh with an even coating of the mixture. Place the thighs along the bottom of the slow cooker.
3. Cover the cooker and set it to low. Cook for around 7 to 8 hours, or until the internal temperature of the chicken reaches 165°F on a meat thermometer and the juices run clear and serve.

Nutrition: Calories: 29 | Total Fat: 14g | Total Carbs: 3g | Sugar: 0g | Fiber: 0 | Protein: 43g | Sodium: 1,017mg

462. Chicken & Apple Cider Chili

Preparation Time: 15 minutes
Cooking Time: 7 to 8 hours
Servings: 4

Ingredients:

- 3 cups chopped cooked chicken (see Basic "Rotisserie" Chicken)
- 1 medium onion, chopped
- 1 (15-ounce) can diced tomatoes
- 3 cups Chicken Bone Broth or store-bought chicken broth
- 1 cup apple cider
- 2 bay leaves
- 1 tablespoon extra-virgin olive oil
- 2 teaspoons garlic powder
- 1 teaspoon chili powder
- 1 teaspoon sea salt
- ½ teaspoon ground cumin
- ¼ teaspoon ground cinnamon
- Pinch cayenne pepper
- Freshly ground black pepper
- ¼ cup apple cider vinegar

Directions:

1. In your slow cooker, combine the chicken, onion, tomatoes, broth, cider, bay leaves, olive oil, garlic powder, chili powder, salt, cumin, cinnamon cayenne, and season with black pepper.

2. Cover the cooker and set it to low. Cook for 7 to 8 hours.
3. Remove and discard the bay leaves. Stir in the apple cider vinegar until well blended and served.

Nutrition: Calories: 469 | Total Fat: 8g | Total Carbs: 46g | Sugar: 13g | Fiber: 9g | Protein: 51g | Sodium: 1,047mg

463. Buffalo Chicken Lettuce Wraps

Preparation Time: 15 minutes
Cooking Time: 7 to 8 hours
Servings: 4
Ingredients:
- 1 tablespoon extra-virgin olive oil
- 2 pounds boneless, skinless chicken breast
- 2 cups Vegan Buffalo Dip
- 1 cup water
- 8 to 10 romaine lettuce leaves
- ½ red onion, thinly sliced
- 1 cup cherry tomatoes, halved

Directions:
1. Coat the bottom of the slow cooker with olive oil.
2. Add the chicken, dip, and water, and stir to combine.
3. Cover the cooker and set it to low. Cook for around 7 to 8 hours, or until the internal temperature reaches 165°F on a meat thermometer and the juices run clear.
4. Shred the chicken using a fork, then mix it into the dip in the slow cooker.
5. Divide the meat mixture among the lettuce leaves. Top with onion and tomato, and serve.

Nutrition: Calories: 437 | Total Fat: 18g | Total Carbs: 18g | Sugar: 8g | Fiber: 4g | Protein: 49 | Sodium: 993mg

464. Cilantro-Lime Chicken Drumsticks

Preparation Time: 15 minutes
Cooking Time: 2 to 3 hours
Servings: 4
Ingredients:
- ¼ cup fresh cilantro, chopped
- 3 tablespoons freshly squeezed lime juice
- ½ teaspoon garlic powder
- ½ teaspoon sea salt
- ¼ teaspoon ground cumin
- 3 pounds' chicken drumsticks

Directions:
1. In a bowl, mix together the cilantro, lime juice, garlic powder, salt, and cumin to form a paste.
2. Put the drumsticks in the slow cooker. Spread the cilantro paste evenly on each drumstick.
3. Cover the cooker and set it to high. Cook for 2 to 3 hours, or until the internal temperature of the chicken reaches 165°F on a meat thermometer and the juices run clear and serve (see Tip).

Nutrition: Calories: 417 | Total Fat: 12g | Total Carbs: 1g | Sugar: 1g | Fiber: 1g | Protein: 71g | Sodium: 591mg

465. Coconut-Curry-Cashew Chicken

Preparation Time: 15 minutes
Cooking Time: 7 to 8 hours
Servings: 4
Ingredients:
- 1½ cups Chicken Bone Broth
- 1 (14-ounce) can of full-fat coconut milk
- 1 teaspoon garlic powder
- 1 tablespoon red curry paste
- 1 teaspoon sea salt
- ½ teaspoon freshly ground black pepper
- ½ teaspoon coconut sugar
- 2 pounds boneless, skinless chicken breasts
- 1½ cup unsalted cashews
- ½ cup diced white onion

Directions:
1. In a bowl, combine the broth, coconut milk, garlic powder, red curry paste, and salt, pepper, and coconut sugar. Stir well.
2. Put the chicken, cashews, and onion in the slow cooker. Pour the coconut milk mixture on top.

3. Cover the cooker and set it to low. Cook for around 7 to 8 hours, or until the internal temperature of the chicken reaches 165°F on a meat thermometer and the juices run clear.
4. Shred the chicken using a fork, then mixed it into the cooking liquid. You can also remove the chicken from the broth and chop it with a knife into bite-size pieces before returning it to the slow cooker. Serve.

Nutrition: Calories: 714 | Total Fat: 43g | Total Carbs: 21g | Sugar: 5g | Fiber: 3g | Protein: 57g | Sodium: 1,606mg

466. Turkey & Sweet Potato Chili

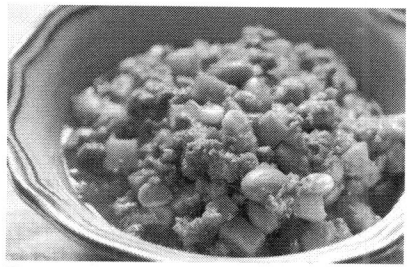

Preparation Time: 15 minutes
Cooking Time: 4 to 6 hours
Servings: 4
Ingredients:
- 1 tablespoon extra-virgin olive oil
- 1-pound ground turkey
- 3 cups sweet potato cubes
- 1 (28-ounce) can diced tomatoes
- 1 red bell pepper, diced
- 1 (4-ounce) can Hatch green chiles
- ½ medium red onion, diced
- 2 cups broth of choice
- 1 tablespoon chili powder
- 1 teaspoon garlic powder
- 1 teaspoon cocoa powder
- 1 teaspoon ground cumin
- 1 teaspoon sea salt
- ½ teaspoon ground cinnamon
- Pinch cayenne pepper

Directions:
1. In your slow cooker, combine the olive oil, turkey, sweet potato cubes, tomatoes, bell pepper, chiles, onion, broth, lime juice, chili powder, garlic powder, cocoa powder, cumin, salt, cinnamon, and cayenne. Using a large spoon, break up the turkey into smaller chunks as it combines with the other ingredients.
2. Cover the cooker and set it to low. Cook for 4 to 6 hours.
3. Stir the chili well, continuing to break up the rest of the turkey, and serve.

Nutrition: Calories: 38 | Total Fat: 12 | Total Carbs: 38 | Sugar: 12 | Fiber: 6g | Protein: 30g | Sodium: 1,268mg

467. Moroccan Turkey Tagine

Preparation Time: 15 minutes
Cooking Time: 7 to 8 hours
Servings: 4
Ingredients:
- 4 cups boneless, skinless turkey breast chunks
- 1 (14 oz.) can diced tomatoes
- 1 (14 oz.) can chickpeas, drained
- 2 large carrots, finely chopped
- ½ cup dried apricots
- ½ red onion, chopped
- 2 tablespoons raw honey
- 1 tablespoon tomato paste
- 1 teaspoon garlic powder
- 1 teaspoon ground turmeric
- ½ teaspoon sea salt
- ¼ teaspoon ground ginger
- ¼ teaspoon ground coriander
- ¼ teaspoon paprika
- ½ cup water
- 2 cups broth of choice
- Freshly ground black pepper

Directions:
1. In your slow cooker, combine the turkey, tomatoes, chickpeas, carrots, apricots, onion, honey, tomato paste, garlic powder, turmeric, salt, ginger, coriander, paprika, water, and broth, and season with pepper. Gently stir to blend the ingredients.
2. Cover the cooker and set it to low. Cook for 7 to 8 hours and serve.

Nutrition: Calories: 428 | Total Fat: 5 | Total Carbs: 46g | Sugar: 25g | Fiber: 8g | Protein: 49g | Sodium: 983mg

468. Turkey Sloppy Joes

Preparation Time: 15 minutes
Cooking Time: 4 to 6 hours
Servings: 4
Ingredients:
- 1 tablespoon extra-virgin olive oil
- 1-pound ground turkey
- 1 celery stalk, minced
- 1 carrot, minced
- ½ medium sweet onion, diced
- ½ red bell pepper, finely chopped
- 6 tablespoons tomato paste
- 2 tablespoons apple cider vinegar
- 1 tablespoon maple syrup
- 1 teaspoon Dijon mustard
- 1 teaspoon chili powder
- ½ teaspoon garlic powder
- ½ teaspoon sea salt
- ½ teaspoon dried oregano

Directions:
1. In your slow cooker, combine the olive oil, turkey, celery, carrot, onion, red bell pepper, tomato paste, vinegar, maple syrup, mustard, chili powder, garlic powder, salt, and oregano. Using a large spoon, break up the turkey into smaller chunks as it combines with the other ingredients.
2. Cover the cooker and set it to low. Cook for 4 to 6 hours, stir thoroughly and serve.

Nutrition: Calories: 251 | Total Fat: 12g | Total Carbs: 14g | Sugar: 9g | Fiber: 3g | Protein: 24g | Sodium: 690mg

469. Turkey Meatballs with Spaghetti Squash

Preparation Time: 15 minutes
Cooking Time: 7 to 8 hours
Servings: 4
Ingredients:
- 1 spaghetti squash, halved lengthwise and seeded
- For the Sauce:
- 1 (15-ounce) can diced tomatoes
- ½ teaspoon garlic powder
- ½ teaspoon dried oregano
- ½ teaspoon sea salt
- For the Meatballs:
- 1-pound ground turkey
- 1 large egg, whisked
- ½ small white onion, minced
- 1 teaspoon garlic powder
- ½ teaspoon sea salt
- ½ teaspoon dried oregano
- ½ teaspoon dried basil leaves
- Freshly ground black pepper

Directions:
1. Place the squash halves in the bottom of your slow cooker, cut-side down.
2. To make the Sauce:
3. Pour the diced tomatoes around the squash in the bottom of the slow cooker.
4. Sprinkle in the garlic powder, oregano, and salt.
5. To make the meatballs:
6. In a medium bowl, mix the turkey, egg, onion, garlic powder, salt, oregano, and basil, and season with pepper. Form the turkey mixture into 12 balls, and place them in the slow cooker around the spaghetti squash.
7. Cover the cooker and set it to low. Cook for 6 to 7 hours.
8. Transfer the squash to a work surface, and use a fork to shred it into spaghetti-like strands. Combine the strands with the tomato sauce, top with the meatballs, and serve.

Nutrition: Calories: 253 | Total Fat: 8 | Total Carbs: 22g | Sugar: 4g | Fiber: 1g | Protein: 24g | Sodium: 948mg

470. Chimichurri Turkey

Preparation Time: 15 minutes
Cooking Time: 7 to 8 hours
Servings: 4
Ingredients:
- 1 (2-to 3-pound) whole, boneless turkey breast

- 2 cups Chimichurri Sauce (double the recipe)
- ½ cup broth of choice

Directions:
1. Put the turkey in the slow cooker. Pour on the sauce and broth.
2. Cover the cooker and set it to low. Cook for 6 to 7 hours, or until the internal temperature of the turkey reaches 165°F on a meat thermometer and the juices run clear and serve.

Nutrition: Calories: 776|Total Fat: 59g|Total Carbs: 14g|Sugar: 4g|Fiber: 6|Protein: 60g|Sodium: 1,128mg

471. Balsamic-Glazed Turkey Wings

Preparation Time: 15 minutes
Cooking Time: 7 to 8 hours
Servings: 4
Ingredients:
- 1¼ cups balsamic vinegar
- 2 tablespoons raw honey
- 1 teaspoon garlic powder
- 2 pounds' turkey wings

Directions:
1. In a bowl, put together the vinegar, honey, and garlic powder, then mix.
2. Put the wings in the bottom of the slow cooker, and pour the vinegar sauce on top.
3. Cover the cooker and set it to low. Cook for 7 to 8 hours.
4. Baste the wings with the sauce from the bottom of the slow cooker and serve.

Nutrition: Calories: 501|Total Fat: 25g|Sugar: 9g|Fiber: 0g| Protein: 47g| Sodium: 162mg

472. Slow Cooker Chicken Fajitas

Preparation Time: 15 minutes
Cooking Time: 7 to 8 hours
Servings: 4
Ingredients:
- 1 (14.5-ounce) can diced tomatoes
- 1 (4-ounce) can Hatch green chills
- 1½ teaspoons garlic powder
- 2 teaspoons chili powder
- 1½ teaspoons ground cumin
- 1 teaspoon paprika
- 1 teaspoon sea salt
- Juice of 1 lime
- Pinch cayenne pepper
- Freshly ground black pepper
- 1 red bell pepper, seeded and sliced
- 1 green bell pepper, seeded and sliced
- 1 yellow bell pepper, seeded and sliced
- 1 large onion, sliced
- 2 pounds boneless, skinless chicken breast

Directions:
1. In a medium bowl, put together the diced tomatoes, chiles, garlic powder, chili powder, cumin, paprika, salt, lime juice, and cayenne, and season with black pepper, then mix. Pour half the diced tomato mixture into the bottom of your slow cooker.
2. Layer half the red, green, and yellow bell peppers and half the onion over the tomatoes in the cooker.
3. Place the chicken on top of the peppers and onions.
4. Cover the chicken with the remaining red, green, and yellow bell peppers and onions. Pour the remaining tomato mixture on top.
5. Cover the cooker and set it to low. Cook for around 7 to 8 hours, or until the internal temperature of the chicken reaches 165°F on a meat thermometer and the juices run clear and serve.

Nutrition: Calories: 310|Total Fat: 5g|Total Carbs: 19g|Sugar: 7g|Fiber: 4g|Protein: 46|Sodium: 1,541mg

473. Spicy Pulled Chicken Wraps

Preparation Time: 15 minutes
Cooking Time: 6 to 8 hours
Servings: 4
Ingredients:
- 1 head romaine lettuce
- 1½ tsp. ground cumin
- 1½ c. low-fat, low-sodium chicken broth
- 1 tsp. paprika
- 1 tsp. garlic powder

- 1 lb. skinless, deboned chicken breasts
- 2 tsp. Chili powder

Directions:
1. In a slow cooker, put all together with the ingredients except lettuce and gently stir to combine.
2. Set the slow cooker on low.
3. Cover and cook for about 6-8 hours.
4. Uncover the slow cooker and transfer the breasts to a large plate.
5. With a fork, shred the breasts.
6. Serve the shredded beef over lettuce leaves.

Nutrition: Calories: 150 | Fat: 3.4 g | Carbs: 12 g | Protein: 14 g | Sugars: 7 g | Sodium: 900 mg

474. Orange Chicken Legs

Preparation Time: 10 minutes
Cooking Time: 8 hours
Servings: 4
Ingredients:
- Zest of 1 orange
- Juice of 1 orange
- ¼ cup red vinegar
- A pinch of salt and black pepper
- 4 chicken legs
- 5 garlic cloves, minced
- 1 red onion, cut into wedges
- 7 ounces canned peaches, halved
- ½ cup chopped parsley

Directions:
1. Mix the orange zest with the orange juice, vinegar, salt, pepper, garlic, onion, peaches, and parsley in a slow cooker. Add the chicken, toss, cover, and cook on Low for 8 hours. Divide between plates and serve.
2. Enjoy!

Nutrition: Calories: 251 | Fat: 4 | Fiber: 8 | Carbs: 14 | Protein: 8

475. Slow Cooker Chicken Cacciatore

Preparation Time: 15 minutes
Cooking Time: 10 minutes
Servings: 4
Ingredients:
- ¼ cup good-quality olive oil
- 4 (4-ounce) boneless chicken breasts, each cut into three pieces
- 1 onion, chopped
- 2 celery stalks, chopped
- 1 cup sliced mushrooms
- 2 tablespoons minced garlic
- 1 (28-ounce) can sodium-free diced tomatoes
- ½ cup tomato paste
- 1 tablespoon dried basil
- 1 teaspoon dried oregano
- ⅛ teaspoon red pepper flakes

Directions:
1. Brown the chicken. In a skillet at medium-high heat, warm the olive oil. Add the chicken breasts and brown them, turning them once, about 10 minutes in total.
2. Cook in the slow cooker. Place the chicken in the slow cooker and stir in the onion, celery, mushrooms, garlic, tomatoes, tomato paste, basil, oregano, and red pepper flakes. Cook it on high for approximately 3 to 4 hours or low for 6 to 8 hours, until the chicken is fully cooked and tender.
3. Serve. Divide the chicken and sauce between four bowls and serve it immediately.

Nutrition: Calories: 383 | Total fat: 26g | Total carbs: 11g | Fiber: 4g
Net carbs: 7g | Sodium: 116mg | Protein: 26g

476. Bacon-Wrapped Chicken with Cheddar Cheese

Preparation Time: 10 minutes
Cooking Time: 4 hours
Servings: 6
Ingredients:
- 2 large chicken breasts, each cut into 6 pieces
- 6 slices of streaky bacon, each cut in half width ways
- 4 garlic cloves, crushed
- ½ cup Cheddar cheese, grated
- From the cupboard:
- 1 tablespoon olive oil
- Salt, to taste
- Freshly ground black pepper, to taste

Directions:

1. Grease the insert of the slow cooker with olive oil.
2. Wrap each piece of chicken breast with each half of the bacon slice, and arrange them in the slow cooker. Sprinkle with garlic, salt, and black pepper.
3. Put the lid and then cook on LOW for 4 hours.
4. Set the oven to 350ºF (180ºC).
5. Transfer the cooked bacon-wrapped chicken to a baking dish, then scatter with cheese.
6. Cook in the preheated oven for 5 minutes or until the cheese melts.
7. Take it off from the oven and serve warm.

Nutrition: Calories: 308 Total fat: 20.8g|Total carbs: 2.9g |Fiber: 0g |Net carbs: 2.9g |Protein: 26.1g

477. Slow Cooker Jerk Chicken

Preparation Time: 10 minutes
Cooking Time: 5 hours
Servings: 4
Ingredients:
- chicken drumsticks and 8 chicken wings
- 4 teaspoons (20 g) salt
- 4 teaspoons (9 g) paprika
- 1 teaspoon (2 g) cayenne pepper
- 2 teaspoons (5 g) onion powder
- 2 teaspoons (3 g) dried thyme
- 2 teaspoons (4 g) white pepper
- 2 teaspoons (6 g) garlic powder
- 1 teaspoon (2 g) black pepper

Directions:
1. Put all the spices in a bowl, then mix to make a run for the chicken.
2. Wash the chicken meat in cold water briefly. Place the washed chicken meat into the bowl with the rub, and rub the spices onto the meat thoroughly, including under the skin.
3. Place each piece of chicken covered with the spices into the slow cooker (no liquid required).
4. Set the slow cooker on medium heat, and cook for 5 hours or until the chicken meat falls off the bone.

Nutrition: Calories: 480 |Fat: 30 g |Net Carbohydrates: 4 g |Protein: 45 g

478. Oregano Pork

Preparation Time: 10 minutes
Cooking Time: 8 hours
Servings: 4
Ingredients:
- 2 pounds' pork roast, sliced
- 2 tablespoons oregano, chopped
- ¼ cup balsamic vinegar
- 1 cup tomato paste
- 1 tablespoon sweet paprika
- 1 teaspoon onion powder
- 2 tablespoons chili powder
- 2 garlic cloves, minced
- A pinch of salt and black pepper

Directions:
1. In your slow cooker, combine the roast with the oregano, the vinegar, and the other ingredients, toss, put the lid on and cook on Low for 8 hours.
2. Divide everything between plates and serve.

Nutrition: Calories 300| Fat 5| Fiber 2| Carbs 12, |Protein 24

479. Cauliflower, Coconut Milk, and Shrimp Soup

Preparation Time: five minutes
Cooking Time: 2 hours and fifteen minutes
Servings: 4
Ingredients:
- 1 (13.5-ounce / 383-g) can unsweetened full-fat coconut milk
- 1 cup shrimp, peeled, deveined, tail off, and cooked
- 1 cup water
- 2 cups riced cauliflower
- 2 tablespoons chopped fresh cilantro leaves, divided
- 2 tablespoons red curry paste
- From the cupboard:
- Salt and freshly ground black pepper, to taste

Directions:
1. Put in the riced cauliflower, red curry paste, coconut milk, 1 tablespoon cilantro, water,

then drizzle with salt and black pepper. Combine the mixture to blend well.
2. Place the slow cooker lid on and cook on HIGH for about two hours.
3. Place the shrimp on a clean working surface, then drizzle salt and black pepper to season.
4. Place the shrimp in the slow cooker and cook for fifteen minutes more.
5. Move the soup into a big container and top with the rest of the cilantro leaves before you serve.

Nutrition: calories: 268, total fat: 21.3g, total carbs: 7.8g, fiber: 3.2g, net carbs: 4.6g, protein: 16.1g

LOW SODIUM RECIPES

480. Pasta Primavera

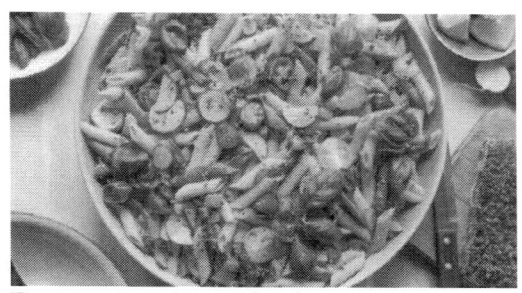

Preparation time: 10 minutes
Cooking time: 25 minutes
Servings: 4

Ingredients:
- 2 cups cauliflower florets, cut into matchsticks
- 16 oz. tortiglioni
- ¼ cup olive oil
- ½ cup chopped fresh green onions
- 1 red bell pepper, thinly sliced
- 4 garlic cloves, minced
- 1 cup grape tomatoes, halved
- 2 tsp. dried Italian seasoning
- ½ lemon, juiced

Directions:
1. In a pot of boiling water, cook the tortiglioni pasta for 8-10 minutes until al dente. Drain and set aside.
2. Heat olive oil in a skillet and sauté onion, cauliflower, and bell pepper for 7 minutes. Mix in garlic and cook until fragrant, 30 seconds.
3. Stir in the tomatoes and Italian seasoning; cook until the tomatoes soften, 5 minutes. Mix in the lemon juice and tortiglioni and adjust the taste with salt and black pepper.
4. Garnish with the Pecorino Romano cheese.

Nutrition: Calories: 381; Protein: 25.3 Grams; Fat: 12.9 Grams; Carbs: 9.7 Grams; Sodium: 48 mg; Cholesterol: 37 mg

481. Tuscan Chicken Linguine

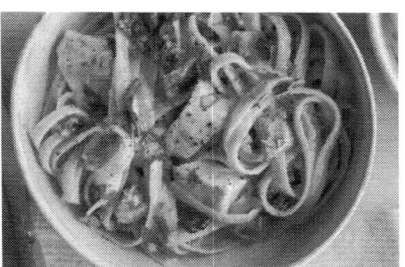

Preparation Time: 10 minutes
Cooking time: 25 minutes
Servings: 4

Ingredients
- 16 oz. linguine
- 2 tbsp. olive oil
- 4 chicken breasts
- 1 medium white onion, chopped
- 1 cup sundried tomatoes in oil, chopped
- 1 red bell pepper, deseeded and chopped
- 5 garlic cloves, minced
- ¾ cup chicken broth
- ¾ cup grated Pecorino Romano cheese
- 1 cup baby kale, chopped Salt and black pepper to taste

Directions
1. In a pot of boiling water, cook the linguine pasta for 8-10 minutes until al dente. Drain and set aside.
2. Heat the olive oil in a large skillet, season the chicken with salt, black pepper, and cook in the oil until golden brown on the outside and cooked within, 7 to 8 minutes.
3. Transfer the chicken to a plate and cut into 4 slices each. Set aside. Add the onion, sundried tomatoes, bell pepper to the skillet and sauté until softened, 5 minutes. Mix in the garlic and cook until fragrant, 1 minute.
4. Deglaze the skillet with the chicken broth and mix in the heavy cream. Simmer for 2

minutes and stir in the Pecorino Romano cheese until melted, 2 minutes.

5. Once the cheese melts, stir in the kale to wilt and adjust the taste with salt and black pepper. Mix in the linguine and chicken until well coated in the sauce. Dish the food and serve warm.

Nutrition: Calories: 281; Protein: 26.3 Grams; Fat: 12.9 Grams; Carbs: 10.7 Grams; Sodium: 90 mg; Cholesterol: 37 mg

482. Classic Beef Lasagna

Preparation time: 20 minutes
Cooking time: 50 minutes
Servings: 4
Ingredients:
- 1 lb lasagna sheets
- 2 tbsp. olive oil
- 1 lb ground beef
- 1 medium white onion, chopped
- 1 tsp. Italian seasoning
- Salt and black pepper to taste
- 1 cup marinara sauce
- ½ cup grated Parmesan cheese

Directions:
1. Preheat oven to 350 F. Warm olive oil in a skillet and add the beef and onion. Cook until the beef is brown, 7-8 minutes.
2. Season with Italian seasoning, salt, and pepper. Cook for 1 minute and mix in the marinara sauce. Simmer for 3 minutes.
3. Spread a layer of the beef mixture in a lightly greased baking sheet and make a first single layer on the beef mixture. Top with a single layer of lasagna sheets.
4. Repeat the layering two more times using the remaining ingredients in the same quantities. Sprinkle with the Parmesan cheese.
5. Bake in the oven until the cheese melts and is bubbly with the sauce, 20 minutes. Remove the lasagna, allow cooling for 2 minutes and dish onto serving plates. Serve warm.

Nutrition: Calories: 291; Protein: 23.3 Grams; Fat: 10.9 Grams; Carbs: 9.6 Grams; Sodium: 110 mg; Cholesterol: 37 mg

483. Spicy Veggie Pasta Bake

Preparation time: 10 minutes
Cooking time: 35 minutes
Servings: 4
Ingredients:
- 16 oz. penne
- 1 tbsp. olive oil
- 1 cup mixed chopped bell peppers
- 1 yellow squash, chopped
- 1 red onion, halved and sliced
- 1 cup sliced white button mushrooms
- Salt and black pepper to taste
- ¼ tsp. red chili flakes
- 1 cup marinara sauce
- 1 cup grated mozzarella cheese
- 1 cup grated Parmesan cheese
- ¼ cup chopped fresh basil

Directions
1. In a pot of boiling water, cook the penne pasta for 8-10 minutes until al dente. Drain and set aside.
2. Heat the olive oil in a cast iron and sauté the bell peppers, squash, onion, and mushrooms. Cook until softened, 5 minutes.
3. Stir in garlic and cook until fragrant, 30 seconds. Season with salt, pepper, and red chili flakes. Mix in marinara sauce and cook for 5 minutes. Stir in the penne and spread the mozzarella and Parmesan cheeses on top. Bake in the oven until the cheeses melt and golden brown on top, 15 minutes. Allow cooling for 2 minutes and dish onto serving plates. Serve warm.

Nutrition: Calories: 281; Protein: 24.3 Grams; Fat: 9.9 Grams; Carbs: 9.6 Grams; Sodium: 130 mg; Cholesterol: 37 mg

484. Parmesan Spaghetti in Mushroom-Tomato Sauce

Preparation time: 10 minutes
Cooking time: 20 minutes
Servings: 4
Ingredients:
- 16 oz. spaghetti, cut in half
- 2 cups mushrooms, chopped

- 1 bell pepper, chopped
- ½ cup yellow onion, chopped
- 3 garlic cloves, minced
- ½ tsp. five-spice powder
- 4 tbsp. fresh parsley, chopped
- 1 tbsp. tomato paste
- 2 ripe tomatoes, chopped
- ½ cup Parmesan cheese, grated
- ¼ cup olive oil
- Salt and black pepper to taste

Directions:
1. Heat olive oil in a skillet over medium heat. Add in mushrooms, bell pepper, onion, and garlic and stir-fry for 4-5 minutes until tender.
2. Mix in salt, black pepper, 2 tbsp. of parsley, five-spice powder, tomato paste, and tomatoes; stir well and cook for 10-12 minutes.
3. In a pot with salted boiling water, add the pasta and cook until al dente, about 8-10 minutes, stirring occasionally.
4. Drain and stir in the vegetable mixture. Serve topped with Parmesan cheese and remaining fresh parsley.

Nutrition: Calories: 341; Protein: 15.3 Grams; Fat: 12.7 Grams; Carbs: 9.7 Grams; Sodium: 127 mg; Cholesterol: 27 mg

485. Mustard Chicken Farfalle

Preparation time: 10 minutes
Cooking time: 30 minutes
Servings: 4

Ingredients:
- 16 oz. farfalle
- 1 tbsp. olive oil
- 4 chicken breasts, cut into strips
- Salt and black pepper to taste
- 1 yellow onion, finely sliced
- 1 yellow bell pepper, sliced
- 1 garlic clove, minced
- 1 tbsp. wholegrain mustard
- 5 tbsp. heavy cream
- 1 cup chopped mustard greens
- 1 tbsp. chopped parsley

Directions:
1. In a pot of boiling water, cook the farfalle pasta for 8-10 minutes until al dente. Drain and set aside.
2. Heat the olive oil in a large skillet, season the chicken with salt, black pepper, and cook in the oil until golden brown, 10 minutes.
3. Set aside. Stir in the onion, bell pepper and cook until softened, 5 minutes. Mix in the garlic and cook until fragrant, 30 seconds.
4. Mix in the mustard and heavy cream; simmer for 2 minutes and mix in the chicken and mustard greens.
5. Allow wilting for 2 minutes and adjust the taste with salt and black pepper. Stir in the farfalle pasta, allow warming for 1 minute and dish the food onto serving plates. Garnish with the parsley and serve warm.

Nutrition: Calories: 281; Protein: 25.7 Grams; Fat: 8.9 Grams; Carbs: 9.7 Grams; Sodium: 98 mg; Cholesterol: 37 mg

486. Italian Mushroom Pizza

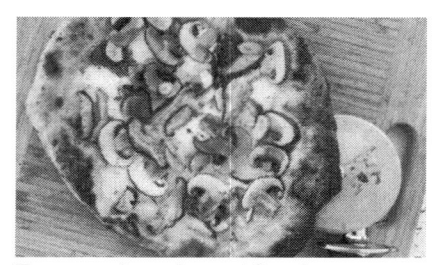

Preparation time: 10 minutes
Cooking time: 35 minutes
Servings: 4

Ingredients:
- For the Crust:
- 2 cups flour
- 1 cup lukewarm water
- 1 pinch of sugar
- 1 tsp. active dry yeast
- ¾ tsp. salt

- For the Topping
- 1 tsp. olive oil
- 2 medium Cremini mushrooms, sliced
- 1 garlic clove, minced
- ½ cup sugar-free tomato sauce

- 1 tsp. sugar 1 bay leaf
- 1 tsp. dried oregano
- 1 tsp dried basil
- Salt and black pepper to taste
- ½ cup grated mozzarella cheese
- ½ cup grated Parmesan cheese
- 6 black olives, pitted and sliced

Directions:
1. Sift the flour and salt in a bowl and stir in yeast. Mix lukewarm water, olive oil, and sugar in another bowl.
2. Add the wet mixture to the dry mixture and whisk until you obtain a soft dough. Place the dough on a lightly floured work surface and knead it thoroughly for 4-5 minutes until elastic.
3. Transfer the dough to a greased bowl. Cover with cling film and leave to rise for 50-60 minutes in a warm place until doubled in size.
4. Roll out the dough to a thickness of around 12 inches. Preheat the oven to 400 F. Line a pizza pan with parchment paper.
5. Heat the olive oil in a medium skillet and sauté the mushrooms until softened, 5 minutes. Stir in the garlic and cook until fragrant, 30 seconds.
6. Mix in the tomato sauce, sugar, bay leaf, oregano, basil, salt, and black pepper. Cook for 2 minutes and turn the heat off.
7. Spread the sauce on the crust, top with the mozzarella and Parmesan cheeses, and then, the olives.
8. Bake in the oven until the cheeses melts, 15 minutes. Remove the pizza, slice, and serve warm.

Nutrition: Calories: 386; Protein: 22.6 Grams; Fat: 10.6 Grams; Carbs: 9.7 Grams; Sodium: 130 mg; Cholesterol: 35 mg

487. Chicken Bacon Ranch Pizza

Preparation time: 10 minutes
Cooking time: 35 minutes
Servings: 4

Ingredients:
- For the Crust:
- 2 cups flour
- 1 cup lukewarm water
- 1 pinch of sugar
- 1 tsp. active dry yeast
- ¾ tsp. salt
- 2 tbsp. olive oil
- For the ranch sauce
- 1 tbsp. butter
- 2 garlic cloves, minced
- 1 tbsp. cream cheese
- ¼ cup half and half
- 1 tbsp. dry Ranch seasoning mix
- For the Topping:
- 3 bacon slices, chopped
- 2 chicken breasts
- Salt and black pepper to taste
- 1 cup grated mozzarella cheese
- 6 fresh basil leaves

Directions
1. Sift the flour and salt in a bowl and stir in yeast. Mix lukewarm water, olive oil, and sugar in another bowl.
2. Add the wet mixture to the dry mixture and whisk until you obtain a soft dough. Place the dough on a lightly floured work surface and knead it thoroughly for 4-5 minutes until elastic.
3. Transfer the dough to a greased bowl. Cover with cling film and leave to rise for 50-60 minutes in a warm place until doubled in size.
4. Roll out the dough to a thickness of around 12 inches. Preheat the oven to 400 F. Line a pizza pan with parchment paper.
5. In a bowl, mix the sauce's ingredients butter, garlic, cream cheese, half and half, and ranch mix. Set aside. Heat a grill pan over medium heat and cook the bacon until crispy and brown, 5 minutes.
6. Transfer to a plate and set aside. Season the chicken with salt, pepper and grill in the pan on both sides until golden brown, 10 minutes.
7. Remove to a plate, allow cooling and cut into thin slices. Spread the ranch sauce on the pizza crust, followed by the chicken and bacon, and then, mozzarella cheese and basil. Bake for 5 minutes or until the cheese melts. Slice and serve warm.

Nutrition: Calories: 351; Protein: 25.3 Grams; Fat: 12.4 Grams; Carbs: 8.7 Grams; Sodium: 140 mg; Cholesterol: 35 mg

488. Fall Baked Vegetable with Rigatoni

Preparation time: 10 minutes
Cooking time: 35 minutes
Servings: 6
Ingredients
- 1 lb pumpkin, chopped
- 1 zucchini, chopped
- 2 tbsp. grated Pecorino-Romano cheese
- 1 onion, chopped
- 1 lb rigatoni
- 2 tbsp. olive oil
- Salt and black pepper to taste
- ½ tsp. garlic powder
- ½ cup dry white wine

Directions
1. Preheat oven to 420 F. Combine zucchini, pumpkin, onion, and olive oil in a bowl. Arrange on a lined aluminum foil sheet and season with salt, pepper, and garlic powder.
2. Bake for 30 minutes until tender. In a pot of boiling water, cook rigatoni for 8-10 minutes until al dente. Drain and set aside. In a food processor, place ½ cup of the roasted veggies and wine and pulse until smooth.
3. Transfer to a skillet over medium heat. Stir in rigatoni and cook until heated through. Top with the remaining roasted vegetables and Pecorino cheese to serve.

Nutrition: Calories: 378; Protein: 35.3 Grams; Fat: 10.9 Grams; Carbs: 8.7 Grams; Sodium: 160 mg; Cholesterol: 28 mg

489. Walnut Pesto Pasta

Preparation time: 10 minutes
Cooking time: 10 minutes
Servings: 4
Ingredients
- 8 oz. whole-wheat pasta
- ¼ cup walnuts, chopped
- 3 garlic cloves, finely minced
- ½ cup fresh dill, chopped
- ¼ cup grated Parmesan cheese
- 3 tbsp. extra-virgin olive oil

Directions
1. Cook the whole-wheat pasta to pack instructions, drain and let it cool.
2. Place the olive oil, dill, garlic, Parmesan cheese, and walnuts in a food processor and blend for 15 seconds or until paste forms.
3. Pour over the cooled pasta and toss to combine. Serve immediately.

Nutrition: Calories: 361; Protein: 25.3 Grams; Fat: 12.9 Grams; Carbs: 9.7 Grams; Sodium: 120 mg; Cholesterol: 27 mg

490. Beef Carbonara

Preparation time: 10 minutes
Cooking time: 20 minutes
Servings: 4
Ingredients:
- 16 oz. linguine
- 4 bacon slices, chopped
- 1 ¼ cups heavy whipping cream
- ¼ cup mayonnaise
- Salt and black pepper to taste
- 4 egg yolks
- 1 cup grated Parmesan cheese

Directions:
1. In a pot of boiling water, cook the linguine pasta for 8-10 minutes until al dente. Drain and set aside.
2. Add the bacon to a skillet and cook over medium heat until crispy, 5 minutes. Set aside. Pour heavy cream into a pot and allow simmering for 5 minutes.
3. Whisk in mayonnaise and season with salt and pepper. Cook for 1 minute and spoon 2 tablespoons of the mixture into a medium bowl. Allow cooling and mix in the egg yolks. Pour the mixture into the pot and mix quickly.
4. Stir in Parmesan and fold in the pasta. Garnish with more Parmesan. Cook for 1 minute to warm the pasta.

Nutrition: Calories: 361; Protein: 19.3 Grams; Fat: 11.9 Grams; Carbs: 10.7 Grams; Sodium: 128 mg; Cholesterol: 24 mg

491. Coconut Flour Pizza

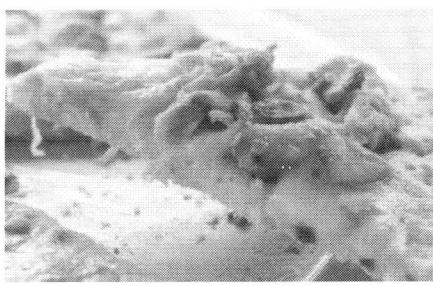

Preparation time: 10 minutes
Cooking Time: 35 minutes
Servings: 4
Ingredients
- 2 tablespoons psyllium husk powder
- ¾ cup coconut flour
- 1 teaspoon garlic powder
- ½ teaspoon salt
- ½ teaspoon baking soda
- 1 cup boiling water
- 1 teaspoon apple cider vinegar

- Toppings:
- 3 tablespoons tomato sauce
- 1½ oz. Mozzarella cheese
- 1 tablespoon basil, freshly chopped

Directions
1. Preheat the oven to 350 degrees f and grease a baking sheet. Mix coconut flour, salt, psyllium husk powder, and garlic powder until fully combined.
2. Add eggs, apple cider vinegar, and baking soda and knead with boiling water. Place the dough out on a baking sheet and top with the toppings.
3. Transfer in the oven and bake for about 20 minutes. Dish out and serve warm.

Nutrition: Calories 308 Total fat: 20.8g | Total carbs: 2.9g | Fiber: 0g | Net carbs: 2.9g | Protein: 26.1g

492. Keto Pepperoni Pizza

Preparation time: 40 minutes
Cooking time: 10 minutes
Servings: 4
Ingredients
- Crust
- 6 oz. mozzarella cheese, shredded
- 4 eggs
- Topping
- 1 teaspoon dried oregano
- 1½ oz. pepperoni
- 3 tablespoons tomato paste
- 5 oz. mozzarella cheese, shredded
- Olives

Directions:
1. Preheat the oven to 400 degrees F and grease a baking sheet. Whisk together eggs and cheese in a bowl and spread on a baking sheet.
2. Transfer in the oven and bake for about 15 minutes until golden. Remove from the oven and allow it to cool.
3. Increase the oven temperature to 450 degrees F. spread the tomato paste on the crust and top with oregano, pepperoni, cheese, and olives on top.
4. Bake for another 10 minutes and serve hot.

Nutrition: Calories: 480 | Fat: 30 g | Net Carbohydrates: 4 g | Protein: 45 g

493. Fresh Bell Pepper Basil Pizza

Preparation time: 25 minutes
Cooking Time: 10 minutes
Servings: 3
Ingredients:
- Pizza Base
- ½ cup almond flour
- 2 tablespoons cream cheese
- 1 teaspoon Italian seasoning
- ½ teaspoon black pepper
- 6 ounces mozzarella cheese
- 2 tablespoons psyllium husk
- 2 tablespoons fresh Parmesan cheese
- 1 large egg
- ½ teaspoon salt
- Toppings
- 4 ounces cheddar cheese, shredded
- ¼ cup Marinara sauce
- 2/3 medium bell pepper
- 1 medium vine tomato

- 3 tablespoons basil, fresh chopped

Directions:
1. Preheat the oven to 400 degrees F and grease a baking dish. Microwave mozzarella cheese for about 30 seconds and top with the remaining pizza crust.
2. Add the remaining pizza ingredients to the cheese and mix together. Flatten the dough and transfer in the oven.
3. Bake for about 10 minutes and remove pizza from the oven. Top the pizza with the toppings and bake for another 10 minutes.
4. Remove pizza from the oven and allow to cool.

Nutrition: Calories: 381; Protein: 25.3 Grams; Fat: 12.9 Grams; Carbs: 9.7 Grams; Cholesterol: 37 mg

494. Basil & Artichoke Pizza

Preparation time: 1 hour
Cooking time: 20 minutes
Servings: 4
Ingredients:
- 1 cup canned passata
- 2 cups flour
- 1 cup lukewarm water
- 1 pinch of sugar
- 1 tsp. active dry yeast
- ¾ tsp. salt 2 tbsp. olive oil
- 1 ½ cups frozen artichoke hearts
- ¼ cup grated Asiago cheese
- ½ onion, minced
- 3 garlic cloves, minced
- 1 tbsp. dried oregano
- 1 cup sun-dried tomatoes, chopped
- ½ tsp. red pepper flakes
- 5-6 basil leaves, torn

Directions:
1. Sift the flour and salt in a bowl and stir in yeast. Mix lukewarm water, olive oil, and sugar in another bowl.
2. Add the wet mixture to the dry mixture and whisk until you obtain a soft dough. Place the dough on a lightly floured work surface and knead it thoroughly for 4-5 minutes until elastic.
3. Transfer the dough to a greased bowl. Cover with cling film and leave to rise for 50-60 minutes in a warm place until doubled in size.
4. Roll out the dough to a thickness of around 12 inches. Preheat oven to 400 F. Warm oil in a saucepan over medium heat and sauté onion and garlic for 3-4 minutes.
5. Mix in tomatoes and oregano and bring to a boil. Decrease the heat and simmer for another 5 minutes.
6. Transfer the pizza crust to a baking sheet. Spread the sauce all over and top with artichoke hearts and sun-dried tomatoes.
7. Scatter the cheese and bake for 15 minutes until golden. Top with red pepper flakes and basil leaves and serve sliced.

Nutrition: Calories: 372; Protein: 22.3 Grams; Fat: 11.9 Grams; Carbs: 9.2 Grams; Sodium: 80 mg; Cholesterol: 37 mg

495. Spanish-Style Pizza de Jarmon

Preparation time: 10 minutes
Cooking time: 35 minutes
Servings: 4
Ingredients:
- For the crust
- 2 cups flour
- 1 cup lukewarm water
- 1 pinch of sugar
- 1 tsp. active dry yeast
- ¾ tsp. salt
- 2 tbsp. olive oil
- For the topping
- ½ cup tomato sauce
- ½ cup sliced mozzarella cheese
- 4 oz. jamon serrano, sliced
- 7 fresh basil leaves

Directions:
1. Sift the flour and salt in a bowl and stir in yeast. Mix lukewarm water, olive oil, and sugar in another bowl.
2. Add the wet mixture to the dry mixture and whisk until you obtain a soft dough. Place the dough on a lightly floured work surface and knead it thoroughly for 4-5 minutes until elastic.

3. Transfer the dough to a greased bowl. Cover with cling film and leave to rise for 50-60 minutes in a warm place until doubled in size.
4. Roll out the dough to a thickness of around 12 inches. Preheat the oven to 400 F. Line a pizza pan with parchment paper.
5. Spread the tomato sauce on the crust. Arrange the mozzarella slices on the sauce and then the jamon serrano. Bake for 15 minutes or until the cheese melts.
6. Remove from the oven and top with the basil. Slice and serve warm.

Nutrition: Calories: 361; Protein: 24 Grams; Fat: 12.7 Grams; Carbs: 9.7 Grams; Sodium: 180 mg; Cholesterol: 37 mg

496. Curry Chicken Pockets

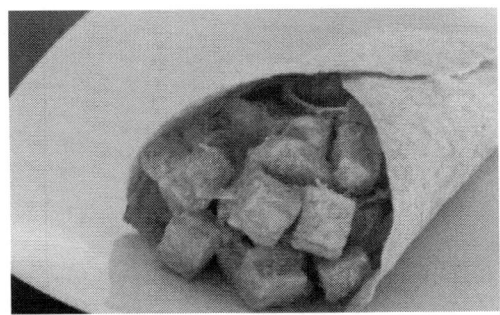

Preparation time: 10 minutes
Cooking time: 25 minutes
Servings: 4
Ingredients:
- 2 Cups Chicken, Cooked & Chopped
- ½ Cup Celery, Chopped
- 1/3 Cup Ricotta Cheese, Part Skim
- 1/ Cup Carrot, Shredded
- 1 Teaspoon Curry Powder
- 1 Tablespoon Apricot Preserved
- 10 Ounces Refrigerated Pizza Dough

- ¼ Teaspoon Ground Cinnamon

Directions:
1. Mix your carrot, ricotta, preserves, celery, chicken, cinnamon, salt and curry powder.
2. Spread the pizza dough and slice it into six equal squares.
3. Divide your mixture between each one, and then fold the corners of each towards the center and pinch them together. Put them on the baking sheet, baking at 375 for fifteen minutes. They should turn golden brown.
4. Allow them to cool before serving warm.

Nutrition: Calories: 415; Protein: 31.2 Grams; Fat: 32.7 Grams; Carbs: 14.7 Grams; Sodium: 77 mg; Cholesterol: 4.1 mg

497. Fajita Style Chili

Preparation time: 10 minutes
Cooking time: 5 hours
Servings: 4
Ingredients:
- 1 Teaspoon Fajita Seasoning
- 1 Tablespoon Chili Powder
- 2 lbs. Chicken Breasts, Boneless & Cubed
- ½ Teaspoon Cumin, Ground
- 2 Cloves Garlic, Minced
- Nonstick Cooking Spray as Needed
- 2 Cans (14.5 Ounces Each) Tomatoes, Diced
- ½ Green Bell Pepper, Julienned
- ½ Red Bell Pepper, Julienned
- ½ Yellow Bell Pepper, Julienned
- ½ Onion, Sliced
- 15 Ounces White Kidney Beans, Rinsed & Drained (Canned)
- 3 Tablespoons Sour Cream
- 3 Tablespoon Cheddar Cheese, Shredded & Reduced Fat
- 3 Tablespoons Guacamole

Directions:
1. Mix your chicken with fajita seasoning, garlic, cumin, and chili powder.
2. Grease a skillet and place it over medium heat. Add in your chicken, cooking until its golden brown.
3. Transfer it to a slow cooker, and then add in your tomatoes with their juices, vegetables, and beans. Cover, and cook on low for five hours.
4. Garnish with guacamole, cheese and sour cream before serving warm.

Nutrition: Calories: 495; Protein: 67.4 Grams; Fat: 11.5 Grams; Carbs: 10.2 Grams; Sodium: 112 mg; Cholesterol: 183 mg

498. Fun Fajita Wraps

Preparation time: 10 minutes
Cooking time: 10 minutes
Servings: 4
Ingredients:
- Nonstick Cooking Spray
- ¼ Teaspoon Garlic Powder
- ½ Teaspoon Chili Powder
- 12 Ounces Chicken Breasts, Skinless & Sliced into Strips
- 1 Green Sweet Pepper, Seeded & Sliced into Strips
- 2 Tortilla, 10 Inches & Whole Wheat
- 2 Tablespoons Ranch Salad Dressing, Reduced Calorie
- ½ Cup Salsa
- 1/3 Cup Cheddar Cheese, Shredded & Reduced Fat

Directions:
1. Mix your chicken strips with chili powder and garlic powder. Heat a skillet and grease with cooking spray. Place it over medium heat, and add in your sweet pepper and chicken. Cook for six minutes.
2. Toss your salad dressing in, and divide between tortillas.
3. Top with salsa and cheese, and roll your tortilla before slicing them in half. Serve warm.

Nutrition: Calories: 245, Protein: 38.5 Grams, Fat: 16.4 Grams, Carbs: 8.7 Grams, Sodium: 71 mg, Cholesterol: 143 mg

499. Classic Chicken Noodle Soup

Preparation time: 10 minutes
Cooking time: 20 minutes
Serves: 4
Ingredients:
- 1 Teaspoon Olive Oil
- 1 Cup Onion, Chopped
- 3 Cloves Garlic, Minced
- 1 Cup Celery, Chopped
- 1 Cup Carrots, Sliced & Peeled
- 4 Cups Chicken Broth
- 4 Ounces Linguini, Dried & Broken
- 1 Cup Chicken Breast, Cooked & Chopped
- 2 Tablespoons Parsley, Fresh

Directions:
1. Put a saucepan over medium heat, and heat up your oil. Stir in your onion and garlic, cooking until soften.
2. Add your celery and carrots. Cook for three minutes before adding your broth. Allow it to come to a boil before reducing it to simmer. Cook for five minutes before adding in your linguini.
3. Bring it to a boil and reduce the heat to simmer. Cook for ten more minutes.
4. Add in your parsley and chicken, and then cook until heated all the way through. Serve warm.

Nutrition: Calories: 381; Protein: 25.3 Grams; Fat: 12.9 Grams; Carbs: 9.7 Grams; Sodium: 80 mg; Cholesterol: 37 mg

500. Open Face Egg and Bacon Sandwich

Preparation time: 10 minutes
Cooking Time: 20 minutes
Servings: 1
Ingredients:
- ¼ oz. reduced fat cheddar, shredded
- ½ small jalapeno, thinly sliced
- ½ whole grain English muffin, split
- 1 large organic egg
- 1 thick slice of tomato
- 1-piece turkey bacon
- 2 thin slices red onion
- 4-5 sprigs fresh cilantro
- Cooking spray
- Pepper to taste

Directions:
1. On medium fire, place a skillet, cook bacon until crisp tender and set aside. In same skillet, drain oils, and place ½ of English muffin and heat for at least a minute per side.
2. Transfer muffin to a serving plate. Coat the same skillet with cooking spray and fry egg to desired doneness.

3. Once cooked, place egg on top of muffin. Add cilantro, tomato, onion, jalapeno and bacon on top of egg.
4. Serve and enjoy.

Nutrition: Calories: 381; Protein: 25.3 Grams; Fat: 12.9 Grams; Carbs: 9.7 Grams; Sodium: 80 mg; Cholesterol: 37 mg

501. Tuscan Stew

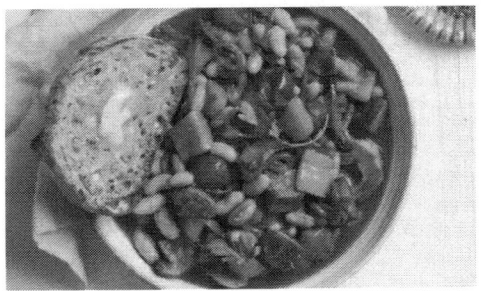

Preparation time: 10 minutes
Cooking time: 1 hour and 30 minutes
Servings: 6

Ingredients:
- Croutons:
- 1 Tablespoons Olive Oil
- 1 Slice Bread, Whole Grain & Cubed
- 2 Cloves Garlic, Quartered
- Soup:
- 2 Cups White Beans, Soaked Overnight & Drained
- 6 Cups Water
- ½ Teaspoon Sea Salt, Divided
- 1 Cup Yellow Onion, Chopped
- 2 Tablespoons Olive Oil
- 3 Carrots, Peeled & Chopped
- 6 Cloves Garlic, Chopped
- ¼ Teaspoon Ground Black Pepper
- 1 Tablespoons Rosemary, Fresh & Chopped
- 1 ½ Cups Vegetable Stock

Directions:
1. Add your oil to a skillet and heat it, and then cook your garlic for a minute. It should become fragrant. Allow it to sit for ten minutes before removing your garlic from the oil.
2. Return the pan with the oil to heat and then throw in your bread cubes. Cook for five minutes. They should be golden, and then set them to the side.
3. Mix your salt, water, bay leaf and white beans in the pot, boiling on high heat before reducing to a simmer.
4. Cover the beans and cook for one hour to one hour and ten minutes. They should be al dente.
5. Drain the beans, but reserve a half a cup of the cooking liquid. Discard the bay leaf, and transfer your beans to a bowl.
6. Mix the reserved liquid with ½ cup of beans, returning it to a boil. Mash with a fork to form a paste, and then place the pot on the stove. Heat the oil using the pot.
7. Add in your onions and carrots. Cook for seven minutes and add garlic, and then cook for a minute more. Add in your rosemary, salt, pepper, stock and bean mixture.
8. Allow it to come to a boil and then reduce the heat to let it simmer. Let it simmer for five minutes, and then top with croutons. Garnish with rosemary sprigs and enjoy.

Nutrition: Calories: 307; Protein: 16 Grams; Fat: 7 Grams; Carbs: 45 Grams; Sodium: 163 mg; Cholesterol: 68 mg

502. Tenderloin Fajitas

Preparation time: 10 minutes
Cooking time: 25 minutes
Servings: 8

Ingredients:
- ¼ Teaspoon Garlic Powder
- ¼ Teaspoon Ground Coriander
- 1 Tablespoon Chili Powder
- ½ Teaspoon Paprika
- ½ Teaspoon Oregano
- 1 lb. Pork Tenderloin, Sliced into Strips
- 8 Flour Tortillas, Whole Wheat & Warned
- 1 Small Onion, Sliced
- ½ Cup Cheddar Cheese, Shredded
- 4 Tomatoes, Diced
- 1 Cup Salsa
- 4 Cups Lettuce, Shredded

Directions:

1. Preheat a grill to 400, and then mix your coriander, garlic, oregano, paprika, and coriander in a bowl. Add in the pork slices, making sure they're well coated.
2. Arrange your pork and onions on a grilling grate, grilling for five minutes per side.
3. Stuff the tortillas with the mixture, topping with two tablespoons tomatoes, a tablespoon of cheese, ½ cup shredded lettuce and two tablespoons of salsa. Fold your tortillas and serve warm.

Nutrition: Calories: 250; Protein: 44 Grams; Fat: 9.8 Grams; Carbs: 21.1 Grams; Sodium: 71 mg; Cholesterol: 22 mg

503. Peanut Sauce Chicken Pasta

Preparation Time: 10 minutes
Cooking time: 20 minutes
Servings: 4

Ingredients:
- 2 Teaspoons Olive Oil
- 6 Ounces Spaghetti, Whole Wheat
- 10 Ounces Snap Peas, Fresh & Trimmed & Sliced into Strips
- 2 Cups Carrots, Julienned
- 2 Cups Chicken, Cooked & Shredded
- 1 Cup Thai Peanut Sauce
- 1 Cucumber, Halved Lengthwise & Sliced Diagonally
- Cilantro, Fresh & Chopped

Directions:
1. Start by cooking spaghetti as the package instructs, and then drain them and rinse the noodles using cold water.
2. Heat your greased skillet using oil, placing it over medium heat.
3. Once it's hot, add in your snap peas and carrot. Cook for eight minutes, and stir in your spaghetti, chicken and peanut sauce. Toss well, and garnish with cucumber and cilantro.

Nutrition: Calories: 403; Protein: 31 Grams; Fat: 15 Grams; Carbs: 43 Grams; Sodium: 132 mg; Cholesterol: 42 mg

504. Chicken Cherry Wraps

Preparation time: 10 minutes
Cooking time: 10 minutes
Serves: 4

Ingredients:
- ¼ Teaspoon Sea Salt, Fine
- ¼ Teaspoon Black Pepper
- 2 Teaspoons Olive oil
- ¾ lb. Chicken Breasts, Boneless & Cubed
- 1 Teaspoon Ginger, Ground
- 1 ½ Cups Carrots, Shredded
- 1 ¼ Cup Sweet Cherries, Fresh, Pitted & Chopped
- 4 Green Onions, Chopped
- 2 Tablespoons Rice Vinegar
- 1/3 Cup Almonds, Chopped Roughly
- 2 Tablespoons Rice Vinegar
- 2 Tablespoons Teriyaki Sauce, Low Sodium
- 1 Tablespoon Honey Raw
- 8 Large Lettuce Leaves

Directions:
1. Season your chicken using ginger, salt and pepper.
2. Get out a skillet, placing over medium heat and adding in your oil. Once your oil is hot cook your chicken for five minutes.
3. Throw in your cherries, green onions, carrots and almonds.
4. Add in your vinegar, teriyaki and honey before making sure it's mixed well, and your chicken is cooked all the way through.
5. Spread this on lettuce leaves to serve.

Nutrition: Calories: 257; Protein: 21 Grams; Fat: 10 Grams; Carbs: 21 Grams; Sodium: 81 mg; Cholesterol: 47 mg

505. Easy Barley Soup

Preparation time: 10 minutes
Cooking time: 20 minutes
Servings: 4

Ingredients:
- 1 Tablespoon Olive Oil
- 1 Onion, Chopped
- 5 Carrots, Chopped
- 2/3 Cup Barley, Quick Cooking

- 6 Cups Chicken Broth, Reduced Sodium
- ½ Teaspoon Black Pepper
- 2 Cups Baby Spinach, Fresh
- 2 Cups Turkey Breast, Cooked & Cubed

Directions:
1. Start by getting a saucepan and heat your oil over medium high heat.
2. Stir in your carrots and onion and sauté for five minutes before adding in your barley and broth. Bring it to a boil before reducing too low to simmer. Cook for fifteen minutes.
3. Stir in your pepper, spinach and turkey. Mix well before serving.

Nutrition: Calories: 208; Protein: 21 Grams; Fat: 4 Grams; Carbs: 23 Grams; Sodium: 62 mg; Cholesterol: 37 mg

506. Cauliflower Lunch Salad

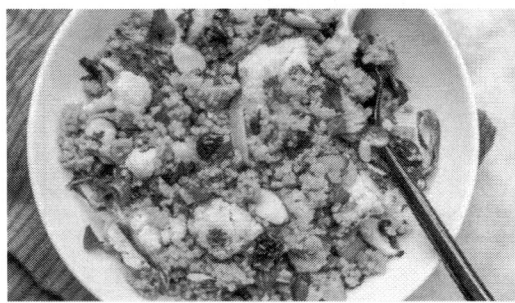

Preparation time: 2 hours
Cooking time: 10 minutes
Servings: 4

Ingredients:
- 1/3 cup low-sodium veggie stock
- 2 tablespoons olive oil
- 6 cups cauliflower florets, grated
- Black pepper to the taste
- ¼ cup red onion, chopped
- 1 red bell pepper, chopped
- Juice of ½ lemon
- 1 teaspoon mint, chopped
- 1 tablespoon cilantro, chopped

Directions:
1. Heat-up a pan with the oil over medium-high heat, add cauliflower, pepper and stock, stir, cook within 10 minutes, transfer to a bowl, and keep in the fridge for 2 hours.
2. Mix cauliflower with olives, onion, bell pepper, black pepper, mint, and cilantro, and lemon juice, toss to coat, and serve.

Nutrition: Calories: 102; Carbs: 3g; Fat: 10g; Protein: 0g; Sodium 97 mg

507. Cheesy Black Bean Wraps

Preparation time: 5 minutes
Cooking time: 10 minutes
Servings: 6

Ingredients:
- 2 Tablespoons Green Chili Peppers, Chopped
- 4 Green Onions, Diced
- 1 Tomato, Diced
- 1 Tablespoon Garlic, Chopped
- 6 Tortilla Wraps, Whole Grain & Fat Free
- ¾ Cup Cheddar Cheese, Shredded
- ¾ Cup Salsa
- 1 ½ Cups Corn Kernels
- 3 Tablespoons Cilantro, Fresh & Chopped
- 1 ½ Cup Black Beans, Canned & Drained

Directions:
1. Toss your chili peppers, corn, black beans, garlic, tomato, onions and cilantro in a bowl.
2. Heat the mixture in a microwave for a minute, and stir for a half a minute.
3. Spread the two tortillas between paper towels and microwave for twenty seconds. Warm the remaining tortillas the same way, and add a half a cup of bean mixture, two tablespoons of salsa and two tablespoons of cheese for each tortilla. Roll them up before serving.

Nutrition: Calories: 341; Protein: 19 Grams; Fat: 11 Grams; Carbs: 36.5 Grams; Sodium: 141 mg; Cholesterol: 0 mg

GRAIN FREE RECIPES

508. Vegan-Friendly Banana Bread

Preparation Time: 15 minutes
Cooking Time: 40 minutes
Servings: 4-6
Ingredients:
- 2 ripe bananas, mashed
- 1/3 cup brewed coffee
- 3 tbsp. chia seeds
- 6 tbsp. water
- ½ cup soft vegan butter
- ½ cup maple syrup
- 2 cups flour
- 2 tsp. baking powder
- 1 tsp. cinnamon powder
- 1 tsp. allspice
- ½ tsp. salt

Directions:
1. Set oven at 350F.
2. Bring the chia seeds to a small bowl, then soak it with 6 tbsp of water. Stir well and set aside.
3. In a mixing bowl, mix the vegan butter and maple syrup with a hand mixer until it turns fluffy. Add the chia seeds along with the mashed bananas.
4. Mix well, and then add the coffee.
5. Meanwhile, sift all the dry ingredients (flour, baking powder, cinnamon powder, spice, and salt) and gradually add the wet ingredients into the bowl.
6. Combine the ingredients well, and then pour over a baking pan lined with parchment paper.
7. Place in the oven to bake for at least 30-40 minutes, or until the toothpick comes out clean after inserting in the bread.
8. Allow the bread to cool before serving.

Nutrition Calories: 371 kca|Protein: 5.59 |Fat: 16.81 g |Carbohydrates: 49.98 g

509. Mango Granola

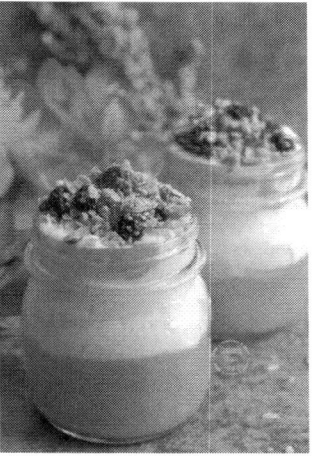

Preparation Time: 10 minutes
Cooking Time: 30 minutes
Servings: 4
Ingredients:
- 2 cups rolled oats
- 1 cup dried mango, chopped
- ½ cup almonds, roughly chopped
- ½ cup dates, roughly chopped
- 3 tbsp. sesame seeds
- 2 tsp. cinnamon

- 2 tbsp. coconut oil
- 2 tbsp. water

Directions:
1. Set oven at 320F
2. Put the oats, almonds, sesame seeds, dates, and cinnamon in a large bowl, then mix well.
3. Meanwhile, heat a saucepan over medium heat, pour in the agave syrup, coconut oil, and water.
4. Stir and let it cook for at least 3 minutes or until the coconut oil has melted.
5. Gradually pour the syrup mixture into the bowl with the oats and stir well, ensuring that all the ingredients are coated with the syrup.
6. Transfer the granola to a baking sheet lined with parchment paper and place it in the oven to bake for 20 minutes.
7. After 20 minutes, take off the tray from the oven and lay the chopped dried mango on top. Put back in the range, then bake again for another 5 minutes.

8. Let the granola cool to room temperature before serving or placing it in an airtight container for storage. The shelf life of the granola will last up to 2-3 weeks.

Nutrition: Calories: 434 kca | Protein: 13.16 | Fat: 28.3 g | Carbohydrates: 55.19 g

510. Tomato Omelet

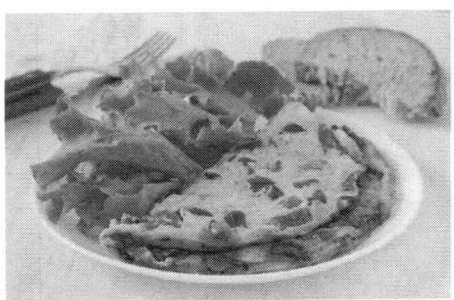

Preparation Time: 2 minutes
Cooking Time: 8 minutes
Servings: 1
Ingredients:
- 2 Eggs
- ½ cup Basil, fresh
- ½ cup Cherry tomatoes
- 1 tsp. Black pepper
- ¼ cup Cheese, any type, shredded
- ½ tsp. Salt

Directions:
1. Cut the tomatoes into quarters. Fry the tomatoes for 3 hours. Set the tomatoes off to the side. Add the salt and pepper to the eggs in a small bowl and beat together well. Pour the mix of beaten egg into the pan and use a spatula to gently work around the edges under the omelet, letting the eggs fry unmoved for three minutes. When just the center third of the egg mix is still runny, add on the basil, tomatoes, and cheese. Fold over half of the omelet onto the other half. Cook two more minutes and serve.

Nutrition: Calories 342 8 grams' carbs | 20 grams' protein | 25.3 grams' fat

511. Sautéed Veggies on Hot Bagels

Preparation Time: 10 minutes
Cooking Time: 16 minutes
Servings: 2
Ingredients:
- 1 yellow squash, diced
- 1 zucchini, sliced thin
- ½ onion, sliced thin
- 2 pcs. tomatoes, sliced
- 1 clove of garlic, chopped
- salt and pepper to taste
- 1 tbsp. olive oil
- 2 pcs. vegan bagels
- vegan butter for spread

Directions:
1. Heat the olive oil to medium temperature in a cast-iron skillet.
2. Lower the heat to medium-low and sauté the onions for 10 minutes or until the onions start to brown.
3. Turn the heat again to medium and then add the diced squash and zucchini to the pan and cook for 5 minutes. Add the clove of garlic and cook for another minute.
4. Throw the tomato slices into the pan and cook for 1 minute. Season with pepper and salt and turn off the heat.
5. Toast the bagels and cut them in half.
6. Spread the bagels lightly with butter and serve with the sautéed veggies on top.

Nutrition Calories: 375 kca | Protein: 14.69 | Fat: 11.46 g | Carbohydrates: 54.61 g

512. Coco-Tapioca Bowl

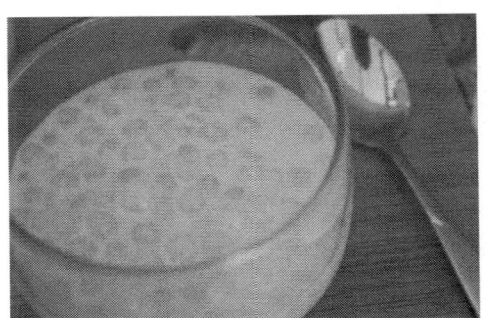

Preparation Time: 10 minutes
Cooking Time: 20 minutes
Servings: 2
Ingredients:
- ¼ cup tapioca pearls, small sized
- 1 can light coconut milk

- ¼ cup maple syrup
- 1 ½ tsp. lemon juice
- ½ cup unsweetened coconut flakes, toasted
- 2 cups water

Directions:
1. Place the tapioca in a saucepan and pour over the 2 cups of water. Let it stand for at least 30 minutes.
2. Pour in the coconut milk and syrup and heat the saucepan over medium temperature. Bring to a boil while stirring constantly.
3. Add the lemon juice and stir and then garnish with coconut flakes.

Nutrition Calories: 309 kca | Protein: 3.93 | Fat: 9.02 g | Carbohydrates: 54.55 g

513. Choco-Banana Oats

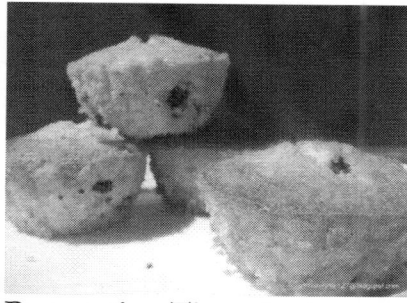

Preparation Time: 5 minutes
Cooking Time: 8 minutes
Servings: 2
Ingredients:
- 2 cups oats
- 2 cups almond milk
- ¾ cup water
- 2 ripe bananas, sliced
- ¼ tsp. Vanilla
- ¼ tsp. almond extract
- 2 tbsp. agave nectar
- 1/8 tsp. cinnamon
- 1/8 tsp. salt
- 1/3 cup toasted walnuts, chopped
- 2 tbsp. vegan chocolate chips, semisweet

Directions:
1. In a large saucepan, pour the almond milk, water, bananas, vanilla, and almond extract. Add the salt, stir, and heat over high temperatures.
2. Mix the oats in the pan along with the unsweetened cocoa powder, 1 tbsp. Agave nectar and lower the temperature to medium. Cook for 7-8 minutes, or until the oats are cooked to your liking. Stir frequently.
3. Scoop the cooked oats into serving bowls and garnish with the chopped walnuts, chocolate chips, and drizzle with the remaining agave nectar.

Nutrition Calories: 522 kca | Protein: 30.17 | Fat: 27.01 g | Carbohydrates: 79.09 g

514. Keto Chicken Enchiladas

Preparation Time: 10 minutes
Cooking Time: 25 minutes
Servings: 6
Ingredients:
- 2 cups gluten-free enchilada sauce
- Chicken
- 1 tablespoon Avocado oil
- 4 cloves Garlic (minced)
- 3 cups Shredded chicken (cooked)
- ¼ cup Chicken broth
- ¼ cup fresh cilantro (chopped)
- Assembly
- 12 Coconut tortillas
- 3/4 cup Colby jack cheese (shredded)
- ¼ cup Green onions (chopped)

Direction:
1. Warm oil at medium to high heat in a large pan. Add the chopped garlic and cook until fragrant for about a minute.
2. Add rice, 1 cup enchilada sauce (half the total), chicken, and coriander. Simmer for 5 minutes.
3. In the meantime, heat the oven to 3750 F. Grease a 9x13 baking dish.
4. In the middle of each tortilla, place ¼ cup chicken mixture. Roll up and place seam side down in the baking dish.
5. Pour the remaining cup of enchilada sauce over the enchiladas. Sprinkle with shredded cheese.
6. Bake for 10 to 12 minutes. Sprinkle with green onions.

Nutrition : Calories: 349 | **Fat:** 19g | **Net Carbs:** 9g | **Protein:** 31g

515. Roasted Whole Chicken

Preparation Time: 20 minutes
Cooking Time: 1 and 32 minutes
Servings: 6
Ingredients:
- 10 tablespoons unsalted butter
- 3 garlic cloves, minced
- 1 (3-pounds) grass-fed whole chicken, neck, and giblets removed
- Salt and ground black pepper, as required

Directions:
1. Preheat the oven to 4000F. Arrange an oven rack into the lower portion of the oven.
2. Grease a large baking dish.
3. Place the butter and garlic in a small pan over medium heat and cook for about 1-2 minutes.
4. Remove the pan from heat and let it cool for about 2 minutes.
5. Season the inside and outside of the chicken evenly with salt and black pepper.
6. Arrange the chicken into a prepared baking dish, breast side up.
7. Pour the garlic butter over and inside of the chicken.
8. Bake for about 1-1½ hours, basting with the pan juices every 20 minutes.
9. Remove from oven and place the chicken onto a cutting board for about 5-10 minutes before carving.
10. Cut into desired size pieces and serve.

Nutrition: Calories: 772 | Fat: 39.1g | Net Carbs: 0.7g | Protein: 99g

516. Mustard Pork Mix

Preparation Time: 10 minutes
Cooking Time: 35 minutes
Servings: 4
Ingredients:
- 2 shallots, chopped
- 1-pound pork stew meat, cubed
- 2 garlic cloves, minced
- 2 tablespoons olive oil
- ¼ cup Dijon mustard
- 2 tablespoons chives, chopped
- 1 teaspoon cumin, ground
- 1 teaspoon rosemary, dried
- Pinch of sea salt
- Pinch black pepper

Directions:
1. Warm a pan with the oil on medium-high heat, add the shallots and sauté for 5 minutes.
2. Put the meat and brown for a further 5 minutes.
3. Put the rest of the ingredients, toss, and cook on medium heat for 25 minutes more.
4. Divide the mix between plates and serve.

Nutrition: Calories 280 | Fat 14.3 | Fiber 6 | Carbs 11.8 | Protein 17

517. Pork with Chili Zucchinis and Tomatoes

Preparation Time: 10 minutes
Cooking Time: 35 minutes
Servings: 4
Ingredients:
- 2 tomatoes, cubed
- 2 pounds' pork stew meat, cubed
- 4 scallions, chopped
- 2 tablespoons olive oil
- 1 zucchini, sliced
- Juice of 1 lime
- 2 tablespoons chili powder
- ½ tablespoons cumin powder
- Pinch of sea salt
- Pinch black pepper

Directions:
1. Warm a pan with the oil on medium heat, add the scallions and sauté for 5 minutes.
2. Add the meat and brown for 5 minutes more.
3. Add the tomatoes and the other ingredients, toss, cook over medium heat for 25 minutes more, divide between plates and serve.

Nutrition: Calories 300 | Fat 5 | Fiber 2 | Carbs 12 | Protein 14

518. Pork with Thyme Sweet Potatoes

Preparation Time: 10 minutes

Cooking Time: 35 minutes
Servings: 4
Ingredients:
- 2 sweet potatoes, cut into wedges
- 4 pork chops
- 3 spring onions, chopped
- 1 tablespoon thyme, chopped
- 2 tablespoons olive oil
- 4 garlic cloves, minced
- Pinch of sea salt
- Pinch black pepper
- ½ cup vegetable stock
- ½ tablespoon chives, chopped

Directions:
1. In a roasting pan, combine the pork chops with the potatoes and the other ingredients, toss gently, and cook at 390 degrees F for 35 minutes.
2. Divide everything between plates and serve.

Nutrition: Calories 210 | Fat 12.2 | Fiber 5.2 | Carbs 12 | Protein 10

519. Pork with Pears and Ginger

Preparation Time: 10 minutes
Cooking Time: 35 minutes
Servings: 4
Ingredients:
- 2 green onions, chopped
- 2 tablespoons avocado oil
- 2 pounds' pork roast, sliced
- ½ cup coconut aminos
- 1 tablespoon ginger, minced
- 2 pears, cored and cut into wedges
- ¼ cup vegetable stock
- 1 tablespoon chives, chopped

Directions:
1. Warm a pan with the oil on medium heat, add the onions and the meat, and brown for 2 minutes on each side.
2. Add the rest of the ingredients, toss gently, and bake at 390 degrees F for 30 minutes.
3. Divide the mix between plates and serve.

Nutrition: Calories 220 | Fat 13.3 | Fiber 2 | Carbs 16.5 | Protein 8

520. Parsley Pork and Artichokes

Preparation Time: 10 minutes
Cooking Time: 35 minutes
Servings: 4
Ingredients:
- 2 tbsp. balsamic vinegar
- 1 cup canned artichoke hearts, drained
- 2 tbsp. olive oil
- 2 lb. pork stew meat, cubed
- 2 tbsp. parsley, chopped
- 1 tsp. cumin, ground
- 1 tsp. turmeric powder
- 2 garlic cloves, minced
- Pinch of sea salt
- Pinch black pepper

Directions:
1. Warm a pan with the oil on medium heat, add the meat, and brown for 5 minutes.
2. Add the artichokes, the vinegar, and the other ingredients, toss, cook over medium heat for 30 minutes, divide between plates and serve.

Nutrition: Calories 260 | Fat 5 | Fiber 4 | Carbs 11 | Protein 20

521. Pork with Mushrooms and Cucumbers

Preparation Time: 10 minutes
Cooking Time: 25 minutes
Servings: 4
Ingredients:
- 2 tablespoons olive oil
- ½ teaspoon oregano, dried
- 4 pork chops
- 2 garlic cloves, minced
- Juice of 1 lime
- ¼ cup cilantro, chopped
- Pinch of sea salt
- Pinch black pepper
- 1 cup white mushrooms, halved
- 2 tablespoons balsamic vinegar

Directions:

1. Warm a pan with the oil on medium heat, add the pork chops, and brown for 2 minutes on each side.
2. Put the rest of the ingredients, toss, cook on medium heat for 20 minutes, divide between plates and serve.

Nutrition: Calories 220| Fat 6| Fiber 8| Carbs 14.2|Protein20

MEAL PLANS

28 Days Meal Plan

28 DAYS	BREAKFAST	LUNCH	DINNER
WEEK 1			
Day 1	Mediterranean Frittata	Strawberries and Cream Trifle	Pan-Seared Halibut with Citrus Butter Sauce
Day 2	Maple Oatmeal	Maple Toast and Eggs	Sole Asiago
Day 3	Tomato Omelet	Sweet Onion and Egg Pie	Cheesy Garlic Salmon
Day 4	Tuna & Sweet Potato Croquettes	Mini Breakfast Pizza	Stuffed Chicken Breasts
Day 5	Quinoa & Veggie Croquettes	Chicken Muffins	Spicy Pork Chops
Day 6	Turkey Burgers	Pumpkin Pancakes	Almond Breaded Chicken Goodness
Day 7	Salmon Burgers	Cauliflower and Chorizo	Garlic Lamb Chops
WEEK 2			
Day 8	Veggie Balls	Carrot Bread	Mushroom Pork Chops
Day 9	Coconut & Banana Cookies	Fruity Muffins	Mediterranean Pork
Day 10	Fennel Seeds Cookies	Edamame Omelet	Brie-Packed Smoked Salmon
Day 11	Hash Browns	Almond Mascarpone Dumplings	Blackened Tilapia
Day 12	Sun-Dried Tomato Garlic Bruschetta	Raisin Bran Muffins	Salsa Chicken Bites
Day 13	Almond Scones	Apple Bread	Tomato & Tuna Balls
Day 14	Oven-Poached Eggs	Zucchini Bread	Fennel & Figs Lamb
WEEK 3			
Day 15	Cranberry and Raisins Granola	Sweetened Brown Rice	Tamari Steak Salad
Day 16	Spicy Marble Eggs	Cornmeal Grits	Blackened Chicken
Day 17	Almond Pancakes with Coconut Flakes	Grapefruit-Pomegranate Salad	Mediterranean Mushroom Olive Steak
Day 18	Bake Apple Turnover	Oatmeal-Raisin Scones	Buttery Scallops
Day 19	Breakfast Arrozcaldo	Yogurt Cheese and Fruit	Brussels sprouts and Garlic Aioli

Day 20	Apple Bruschetta with Almonds and Blackberries	Chicken & Cabbage Platter	Broccoli Bites
Day 21	Mushroom Crêpes	Balsamic Chicken and Vegetables	Bacon Burger Cabbage Stir Fry
WEEK 4			
Day 22	Oat Porridge with Cherry & Coconut	Onion Bacon Pork Chops	Bacon Cheeseburger
Day 23	Gingerbread Oatmeal Breakfast	Caramelized Pork Chops	Cauliflower Mac & Cheese
Day 24	Apple, Ginger, and Rhubarb Muffins	Chicken Bacon Quesadilla	Mushroom & Cauliflower Risotto
Day 25	Anti-Inflammatory Breakfast Frittata	Rosemary Roasted Pork with Cauliflower	Pita Pizza
Day 26	Breakfast Sausage and Mushroom Casserole	Grilled Salmon and Zucchini with Mango Sauce	Skillet Cabbage Tacos
Day 27	Yummy Steak Muffins	Beef and Broccoli Stir-Fry	Taco Casserole
Day 28	White and Green Quiche	Parmesan-Crusted Halibut with Asparagus	Creamy Chicken Salad

Vegan Meal Plan

14 DAYS	BREAKFAST	LUNCH	DINNER
WEEK 1			
Day 1	Maple Oatmeal	Loaded Kale Salad	Lentils with Tomatoes and Turmeric
Day 2	Mediterranean Frittata	Avocado Kale Salad	Whole-Wheat Pasta with Tomato-Basil Sauce
Day 3	Quinoa & Veggie Croquettes	Broccoli Sweet Potato Chickpea Salad	Fried Rice with Kale
Day 4	Veggie Balls	Broccoli, Kelp, And Feta Salad	Nutty and Fruity Garden Salad
Day 5	Fennel Seeds Cookies	Cauliflower & Lentil Salad	Roasted Root Vegetables
Day 6	Sun-Dried Tomato Garlic Bruschetta	Cherry Tomato Salad with Soy Chorizo	Stir-Fried Brussels Sprouts and Carrots
Day 7	Coconut & Banana Cookies	French Style Potato Salad	Curried Veggies and Poached Eggs
WEEK 2			
Day 8	Hash Browns	Kale Salad with Tahini Dressing	Braised Kale
Day 9	Mushroom Crêpes	Almond-Goji Berry Cauliflower Salad	Braised Leeks, Cauliflower and Artichoke Hearts

Day 10	Oven-Poached Eggs	Mango Salad with Peanut Dressing	Celery Root Hash Browns
Day 11	Anti-Inflammatory Breakfast Frittata	Niçoise Salad	Braised Carrots 'n Kale
Day 12	Spicy Marble Eggs	Penne Pasta Salad	Stir-Fried Gingery Veggies
Day 13	Bake Apple Turnover	Maple Rice	Cauliflower Fritters
Day 14	Almond Pancakes with Coconut Flakes	Rainbow Vegetable Bowl	Stir-Fried Squash

Paleo Meal Plan

14 DAYS	BREAKFAST	LUNCH	DINNER
WEEK 1			
Day 1	Oven-Poached Eggs	Strawberries and Cream Trifle	Pan-Seared Halibut with Citrus Butter Sauce
Day 2	Turkey Burgers	Maple Toast and Eggs	Sole Asiago
Day 3	Anti-Inflammatory Breakfast Frittata	Sweet Onion and Egg Pie	Cheesy Garlic Salmon
Day 4	Mediterranean Frittata	Mini Breakfast Pizza	Stuffed Chicken Breasts
Day 5	Spicy Marble Eggs	Chicken Muffins	Spicy Pork Chops
Day 6	Quinoa & Veggie Croquettes	Pumpkin Pancakes	Almond Breaded Chicken Goodness
Day 7	Tuna & Sweet Potato Croquettes	Cauliflower and Chorizo	Garlic Lamb Chops
WEEK 2			
Day 8	Veggie Balls	Carrot Bread	Mushroom Pork Chops
Day 9	Salmon Burgers	Fruity Muffins	Mediterranean Pork
Day 10	Fennel Seeds Cookies	Edamame Omelet	Brie-Packed Smoked Salmon
Day 11	Sun-Dried Tomato Garlic Bruschetta	Almond Mascarpone Dumplings	Blackened Tilapia
Day 12	Coconut & Banana Cookies	Raisin Bran Muffins	Salsa Chicken Bites
Day 13	Hash Browns	Apple Bread	Tomato & Tuna Balls
Day 14	Mushroom Crêpes	Zucchini Bread	Fennel & Figs Lamb

Keto Meal Plan

14 DAYS	BREAKFAST	LUNCH	DINNER
WEEK 1			
Day 1	Turkey Burgers	Basic "Rotisserie" Chicken	Pan-Seared Halibut with Citrus Butter Sauce
Day 2	Mediterranean Frittata	Hidden Valley Chicken Dummies	Sole Asiago
Day 3	Spicy Marble Eggs	Chicken Divan	Cheesy Garlic Salmon
Day 4	Quinoa & Veggie Croquettes	Apricot Chicken Wings	Stuffed Chicken Breasts
Day 5	Tuna & Sweet Potato Croquettes	Champion Chicken Pockets	Spicy Pork Chops
Day 6	Veggie Balls	Chicken-Bell Pepper Sauté	Almond Breaded Chicken Goodness
Day 7	Anti-Inflammatory Breakfast Frittata	Avocado-Orange Grilled Chicken	Garlic Lamb Chops
WEEK 2			
Day 8	Salmon Burgers	Honey Chicken Tagine	Mushroom Pork Chops
Day 9	Fennel Seeds Cookies	Roasted Chicken	Mediterranean Pork
Day 10	Sun-Dried Tomato Garlic Bruschetta	Chicken in Pita Bread	Brie-Packed Smoked Salmon
Day 11	Coconut & Banana Cookies	Skillet Chicken with Brussels Sprouts Mix	Blackened Tilapia
Day 12	Hash Browns	Spicy Chipotle Chicken	Salsa Chicken Bites
Day 13	Mushroom Crêpes	Chicken with Fennel	Tomato & Tuna Balls
Day 14	Oven-Poached Eggs	Adobo Lime Chicken Mix	Fennel & Figs Lamb

Mediterranean Meal Plan

14 DAYS	BREAKFAST	LUNCH	DINNER
WEEK 1			
Day 1	Mediterranean Frittata	Strawberries and Cream Trifle	Pan-Seared Halibut with Citrus Butter Sauce
Day 2	Maple Oatmeal	Maple Toast and Eggs	Sole Asiago
Day 3	Tomato Omelet	Sweet Onion and Egg Pie	Cheesy Garlic Salmon
Day 4	Tuna & Sweet Potato Croquettes	Mini Breakfast Pizza	Stuffed Chicken Breasts
Day 5	Quinoa & Veggie Croquettes	Chicken Muffins	Spicy Pork Chops
Day 6	Turkey Burgers	Pumpkin Pancakes	Almond Breaded Chicken Goodness

Day 7	Salmon Burgers	Cauliflower and Chorizo	Garlic Lamb Chops
WEEK 2			
Day 8	Veggie Balls	Carrot Bread	Mushroom Pork Chops
Day 9	Coconut & Banana Cookies	Fruity Muffins	Mediterranean Pork
Day 10	Fennel Seeds Cookies	Edamame Omelet	Brie-Packed Smoked Salmon
Day 11	Hash Browns	Almond Mascarpone Dumplings	Blackened Tilapia
Day 12	Sun-Dried Tomato Garlic Bruschetta	Raisin Bran Muffins	Salsa Chicken Bites
Day 13	Almond Scones	Apple Bread	Tomato & Tuna Balls
Day 14	Oven-Poached Eggs	Zucchini Bread	Fennel & Figs Lamb

Time Saving Meal Plan

14 DAYS	BREAKFAST	LUNCH	DINNER
WEEK 1			
Day 1	Oven-Poached Eggs	Oats with Berries	Loaded Kale Salad
Day 2	Turkey Burgers	Spinach Avocado Smoothie	Avocado Kale Salad
Day 3	Anti-Inflammatory Breakfast Frittata	Golden Milk	Broccoli Sweet Potato Chickpea Salad
Day 4	Mediterranean Frittata	Granola	Broccoli, Kelp, And Feta Salad
Day 5	Spicy Marble Eggs	Overnight Coconut Chia Oats	Cauliflower & Lentil Salad
Day 6	Quinoa & Veggie Croquettes	Blueberry Hemp Seed Smoothie	Cherry Tomato Salad with Soy Chorizo
Day 7	Tuna & Sweet Potato Croquettes	Spiced Morning Chia Pudding	French Style Potato Salad
WEEK 2			
Day 8	Veggie Balls	Green Smoothie	Kale Salad with Tahini Dressing
Day 9	Salmon Burgers	Oatmeal Pancakes	Almond-Goji Berry Cauliflower Salad
Day 10	Fennel Seeds Cookies	Anti-inflammatory Porridge	Mango Salad with Peanut Dressing
Day 11	Sun-Dried Tomato Garlic Bruschetta	Cherry Smoothie	Niçoise Salad
Day 12	Coconut & Banana Cookies	Gingerbread Oatmeal	Penne Pasta Salad
Day 13	Hash Browns	Roasted Almonds	Maple Rice
Day 14	Mushroom Crêpes	Roasted Pumpkin Seeds	Rainbow Vegetable Bowl

INDEX

4

473.Bruschetta 94

A

Adobo Lime Chicken Mix 159
Almond and Honey Homemade Bar 106
Almond Breaded Chicken Goodness 74
Almond Butter Balls Vegan 241
Almond Chicken Cutlets 168
Almond Cookies 242
Almond Mascarpone Dumplings 57
Almond Pancakes with Coconut Flakes 22
Almond Scones 25
Almond-Goji Berry Cauliflower Salad 193
Almonds and Blueberries Yogurt Snack 102
Anti-Inflammatory Apricot Squares 239
Anti-Inflammatory Breakfast Frittata 14
Anti-Inflammatory Crepes 49
Anti-inflammatory Porridge 37
Apple Bread 58
Apple Bruschetta with Almonds and Blackberries 28
Apple Fritters 237
Apple Pie Smoothie 229
Apple, Ginger, and Rhubarb Muffins 25
Apricot Chicken Wings 154
Artichoke Spinach Dip 129
Asian Cabbage Salad 111
Asian Peanut Cabbage Slaw 121
Athenian Avgolemono Sour Soup 221
Avocado and Egg Sandwich 105
Avocado Banana Smoothie 230
Avocado Brownies 251
Avocado Chocolate Mousse 238
Avocado Hummus 97
Avocado Kale Salad 189
Avocado Milk Whip 232
Avocado Turmeric Smoothie 226
Avocado with Tomatoes and Cucumber 104
Avocado-Orange Grilled Chicken 156

B

Bacon Burger Cabbage Stir Fry 82
Bacon Cheeseburger 82
Bacon-Wrapped Chicken with Cheddar Cheese 264
Bake Apple Turnover 22
Baked Eggs with Portobello Mushrooms 46
Baked Tomato Hake 142
Baked Zucchini Fries 114
Balsamic Chicken and Vegetables 63
Balsamic Scallops 145
Balsamic-Glazed Turkey Wings 261
Banana Almond Smoothie 229
Banana and Kale Smoothie 231
Banana Cherry Smoothie 231
Barbecue Sauce 131
Barbecue Tahini Sauce 131
Basic "Rotisserie" Chicken 153
Basil & Artichoke Pizza 275
Beef & Veggies Chili 182
Beef and Broccoli Stir-Fry 66
Beef Breakfast Casserole 30
Beef Carbonara 273
Beef Meatballs in Tomato Gravy 185
Beef with Asparagus & Bell Pepper 178
Beef with Carrot & Broccoli 176
Beef with Mushroom & Broccoli 176
Beef with Zucchini Noodles 178
Beet and Cherry Smoothie 47
Berry Cheesecake Smoothies 227
Berry Delight 92
Berry Energy bites 93
Berry Ice Pops 248
Berry Parfait 240
Berry-Banana Yogurt 238

BlackBerry & Banana Smoothie	228
Blackened Chicken	79
Blackened Tilapia	77
Blueberry & Chia Flax Seed Pudding	92
Blueberry and Spinach Smoothie	232
Blueberry Crisp	235
Blueberry Hemp Seed Smoothie	35
Blueberry Smoothie	226
Boiled Okra and Squash	95
Bolognese Sauce	132
Boozy Glazed Chicken	171
Braised Carrots 'n Kale	205
Braised Kale	203
Braised Leeks, Cauliflower and Artichoke Hearts	204
Breaded Chicken Fillets	170
Breakfast Arrozcaldo	27
Breakfast Burgers with Avocado Buns	44
Breakfast Cherry Muffins	48
Breakfast Sausage and Mushroom Casserole	23
Breakfast Shakshuka	49
Breakfast Spinach Mushroom Tomato Fry Up	46
Breakfast Stir Fry	50
Brie with Apricot Topping	118
Brie-Packed Smoked Salmon	76
Broccoli Bites	81
Broccoli Sweet Potato Chickpea Salad	189
Broccoli, Kelp, And Feta Salad	190
Brussels sprouts and Garlic Aioli	80
Buffalo Chicken Lettuce Wraps	257
Buffalo Dip	130
Buttery Scallops	80

C

Cajun Chicken & Prawn	160
Candied Dates	92
Caprese Salad Bites	119
Caramelized Pears	248
Caramelized Pork Chops	64
Carrot Bread	55
Carrot Cake	234
Carrot Sticks with Avocado Dip	95
Cashew Cheese	94
Cashew Pesto & Parsley with veggies	214
Cashew Yogurt	128
Cauliflower & Lentil Salad	190
Cauliflower and Chorizo	55
Cauliflower Fried Rice	109
Cauliflower Fritters	206
Cauliflower Hash Brown	206
Cauliflower Lunch Salad	282
Cauliflower Mac & Cheese	82
Cauliflower Rice	116
Cauliflower, Coconut Milk, and Shrimp Soup	265
Celery Root Hash Browns	204
Champion Chicken Pockets	154
Cheese Chips	119
Cheesy Bacon-Wrapped Chicken with Asparagus Spears	172
Cheesy Black Bean Wraps	283
Cheesy Chicken Sun-Dried Tomato Packets	169
Cheesy Garlic Salmon	73
Cheesy Gratin Zucchini	210
Cheesy Ham Quiche	86
Cheesy Tuna Pasta	143
Cherry Smoothie	38
Cherry Tomato Salad with Soy Chorizo	191
Chewy Blackberry Leather	98
Chia Chocolate Pudding	113
Chicken & Apple Cider Chili	256
Chicken & Cabbage Platter	62
Chicken Bacon Quesadilla	64
Chicken Bacon Ranch Pizza	271
Chicken Cherry Wraps	281
Chicken Divan	154
Chicken in Pita Bread	157
Chicken Muffins	54
Chicken Piccata	166
Chicken Scarpariello with Spicy Sausage	167
Chicken with Fennel	159
Chicken-Bell Pepper Sauté	155
Chickpea & Artichoke Mushroom Pâté	129
Chili Shrimp and Pineapple	145
Chili Snapper	151

Chimichurri Turkey	261
Chinese-Orange Spiced Duck Breasts	161
Chipotle Bean Cheesy Dip	133
Choco-Banana Oats	287
Chocolate Bananas	250
Chocolate Cherry Chia Pudding	244
Chocolate Chip Cookies	252
Chocolate Chip Quinoa Granola Bars	236
Chocolate Mousse	242
Chocolate Peanut Butter Protein Balls	118
Cilantro and Parsley Hot Sauce	134
Cilantro-Lime Chicken Drumsticks	257
Cinnamon Apple Chips	250
Cinnamon Fried Bananas	121
Cinnamon Roll Smoothie	225
Citrus Beef with Bok Choy	177
Citrus Salmon on a Bed of Greens	138
Classic Beef Lasagna	268
Classic Chicken Noodle Soup	278
Classic Guacamole Dip	69
Clean Salmon with Soy Sauce	89
Coconut & Banana Cookies	20
Coconut and Chocolate Cream	249
Coconut Chicken Curry with Cauliflower Rice	68
Coconut Flour Pizza	274
Coconut Muffins	243
Coconut Porridge	105
Coconut-Curry-Cashew Chicken	258
Coco-Tapioca Bowl	286
Cod with Bell Pepper	255
Cod with Ginger	140
Coffee Cream	242
Collard Green Wrap	211
Cornmeal Grits	60
Cottage Cheese with Apple Sauce	103
Cranberry and Raisins Granola	26
Creamy Chicken Salad	84
Creamy Queso Dip	70
Crispy Chicken Fingers	41
Cucumber Bites	40
Cucumber Rolls Hors D'oeuvres	103
Curried Beef Meatballs	184
Curried Okra	207
Curried Veggies and Poached Eggs	203
Curry Chicken Pockets	277

D

Dalmatian Cabbage, Potato, And Pea Soup	217, 223
Dark Chocolate Granola Bars	235
Delectable Cookies	101
Delicious Creamy Crab Meat	91
Delicious Roasted Duck	163
Delightful Teriyaki Chicken Under Pressure	173
Dill Haddock	150
Duck Breast and Blackberries Mix	165
Duck Breast Salad	164
Duck Breast with Apricot Sauce	164

E

Easy Barley Soup	282
Easy Chicken Tacos	172
Easy Peach Cobbler	240
Easy Shrimp	90
Edamame Hummus	113
Edamame Omelet	57
Eggplant Gratin	209
Energetic Oat Bars	100
Energy Dates Balls	100
Everything Parmesan Crisps	112
Exquisite Pear and Onion Goose	174

F

Fajita Style Chili	277
Fall Baked Vegetable with Rigatoni	272
Fennel & Figs Lamb	78
Fennel Seeds Cookies	19
Feta and Cauliflower Rice Stuffed Bell Peppers	86
Flavorsome Almonds	98
Flourless Sweet Potato Brownies	246
French Style Potato Salad	192
Fresh Bell Pepper Basil Pizza	275
Fresh Lemon Cream Shake	230
Fried Coconut Shrimp with Asparagus	68
Fried Rice with Kale	201

Fruit Bowl with Yogurt Topping	211
Fruit Cobbler	249
Fruit Salad	251
Fruity Muffins	56
Fun Fajita Wraps	278

G

Garlic Lamb Chops	75
Garlic Soup	222
Garlic-Parmesan Cheesy Chips	126
Ginger Turmeric Protein Bars	103
Gingerbread Oatmeal	38
Gingerbread Oatmeal Breakfast	28
Golden Milk	34
Granola	34
Grapefruit-Pomegranate Salad	61
Greek Chop-Chop Salad	109
Green Beans Greek Style	124
Green Smoothie	36
Green Smoothie with Raspberries	228
Grilled Eggplant Roll-Ups	208
Grilled Salmon and Zucchini with Mango Sauce	65
Ground Beef & Veggies Curry	183
Ground Beef with Cabbage	180
Ground Beef with Cashews & Veggies	181
Ground Beef with Greens & Tomatoes	181
Ground Beef with Veggies	180
Guava Smoothie	227

H

Halibut Curry	140
Halibut Stir Fry	149
Ham and Veggie Frittata Muffins	31
Hash Browns	20
Healthy Breakfast Chocolate Donuts	45
Healthy Halibut Fillets	89
Healthy Turkey Gumbo	160
Hearty Beef and Bacon Casserole	67
Herb And Melon Kefir Smoothie	224
Herb Butter Scallops	70
Hidden Valley Chicken Dummies	153
Homemade Potato Chips	117

Honey Chicken Tagine	156
Honey Crusted Salmon with Pecans	152
Honey-Mustard Lemon Marinated Chicken	166
Hot Tuna Steak	141
Hummus	118

I

Italian Bean Soup	221
Italian Eggplant Pizzas	115
Italian Halibut Chowder	150
Italian Mushroom Pizza	270

K

Kale Salad with Tahini Dressing	193
Kale, Butternut Squash, and Sausage Pasta	120
Kefir And Yogurt Banana Flaxseed Shake	224
Keto Chicken Enchiladas	287
Keto Pepperoni Pizza	274
Key Lime Pie Smoothie	224
Korean Barbecue Tofu	210

L

Lebanese Chicken Kebabs and Hummus	162
Lemon & Garlic Chicken Thighs	256
Lemon and Egg Pasta Soup	218
Lemon Juice Salmon with Quinoa	121
Lemon Vegan Cake	234
Lemon-Caper Trout with Caramelized Shallots	135
Lemony Mackerel	151
Lemony Mussels	141
Lentils with Tomatoes and Turmeric	201
Loaded Kale Salad	188
Low Cholesterol Scalloped Potatoes	123
Low Cholesterol-Low Calorie Blueberry Muffin	94

M

Mango Granola	284
Mango Salad with Peanut Dressing	194
Manhattan-Style Salmon Chowder	137
Maple Oatmeal	24
Maple Rice	196
Maple Toast and Eggs	52
Maple-Mashed Sweet Potatoes	126
Marinated Fish Steaks	142

Marinated Mushrooms	124
Mashed Cauliflower	114
Mashed Sweet Potato Burritos	216
Matcha Mango Smoothie	232
Mediterranean Frittata	14
Mediterranean Mushroom Olive Steak	80
Mediterranean Pork	76
Mediterranean Rolled Baklava with Walnuts	245
Mediterranean Tomato Soup	220
Melting Tuna and Cheese Toasties	122
Mexican Cod Fillets	87
Mini Breakfast Pizza	53
Mini Pepper Nachos	97
Mint Chocolate Chip Ice-cream	246
Moch Mashed Potatoes	125
Moroccan Turkey Tagine	259
Mushroom & Cauliflower Risotto	83
Mushroom Crêpes	21
Mushroom Pork Chops	75
Mustard Chicken Farfalle	270
Mustard Pork Mix	288

N

Niçoise Salad	195
No Dish Summer Medley	125
No-Bake Turmeric Protein Donuts	50
Nutty and Fruity Garden Salad	202
Nutty Pesto Chicken Supreme	163

O

Oat Porridge with Cherry & Coconut	28
Oatmeal Pancakes	37
Oatmeal-Raisin Scones	61
Oats with Berries	33
Olive and Tomato Balls	96
Onion Bacon Pork Chops	63
Open Face Egg and Bacon Sandwich	279
Orange and Maple-Glazed Salmon	139
Orange Chicken Legs	263
Oregano Pork	265
Oven Crisp Sweet Potato	96
Oven-Poached Eggs	13
Overnight Coconut Chia Oats	35

P

Paleo Raspberry Cream Pie	247
Pancetta and Chicken Risotto	174
Pan-Fried Chorizo Sausage	171
Pan-Seared Halibut with Citrus Butter Sauce	72
Pan-Seared Scallops with Lemon-Ginger Vinaigrette	137
Parmesan Spaghetti in Mushroom-Tomato Sauce	269
Parmesan-Crusted Halibut with Asparagus	66
Parsley Pork and Artichokes	290
Parsley Tilapia	254
Party-Time Chicken Nuggets	99
Pasta Primavera	267
Peanut Butter Banana Smoothie	225
Peanut Butter Cup Smoothies	227
Peanut Sauce Chicken Pasta	281
Penne Pasta Salad	195
Pickle Roll-Ups	114
Pineapple Cake	245
Pineapple Ginger Smoothie	47
Pita Pizza	83
Poached Halibut and Mushrooms	148
Pork Chops with Tomato Salsa	187
Pork with Chili Zucchinis and Tomatoes	289
Pork with Lemongrass	186
Pork with Mushrooms and Cucumbers	291
Pork with Olives	186
Pork with Pears and Ginger	290
Pork with Thyme Sweet Potatoes	289
Protein Spinach Shake	230
Protein-Packed Croquettes	99
Pumpkin Pancakes	54
Pumpkin Spiced Almonds	69
Pureed Classic Egg Salad	125

Q

Quinoa & Veggie Croquettes	16, 42
Quinoa and Cauliflower Congee	253

R

Rainbow Vegetable Bowl	196
Raisin Bran Muffins	58

Rajun' Cajun Roll-Ups	112
Raspberry Diluted Frozen Sorbet	243
Raspberry Grapefruit Smoothie	44
Raw Black Forest Brownies	239
Red Bell Pepper Hummus	197
Red Soup, Seville Style	222
Roasted Almonds	39
Roasted Asparagus with Feta Cheese Salad	198
Roasted Bananas	238
Roasted Beets	93
Roasted Bell Pepper Salad with Olives	198
Roasted Broccoli with Peanuts and Kecap Manis	199
Roasted Chicken	157
Roasted Chickpeas	40
Roasted Chili Potatoes	200
Roasted Garden Vegetables	110
Roasted Garlic Dip	128
Roasted Pumpkin Seeds	39
Roasted Root Vegetables	116
Roasted Salmon and Asparagus	138
Roasted Vegetable Soup	219
Roasted Whole Chicken	288
Rosemary Roasted Pork with Cauliflower	65
Rosemary-Lemon Cod	140

S

Salad Bites	108
Salmon & Avocado Toast	104
Salmon and Roasted Peppers	143
Salmon Burgers	18
Salmon Ceviche	139
Salmon in Dill Sauce	254
Salsa Chicken Bites	77
Salsa Verde Chicken	256
Sautéed Garlic Mushrooms	213
Sautéed Veggies on Hot Bagels	286
Savory Breakfast Pancakes	43
Scallops with Mushroom Special	90
Scrambled Eggs with Smoked Salmon	44
Sesame Wings with Cauliflower	67
Sesame-Tuna Skewers	147
Sherbet Pineapple	240
Shrimp and Beets	144
Shrimp and Corn	144
Shrimp Scampi	135
Shrimp with Cinnamon Sauce	136
Shrimp with Linguine	87
Shrimp with Spicy Spinach	136
Simple Mushroom Chicken Mix	88
Simple Salmon with Eggs	89
Simply Vanilla Frozen Greek Yogurt	108
Skillet Cabbage Tacos	83
Skillet Chicken with Brussels Sprouts Mix	158
Slow Cooker Boston Beans	123
Slow Cooker Chicken Cacciatore	263
Slow Cooker Chicken Fajitas	262
Slow Cooker Jerk Chicken	264
Soft Flourless Cookies	101
Sole Asiago	72
Sole with Vegetables	148
Southwest Deviled Eggs	111
Spanish-Style Pizza de Jarmon	276
Special Vegetable Kitchree	215
Spiced Ground Beef	179
Spiced Morning Chia Pudding	36
Spiced Popcorn	40
Spiced Soup with Lentils & Legumes	218
Spicy & Creamy Ground Beef Curry	183
Spicy Almond Chicken Strips with Garlic Lime Tartar Sauce	167
Spicy Chickpeas with Roasted Vegetables	215
Spicy Chipotle Chicken	158
Spicy Keto Chicken Wings	85
Spicy Marble Eggs	15
Spicy Pineapple Smoothie	48
Spicy Pork Chops	74
Spicy Pulled Chicken Wraps	262
Spicy Roasted chickpeas	93
Spicy Veggie Pasta Bake	269
Spinach and Artichoke Dip	122
Spinach Avocado Smoothie	33
Spinach Breakfast	45
Spinach Fritters	41

Spring Soup with Gourmet Grains	217
Squash Spaghetti with Bolognese Sauce	88
Steamed Garlic-Dill Halibut	149
Stir-Fried Asparagus and Bell Pepper	213
Stir-Fried Brussels Sprouts and Carrots	202
Stir-Fried Eggplant	212
Stir-Fried Gingery Veggies	205
Stir-Fried Squash	206
Strawberries and Cream Trifle	52
Strawberry Cheesecake Smoothie	225
Strawberry Granita	237
Strawberry Orange Sorbet	244
Stuffed Chicken Breasts	73
Sun-Dried Tomato Garlic Bruschetta	19
Super Sesame Chicken Noodles	161
Sweet Cherry Almond Chia Pudding	47
Sweet Onion and Egg Pie	53
Sweet Potato Cranberry Breakfast bars	42
Sweet Potato Puree	207
Sweetened Brown Rice	60
Swordfish with Pineapple and Cilantro	146

T

Taco Casserole	84
Tamari Steak Salad	79
Tangy Barbecue Chicken	255
Tenderloin Fajitas	280
Thar She' Salts Peanut Butter Cookies	241
Tomato & Tuna Balls	77
Tomato and Avocado Omelet	32
Tomato and Cabbage Puree Soup	220
Tomato and Mozzarella Bites	117
Tomato Omelet	285
Tomato, Basil, and Cucumber Salad	116
Trout with Chard	147
Tuna & Sweet Potato Croquettes	16

Turkey & Sweet Potato Chili	259
Turkey and Potatoes with Buffalo Sauce	173
Turkey Breast with Fennel and Celery	174
Turkey Burgers	13
Turkey Ham and Mozzarella Pate	170
Turkey Meatballs with Spaghetti Squash	260
Turkey Sloppy Joes	260
Turmeric Chickpea Cakes	102
Tuscan Chicken Linguine	267
Tuscan Chicken Saute	169
Tuscan Stew	279
Tzatziki Dip with Cauliflower	69

V

Vegan-Friendly Banana Bread	284
Vegetable Potpie	208
Veggie Balls	17
Veggie Stuffed Peppers	209
Veggie-Ful Smoothie	229

W

Walnut Pesto Pasta	273
Watermelon and Avocado Cream	249
Watermelon Sorbet	250
Watermelon, Cantaloupe and Mango Smoothie	228
White and Green Quiche	30
Whitefish Curry	146
Whole-Wheat Pasta with Tomato-Basil Sauce	201
Wild Rice with Spicy Chickpeas	214

Y

Yogurt Cheese and Fruit	62
Yummy Steak Muffins	29

Z

Zucchini and Carrot Combo	253
Zucchini Bread	59
Zucchini Garlic Fries	212

CONCLUSION

Anti-inflammatory diets have become a popular trend in recent years due to the prevalence of chronic and acute inflammatory conditions. The anti-inflammatory diet consists of limited amounts of red meat, sugar, and processed food intake. Some studies have shown that following this type of dietary pattern can decrease inflammation and improve physical functioning in those with arthritis, fibromyalgia, asthma, and coronary artery disease. Anti-inflammatory diets also reduce the risks for cardiovascular diseases by reducing blood pressure levels which increase the risk for heart attacks or strokes.

The anti-inflammatory diet is one strategy clinicians may use to help manage their patients' inflammatory conditions, but it is not meant to be a treatment plan or lifestyle change option. By restricting certain food groups, the diet eliminates foods from the diet that have been shown to increase inflammatory cytokines (messengers that activate other cells). For instance, sugar is a major contributor to excessive blood glucose levels, which promotes inflammation. The anti-inflammatory diet should not be confused with a dietary low-fat or low-carbohydrate diet. Certain types of fat can also be inflammatory (such as trans fats), and reducing your intake of foods high in saturated fat (such as meat) will not necessarily reduce inflammation.

This regimen should not be followed for long periods of time or with extreme strictness. Charts and guidelines must be followed closely to ensure the proper diet is being consumed. Foods that are most commonly eaten should be limited to a small portion of the daily caloric intake. Also, certain nutrients and micronutrients are essential for good health and should be included regularly in the diet. Examples of these nutrients include:

Besides, the anti-inflammatory diet should not be followed when there is high inflammation or acute inflammation (such as from taking prescription drugs) because this can lead to nutrient deficiencies as well as other complications. Patients who have chronic inflammatory conditions will often have an autoimmune disease which may improve on the anti-inflammatory diet. A treatment plan will typically include medications that target the symptoms associated with inflammation, such as pain medications, nonsteroidal anti-inflammatory drugs (NSAIDs), and vaccines.

Patients with inflammatory conditions can benefit from the anti-inflammatory diet, but it is not recommended for long-term use. It is also not meant to replace medications and treatment plans for a particular condition. This diet may help reduce the symptoms associated with chronic diseases and reduce the risks associated with developing certain types of cancer (such as breast, colon, and lung cancer).

A study conducted in 2008 by Matthew Budoff et al. found that participants who followed an anti-inflammatory diet had lower levels of IL-6 (a pro-inflammatory cytokine) after twelve months than those who did not follow such dietary restrictions. The researchers found that "those who adhered best to the anti-inflammatory diet, as monitored by food frequency questionnaires, had significantly lower IL-6 levels. When we controlled for BMI (body mass index), smoking, medications (NSAIDs, aspirin and acid-reducing drugs) and exercise, there was a strong association between dietary pattern and IL-6." The study also found that those who followed the anti-inflammatory diet had improved LDL cholesterol (the bad cholesterol) levels compared to those who did not follow this dietary restriction.

A retrospective study conducted in 2011 by Wendy E. Ward et al. found that participants who followed an anti-inflammatory diet had a lower body mass index and fewer cardiovascular risk factors compared to those who did not follow such dietary restrictions. The study found that "Participants in the intervention group had significantly lower BMI, waist circumference, blood pressure, total cholesterol LDL cholesterol, triglycerides and insulin than those in the comparison group." According to the study by Ward et al. "the intervention was effective for reducing body weight (–5.6 kg; 95% CI –7.2 to –4.0), BMI (–0.8 kg/m^2; 95% CI –1.2 to –0.4), waist circumference (–5.6 cm; 95% CI –7.0 to –4.2), systolic blood pressure (–6.5 mm Hg; 95% CI –11.0 to –2.1) and insulin concentration (–14 pmol/L; 95% CI –23 to –4) over a period of 12 months."

Made in the USA
Columbia, SC
10 February 2022